OSTEOSARCOMA

Edited by **Manish Agarwal**

Osteosarcoma
Edited by Manish Agarwal

Published by InTech
Janeza Trdine 9, 51000 Rijeka, Croatia

Publishing Process Manager Ivana Zec

Technical Editor Teodora Smiljanic

Cover Designer InTech Design Team

Additional hard copies can be obtained from orders@intechopen.com

Osteosarcoma, Edited by Manish Agarwal
p. cm.
ISBN 978-953-51-0506-0

For EU product safety concerns:
IN TECH d.o.o., Prolaz Marije Krucifikse Kozulić 3, 51000 Rijeka, Croatia,
info@intechopen.com or visit our website at intechopen.com.

Meet the editor

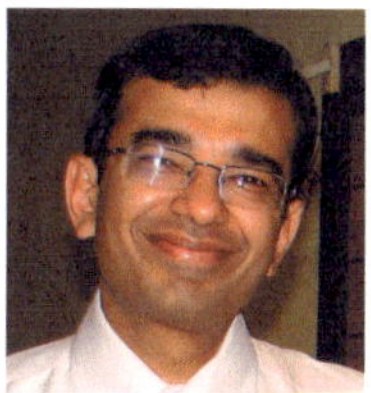

Dr Manish Agarwal is currently a consultant Orthopedic Oncologist at P.D Hinduja National Hospital, Mumbai. He has pioneered the development of the indigenous tumor megaprosthesis system which is used nationally as well as in some centers abroad. He has also pioneered the use of strut allografts for tumor defects, and expandable prostheses in India. Dr. Agarwal helped expand the tissue bank at Tata Memorial Hospital, Mumbai, where he was the associate professor for 10 years. Along with Non Ferrous technology development corporation (NFTDC, Hyderabad) and IIT Mumbai, he has developed an international class tumor prosthetic system, which will shortly undergo clinical trials. He has also done basic research work and phase I trials with traditional herbs for osteosarcoma.

Contents

Preface

Osteosarcoma, is the most common malignant primary bone tumor. Though high grade and potentially lethal, it is highly curable. Though a rare cancer, it predominantly affects children and young adults and being highly curable, the treatment strategy has permanent impact on the life of the patient. A plateau has been reached in its outcome but a lot of research is now being aimed at molecular level to find potential targets for treatment. The dissemination of knowledge coupled with availability of affordable chemotherapeutic drugs and prosthesis have improved the outcomes even in the developing world. The necessity of providing low cost treatment has resulted in innovation in strategy and surgical approach.

Osteosarcoma is to orthopaedic oncology what tuberculosis is to infection. Both have varied spectrum of presentation and can mimic a host of conditions. This book is not meant to be a treatise on osteosarcoma. As the title suggests, it is a fresh look at this disease with an aim to update the existing knowledge on etiology, pathology and workup and to provide a look at the chemotherapeutic and surgical strategy. Importance has also been given to the new research which could potentially change the systemic treatment.

What is also different about this book is that it is online, open access and has been done in a short turnaround time keeping the information very current at time of publication. The authors have published in this field before and many have experience of seeing hundreds of osteosarcomas. This book should be useful to clinicians, researchers as well as students with an interest in the field of osteosarcoma.

Manish Agarwal
Hinduja Hospital, Mumbai,
India

Part 1

Osteosarcoma Workup

1

Histopathology and Molecular Pathology of Bone and Extraskeletal Osteosarcomas

Helen Trihia and Christos Valavanis
"Metaxa" Cancer Hospital, Department of Pathology and Molecular Pathology Unit
Greece

1. Introduction

Osteosarcoma has been recognized for almost two centuries and is the most common primary, non-haemopoietic malignant tumour of the skeletal system. It is thought to arise from primitive mesenchymal bone-forming cells and its histologic hallmark is the production of osteoid. Other cell populations may also be present, as these types of cells may also arise from pluripotential mesenchymal cells, but any area of bone or osteoid synthesized by malignant cells in the lesion establishes the diagnosis of osteosarcoma (Acchiappati et al, 1965).

It accounts for approximately 20% of all primary malignant bone tumours. In the United States, the incidence of osteosarcoma is 400 cases per year (4.8 per million population <20 y). The incidence is slightly higher in blacks than in whites (Huvos et al, 1983), in males than in females. It has a bimodal age distribution and a propensity to develop in adolescents and young adults (Dix et al, 1983; Soloviev, 1969; Wilimas, et al, 1977, Dorfman & Czerniak, 1995), with 60% of tumours occurring in patients younger than 25 years of age and only 13% to 30% in patients older than 40 years (de Santos et al, 1982; Huvos, 1986). Osteosarcoma is very rare in young children (0.5 cases per million per year in children <5y).

Osteosarcoma can occur in any bone, but most tumours originate in the long bones of the appendicular skeleton, near metaphyseal growth plates, especially the distal femur (42%, 75% of which in the distal femur), followed by the proximal tibia (19%, 80% of which in the proximal tibia) and proximal humerus (10%, 90% of which in the proximal humerus) (Goes M, 1952). In the long bones the tumour is most frequently centered in the metaphysis (90%), infrequently in the diaphysis (9%) and rarely in the epiphysis (Tsuneyoshi & Dorfman, 1987). Other significant locations are the skull and jaw (8%) and pelvis (8%) (Benson et al, 1984).

The clinicopathologic features of osteosarcoma form the basis of its classification, most importantly including the histologic features, the biologic potential (grade), relation to bone (intramedullary or surface), multiplicity (solitary and multifocal) and the pre-existing state of underlying bone (primary or secondary).

Osteosarcomas have a wide range of radiographic and histologic appearances. For example, some may be radiolucent or radiodense. Some are confined to the medullary cavity, or originate and grow on the bone surface. Some arise on normal bone (*de novo* osteosarcoma), others arise in the setting of Paget disease or radiation (secondary osteosarcoma). Most arise in genetically normal individuals but rare cases have been seen in patients' various genetic syndromes (such as Rothmund-Thompson, Li Fraumeni and Retinoblastoma gene mutation) (Dick et al, 1982; Hansen et al, 1985; Kozlowski et al, 1980). The vast majority are solitary lesions, although rare cases of multifocal osteosarcomas have been reported (Ackermann, 1948, Amstutz, 1969, Laurent et al, 1973).

According to the mode of growth, osteosarcomas are subdivided into intramedullary and surface osteosarcomas. Intramedullary osteosarcomas are further subdivided into typical intramedullary, telangiectatic and highly differentiated. Surface osteosarcomas are subdivided into periosteal and parosteal osteosarcomas and high-grade surface osteosarcomas. According to the prevalent cell in the neoplastic tissue are subdivided into osteoblastic, chondroblastic, fibroblastic, giant cell, small cell and mixed (McDonald & Budd, 1943).

Most osteosarcomas can be categorized into four major groups: 1) conventional, high grade osteosarcoma and its histologic subtypes (75%-85%), 2) high grade osteosarcoma that arises in a diseased bone (10%), 3) intramedullary, well-differentiated (1%) and 4) surface osteosarcoma (5%-10%).

Bone tumour grading has traditionally been based on a combination of histologic diagnosis and the Broders grading system which assesses cellularity and degree of anaplasia (Broders, 1920; Inwards & Unni, 1995). The 7th edition of the AJCC Cancer Staging Manual recommends a 4-grade system (Edge et al, 2009), with grades 1 and 2, considered as 'low grade' and grades 3 and 4 'high grade'. The 2009 CAP Bone Tumour Protocol recommends a pragmatic approach, based principally on histologic classification. Under this system, central low grade osteosarcoma and parosteal osteosarcoma are considered Grade 1 sarcomas, with periosteal osteosarcoma considered Grade 2, and all other osteosarcomas considered Grade 3 (Dorfman et al, 1998, 2002).

The exact cause of osteosarcoma is unknown. The best known causative association - environmental risk factor is exposure to radiation (Huvos, 1986). Its causal relation was first documented in radium dial painters. Osteosarcoma after therapeutic irradiation is an uncommon complication, and usually develops after approximately 15 (range 3 to 55) years.

Osteosarcoma is known to affect approximately 1% of patients with Paget disease of bone, which reflects a several thousand-fold increase in risk in comparison with that of the general population (Wick et al, 1981).

Osteosarcoma may also arise in sites of previous bone infarction (Mirra et al, 1974), chronic osteomyelitis (Bartkowski & Klenczynski, 1974; Spyra, 1976), pre-existing primary benign bone tumours (osteochondroma, enchondroma, fibrous dysplasia, giant cell tumour, osteoblastoma, aneurysmal bone cyst and unicameral bone cyst) and adjacent to metallic implants (Johnson et al, 1962; Koppers et al, 1977, Ruggieri 1995; Schweitzer & Pirie, 1971; Smith et al, 1986). These secondary osteosarcomas account for only a small percentage of osteosarcomas and their pathogenesis is likely related to chronic cell turnover that is associated to the underlying bone disease.

The diagnosis of osteosarcoma, like all bone-tumours, emphasizes the necessity of close cooperation of all involved disciplines for diagnosis and therapy, including clinicians, radiologists and pathologists, as the correct diagnosis relies on their clinico-pathological appearance.

2. Pathologic features

2.1 Conventional osteosarcoma

Conventional osteosarcoma, is solitary, arises in the medullary cavity of an otherwise normal bone, is of high grade and produces neoplastic bone with or without cartilaginous or fibroblastic components. The gross findings are variable depending on the amount of bone and other components present. It manifests as a large, metaphyseal, intramedullary and tan-gray-white, gritty mass. Tumours that are producing abundant mineralized bone are tan-gray and hard, whereas non-mineralized, cartilaginous components are glistening, gray, and may be mucinous if the matrix is myxoid, or more rubbery if hyaline in nature. It can be necrotic, hemorrhagic and cystic. Intramedullary involvement is often considerable and the tumour usually destroys the overlying cortex and forms an eccentric or circumferential soft tissue component that displaces the periosteum peripherally. In the proximal and distal portions of the tumour the raised periosteum deposits a reactive bone, known as Codman's triangle. In some cases, the tumour grows into the joint space, resulting in coating of the peripheral portions of the articular cartilage by the sarcoma. Solitary or multiple skip metastases appear as intramedullary nodules in the vicinity of or far from the main mass. Furthermore, not all osteosarcomas arise in a solitary fashion, as multiple sites may become apparent within a period of about 6 months (synchronous osteosarcoma), or multiple sites may be noted over a period longer than 6 months (metachronous osteosarcoma). Such multifocal osteosarcoma is decidedly rare, but when it occurs, it tends to be in patients, younger than 10 years.

The diagnosis of osteosarcoma is based on the accurate identification of osteoid. Osteoid is unmineralized bone matrix that histologically appears as eosinophilic, dense, homogeneous, amorphous and curvilinear intercellular material, somewhat refractile. It must be distinguished from other eosinophilic extra-cellular materials such as fibrin and amyloid. Unequivocal discrimination between osteoid and non-osseous collagen may be difficult, or sometimes arbitrary (Fornasier, 1977). Non-osseous collagen tends to be linear, fibrillar and compresses between neoplastic cells. In contrast, osteoid is curvilinear with small nubs, arborisation and what appears to be abortive, lacunae formation. The thickness of the osteoid is highly variable with the 'thinnest' variant referred to as 'filigree', whereas osteoid seams are flat and thick. Osseous matrix has also the predisposition for appositional deposition upon previously existing normal bone trabeculae ('scaffolding').

Conventional osteosarcoma can produce varying amounts of cartilage and/or fibrous tissue. The algorithm is: identify the presence or absence of matrix, and if significant matrix is present, determine the matrix form and therefore subclassify into osteoblastic, chondroblastic, fibroblastic and mixed types, by virtue of the predominance of the neoplastic component.

Histologic subtyping may not always be possible, even with generous sampling. Such lesions are better categorized under the term 'osteogenic sarcoma with no predominant growth pattern'. Furthermore, sub-classification on local recurrence or following chemotherapy or irradiation can provide false results, because treatment can alter tumour appearance.

In addition, osteosarcoma may be of any histologic grade. Some contain highly pleomorphic cells and abundant mitotic figures, whereas others may be difficult to differentiate from benign neoplasms.

2.1.1 Osteoblastic osteosarcoma

Conventional osteosarcoma is usually of the osteoblastic type. In osteoblastic osteosarcoma the predominant matrix is bone and/or osteoid. It contains pleomorphic malignant cells and coarse neoplastic woven bone. The tumour cells are intimately related to the surface of the neoplastic bone, which is woven in architecture, varies in quantity and is deposited as primitive, disorganized trabeculae in a coarse, lace-like pattern, thin, arborising lines of osteoid (filigree) interweaving between neoplastic cells, or broad, large sheets of coalescing , trabeculae, as seen in the sclerosing variant. Depending on its state of mineralization, the bone can be eosinophilic, or basophilic and may have a pagetoid appearance caused by haphazardly deposited cement lines.

2.1.2 Chondroblastic osteosarcoma

Chondroid matrix is predominant in chondroblastic osteosarcoma, intimately associated with non-chondroid elements. The neoplastic chondrocytes are mostly characterized by severe cytologic atypia and reside in lacunar spaces, hyaline matrix or float singly or in cords in myxoid matrix. Myxoid and other forms of cartilage are uncommon, except in the jaws and in the pelvis.

2.1.3 Fibroblastic osteosarcoma

Typically, is composed of fusiform highly pleomorphic malignant cells, arranged in a herringbone or storiform pattern, similar to fibrosarcoma or malignant fibrous histiocytoma, with minimal osseous matrix. Although, the degree of atypia is variable, is frequently severe, with numerous mitoses, including atypical forms. In general, the lack of significant amounts of osteoid, bone or cartilage, relegates them to subtypes of fibroblastic osteosarcoma.

Although, there is a tendency for metastases of osteosarcomas to mimic the primary, exceptions are frequent and is a higher than expected incidence of fibroblastic differentiation in metastases.

2.2 Small cell osteosarcoma

It comprises 1.5% of osteosarcomas, with slight predilection for females and is composed of small cells with variable degree of osteoid production (Sim et al, 1979). According to the predominant cell pattern, tumours are classified to round cell type or short spindle cell type. Nuclei can be very small to medium sized, with scanty amount of cytoplasm, comparable to those of Ewing sarcoma and to large cell lymphoma respectively. The chromatin distribution can be fine or coarse and the mitoses range from 3 to 5/per high power field-HPF. Lace-like osteoid production is always present, although particular care must be taken to differentiate osteoid from fibrin deposits that may be seen among Ewing sarcoma cells.

2.3 Telangiectatic osteosarcoma

When first recognized, telangiectatic osteosarcoma was considered a distinct clinical and pathologic entity (Gaylord, 1903). On the basis of subsequent findings, telangiectatic osteosarcoma was considered a variant of osteosarcoma (Ewing, 1922, 1939).

It is rare, less than 4% of all cases of osteosarcomas and more frequent in the second decade of life. Although, most frequently affects long tubular bones, has also been noted to arise in extraosseous soft tissues in the forearm, thigh and popliteal fossa (Mirra et al, 1993).

Radiographically, is characterized by typically purely lytic destructive process, without matrix mineralization. Clinically, a pathological fracture is present in one fourth of the cases. On gross examination, there is a dominant cystic architecture in the bone medulla. The cystic space is filled incompletely with blood clot, described as 'a bag of blood'. Histologically, the tumour is characterized by dilated, blood-filled or empty spaces, separated by thin septae, simulating aneurysmal bone cyst. The cystic spaces are lined by benign osteoclast-like giant cells, without endothelial lining. The septae are cellular, containing highly malignant, atypical mononuclear tumour cells with high mitotic activity, including atypical mitoses. The amount of osteoid varies, but usually is fine, lace-like and of minimal amount, although it tends to be more prominent in metastatic foci. Therefore, it is imperative that the entire specimen is meticulously examined histologically.

Telangiectatic osteosarcomatous differentiation has been reported in parosteal osteosarcoma (Wines et al,2000), in dedifferentiated chondrosarcoma arising in the background of osteochondroma (Radhi & Loewy, 1999), in association with aneurysmal bone cysts (Adler, 1980; Kyriakos & Hardy, 1991), in osteitis deformans, as well as in cases of malignant phylloedes tumour of the breast (Gradt et al, 1998) and in ovarian sarcomas (Hirakawa et al, 1998).

2.4 Low grade central (well differentiated intraosseous/intramedullary) osteosarcoma

It accounts for 1-2% of all osteosarcomas and is the medullary equivalent to parosteal osteosarcoma (Kurt et al, 1990; Unni et al, 1977). There is a tendency for a slightly older age and slightly longer symptomatology in comparison to the conventional osteosarcoma. It is important to recognize this subtype, since the patient tends to do much better, than those with conventional osteosarcoma. It is a low grade fibroblastic osteosarcoma and is histologically identical to parosteal osteosarcoma.

Histologically, contains long, parallel trabeculae or round islands of woven bone intimately associated with a mildly to moderately cellular population of cytologically bland neoplastic spindle cells with variable amounts of osteoid production. Nuclear enlargement and hyperchromasia are generally evident with occasional mitotic figures (1-2 mitoses per 10 high power fields-HPFs). When involving the medullary canal it may be confused with fibrous dysplasia (FD). Radiologically, FD is homogeneous ('ground glass' appearance), whereas the well differentiated osteosarcoma is less so, and may show trabeculations. Furthermore, a permeative growth pattern into the pre-existing lamellar bone or fatty marrow is diagnostic. Microscopically, the trabeculae of FD tend to be rather short and curled, whereas those of well differentiated osteosarcoma are longer and may be arranged in parallel arrays. Again, cytologic atypia should be sought and is diagnostic if found.

Conventional osteosarcomas often have better differentiated, innocuous 'normalized' areas. These should not be underdiagnosed as low grade osteosarcoma, since biologically they behave accordingly to their more aggressive foci.

Desmoplastic fibromas may infiltrate the bone and can be diagnostically challenging. In these cases, osteoid production should be sought. Radiographic evidence of matrix production is helpful in establishing the correct diagnosis.

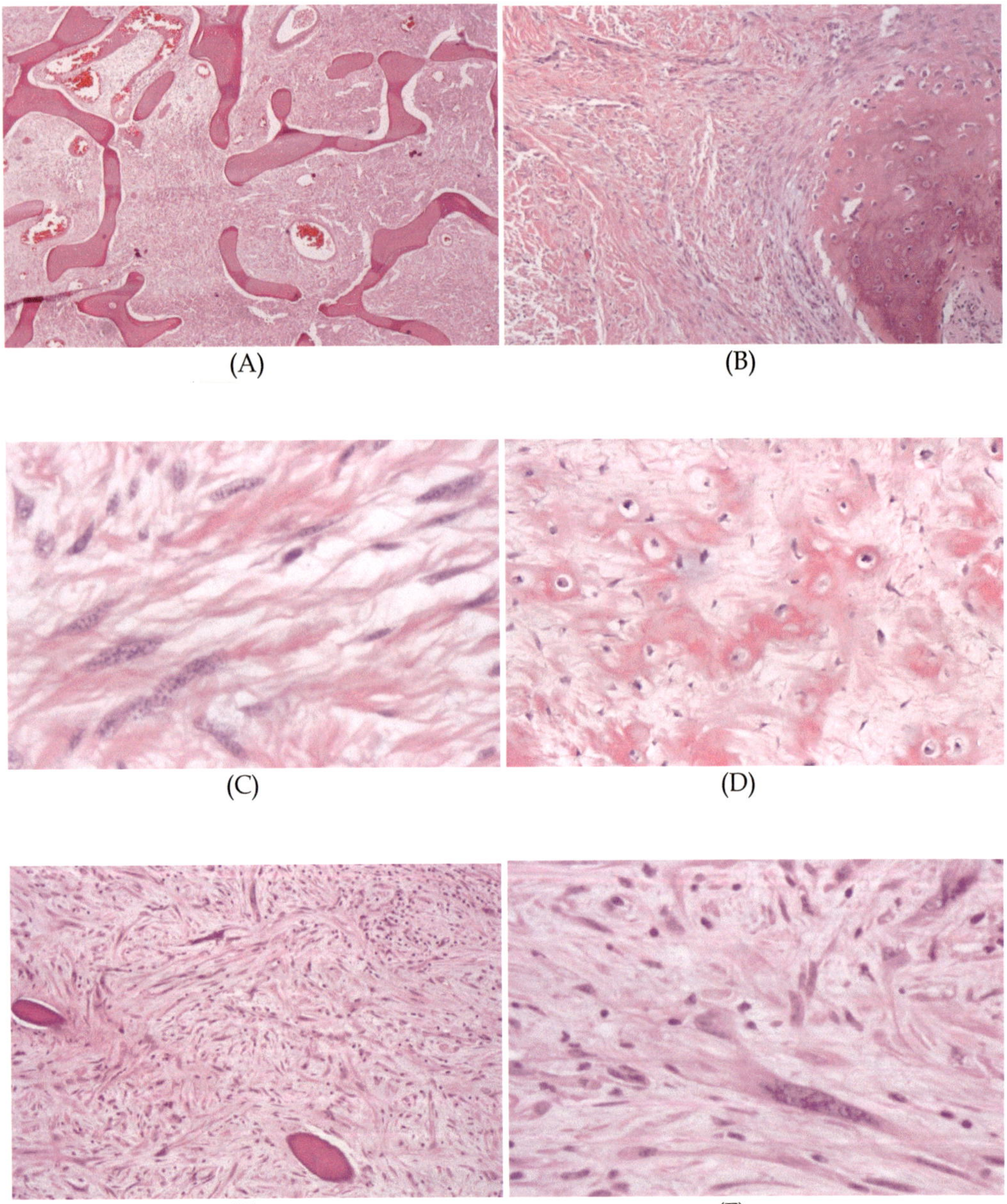

Fig. 1. **(A-D) Intramedullary (central) low grade osteosarcoma** (H&E stain). A. Long parallel neoplastic bony trabeculae associated with spindle cell stroma. B. Hypocellular spindle cell collagenized stroma with osteoid production C. Scattered fusiform cells with nuclear enlargement (high magnification). D. Area of chondroblastic differentiation. **(E, F) Osteosarcoma fibroblastic type** (H&E stain). E. Neoplastic bony trabeculae surrounded by spindle cell stroma exhibiting scattered cytologic atypia prominent at low magnification. F. Prominent cytologic atypia (high magnification)

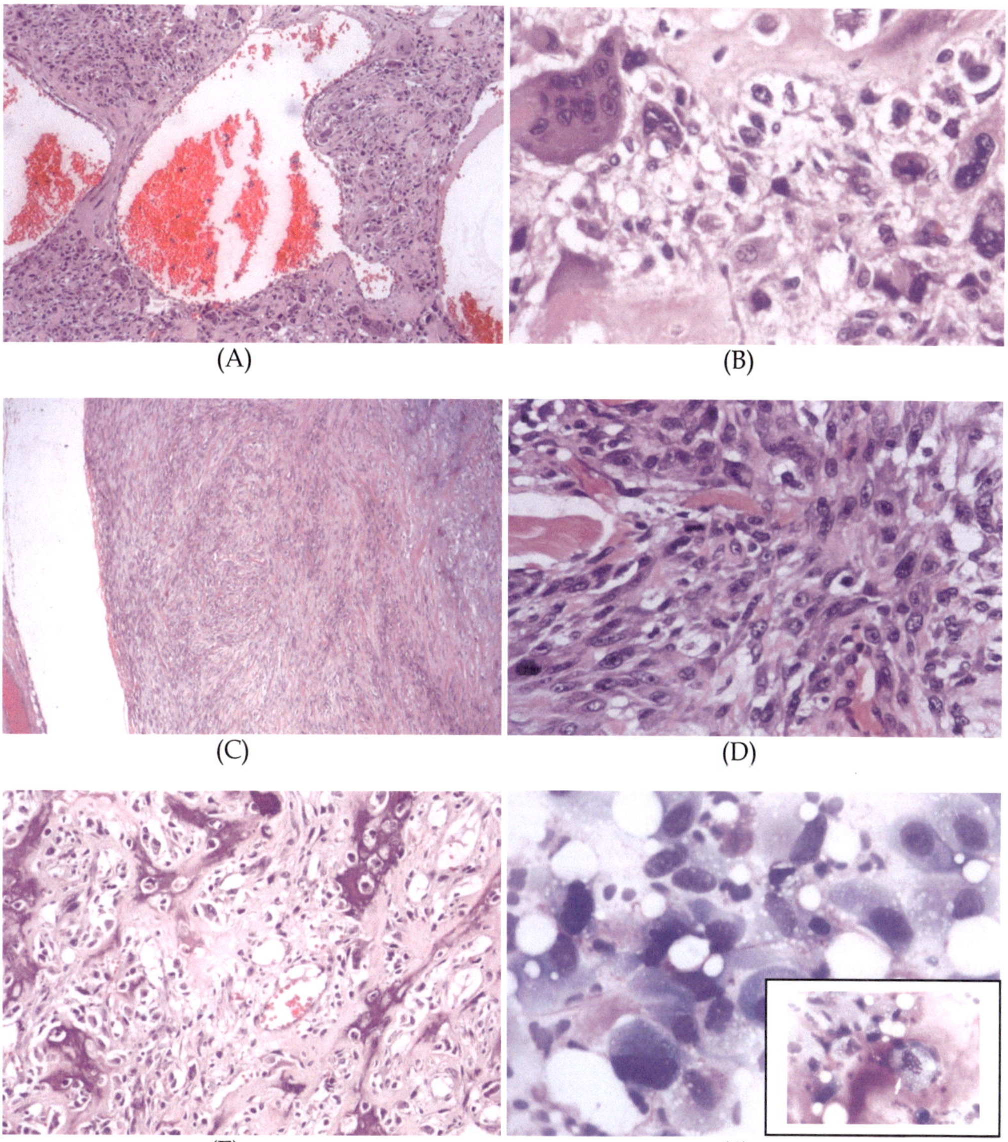

(A) (B)

(C) (D)

(E) (F)

Fig. 2. **(A, B) Telangiectatic osteosarcoma** (H&E stain). (A) Blood-filled cystic spaces, separated by septae with abundant osteoclastic-type giant cells. (B) Giant cell-rich area with high cellular pleomorphism and patchy osteoid formation. **(C-E) Extraskeletal osteosarcoma of the breast**. (C) Well circumscribed margins, peripheral spindle cell component and chondroblastic area (on the right). (D) Highy pleomorphic tumor cells including mitoses. (E) Osteoblastic osteosarcoma area with abundant mineralized osteoid. **(F) Fine needle aspirate from extraskeletal osteosarcoma of the breast** (MGG stain). Cellular smear displaying epithelioid cells with plasmacytoid appearance. (Inset) Enlarged pleomorphic cell with fine cytoplasmic vacuolization, reminiscent of neoplastic chondroblast in association with red-purple amorphous material (reproduced with permission from S. Karger A.G., Medical and Scientific Publishers, first published by Trihia et al, Acta Cytologica, 2007;51:443-450)

2.5 Secondary osteosarcomas

Secondary osteosarcomas are bone forming sarcomas occurring in bones that are affected by preexisting abnormalities, the most common being Paget disease and radiation change.

2.5.1 Paget osteosarcoma

Incidence of sarcomatous change in Paget disease is estimated to 0.7-0.95%, with osteosarcomas representing 50-60% of Paget sarcomas (Haibach et al, 1985; Huvos et al, 1983; Schajowicz et al, 1983). It is more common in men, with median age of 64 years and is usually observed in patients with widespread Paget disease (70%). Most tumours arise in the medulla. Histologically are high grade sarcomas, mostly osteoblastic or fibroblastic. A great number of osteoclast-like giant cells may be found. Telangiectatic and small cell osteosarcomas have been reported.

2.5.2 Post-radiation osteosarcoma

They constitute 3.4-5.5% of all osteosarcomas and 50-60% of radiation-induced sarcomas. It is estimated that the risk of developing osteosarcoma in irradiated bone is 0.03-0.8% (Huvos et al, 1985; Mark et al, 1994). Children treated with high-dose radiotherapy and chemotherapy are at the greater risk, and the prevalence of post-radiation osteosarcomas is increasing as children survive treatment for their malignant tumour. It can develop in any irradiated bone, with most common locations the pelvis and the shoulder. The modified criteria for postradiation cancer initially promulgated in 1948 by Cahan and associates are as follows : (1) the patient received irradiation, (2) the neoplasm occurred in the radiation field, (3) a latent period of years had elapsed, (4) histologic or radiographic evidence for the pre-existent osseous lesion, a benign tumour or non-bone forming malignancy (Cahan et al, 1948).

Histologically, high grade osteosarcomas predominate.

Many of the reported cases of osteosarcoma arising in fibrous dysplasia have also been complicated by radiation therapy.

2.5.3 Osteosarcomas in other benign precursors

Other rare instances of secondary osteosarcomas have included cases arising in association with bone infarcts, endoprostheses and already mentioned fibrous dysplasia. Infarct associated sarcomas as well as malignant tumours at the site of prosthetic replacements (Brien et al, 1990), or at the site of prior fixation, most commonly show the histological pattern of malignant fibrous histiocytoma (MFH), with a minority being osteosarcomas.

2.6 Parosteal osteosarcoma

It is the most common type of osteosarcoma of the bone surface, although it accounts for about 5% of all osteosarcomas, with a slight female predominance (Okada et al, 1995). It is a low grade, slow growing neoplasm, with a predilection for the posterior aspect of the distal femur, where presents as a hard lobulated mass attached to the underlying cortex with a broad base. Histologically, it is a well differentiated fibro-osseous neoplasm, consisting of well formed bony trabeculae embedded in a hypocellular fibrous stroma. The bony trabeculae can be arranged in parallel strands, simulating normal bone and may or may not show osteoblastic rimming. The intertrabecular stroma is hypocellular with minimal atypia, whereas it can be more cellular with moderate cytologic atypia in 20% of cases. About 50% of the tumours will show cartilaginous differentiation, in the form of hypercellular nodules of cartilage within the tumour substance or as a cup on the surface. When present, the cartilage cup is mildly cellular with mild cytologic atypia and lacks the 'columnar' appearance seen in osteochondromas.

About 15% of the tumours will show high grade spindle cell sarcoma (dedifferentiation), more often at the time of recurrence, in the form of osteosarcoma, fibrosarcoma or MFH (Wold et al, 1984).

Its diagnosis can be very difficult and the differential diagnosis has included diverse entities, such as: myositis ossificans, fracture callus, ossifying haematoma, osteochondroma, extraosseous osteosarcoma, parosteal chondroma, desmoplastic fibroma and osteoma. Therefore, parosteal osteosarcoma, like no other tumour, implies the necessity of close cooperation of all involved disciplines for the correct diagnosis.

2.7 Periosteal osteosarcoma

It accounts for less than 2% of all osteosarcomas, more common than high grade surface osteosarcoma, but about one third as common as parosteal osteosarcoma (Unni et al, 1976). Unlike parosteal osteosarcoma, which extends from the cortex like a bony knob, periosteal osteosarcoma tightly encases the bone, like a glove. Unlike other osteosarcomas, it tends to involve the diaphysis. Radiologically, it is a circumferential surface mass, less radiodense than parosteal osteosarcoma. Mineralization occurs as ring-shaped radiodensities or as streaks of reactive bone radiating from the surface. Lesions can be best visualized by MRI scan. A sub-periosteal lesion with a bright white signal is present, indicating its high cartilage content. Histologically, it has the appearance of a moderately differentiated, grade 2/3 chondroblastic osteosarcoma. It consists almost entirely of lobules of cellular, atypical cartilage, with bone formation in the centre of the lobules, separated by thin strands of fibrous tissue. Careful scrutiny of the fibrous component, reveals seams of neoplastic osteoid, usually at the outer surface of the neoplasm, which distinguishes it from surface chondrosarcoma.

2.8 High grade surface osteosarcoma

A high grade, bone-forming malignant tumour, arising from the bone surface, which comprises less than 1% of all osteosarcomas. Histologically, is similar to conventional osteosarcoma. Regions of predominantly osteoblastic, chondroblastic, or fibroblastic differentiation may predominate. However all tumours will show high cytologic atypia and lace-like osteoid. The pattern of osteoid production and the high grade cytologic atypia help to separate it from parosteal osteosarcoma. High grade surface osteosarcoma with chondroblastic differentiation may be confused with periosteal osteosarcoma. The degree of cytologic atypia is greater in high grade surface osteosarcoma and the tumours generally show larger spindle cell areas. Finally, unlike dedifferentiated parosteal osteosarcomas, low grade regions are not found in high grade surface osteosarcomas.

Cortical destruction and invasion into the medullary canal in high-grade juxtacortical (periosteal and high-grade surface) osteosarcomas, is often absent, but when present, is only focal. If extensive, it becomes difficult, if not impossible to distinguish an intramedullary tumour with an eccentric soft tissue component from a surface neoplasm with extensive invasion of the medullary canal.

2.9 Extraskeletal osteosarcomas

Extraskeletal osteosarcomas (EOs) or soft tissue osteosarcomas (STOs) are rare sarcomas arising in extraskeletal somatic soft tissue, in which the neoplastic cells produce osteoid and/or bone matrix, therefore recapitulating the phenotype of osteoblasts. By definition, it is a high grade mesenchymal neoplasm that produces osteoid, bone and chondroid material, shows no evidence of epithelial component and is located in soft tissues, without attachment to bone or periosteum, as determined by X-ray findings or inspection during the operative procedure. It is significantly less frequent than its osseous counterpart. They account for 1.2% of soft tissue sarcomas and 4% of osteosarcomas (Bane et al, 1990; Sordillo et al, 1983). They typically arise in the deep soft tissues of the proximal extremities, with most common locations the deep soft tissues of the thigh and buttocks, followed in descending order by the upper limb, retroperitoneum, trunk, head and neck (Chung & Enzinger, 1987; Lee et al, 1995; Lidang et al, 1998; Sordillo et al, 1983). Fewer than 10% are superficial, originating in the dermis or subcutis. Cases of EOs arising in unusual sites have been reported, such as the breast, larynx, thyroid gland, parotid, abdominal viscera, including esophagus, small intestine, omentum majum, liver, heart, the urogenital system, including urinary bladder, ureter the prostate and the penis, pleura, mediastinum, ectopic thymus, pulmonary artery, pilonidal area and aorta (Baydar, et al, 2009; Burke & Virmani, 1991; Kemmer et al, 2008; Loose et al, 1990; Micolonghi et al, 1984; Piscioli et al, 1985; Shui et al, 2011; Silver & Tavassoli, 1998; Trowell & Arkell, 1976; Young & Rosenberg, 1987; Wegner et al, 2010; Greenwood & Meschter, 1989). Fewer than 300 cases have been reported to date and their aetiology is essentially unknown. Unlike osseous conventional osteosarcoma, it typically occurs in older adults, with a peak incidence in the fifth and sixth decades of life, in contrast with skeletal osteosarcomas that most commonly affect young adults (Sordillo et al, 1983). Males are affected more frequently than females at a ratio of 1.9:1. Some cases have been associated with a history of prior therapeutic irradiation at the site of the tumour (Logue & Cairnduff, 1991) and trauma (Allan & Soule, 1971). In one case report of primary osteosarcoma of the urinary bladder, prolonged treatment with immunosuppressive medications, including cyclophosphamide for active systemic lupus erythematosus (SLE) has been reported (Baydar et al, 2009). The diagnosis is generally delayed and prognosis is poor, with most patients died within months of diagnosis and with a cause-specific survival rate at 5 years less than 25%. Clinically and mammographically can mimic a benign tumour. Like most of soft tissue sarcomas, tumours may appear grossly circumscribed, however they are microscopically infiltrative. Imaging studies usually reveal compact calcifications/variable mineralization within the mass. Primary extraosseous osteosarcoma should always be included in the differential diagnosis, in the view of a well demarcated calcified mass on image analysis. In the case of extraskeletal osteosarcoma of the breast, an underdiagnosis as a calcified fibroadenoma, should be avoided.

STOs are usually large, ranging in size between 5 and 10 cm, well-circumscribed, grossly heterogeneous tumours that exhibit areas of haemorrhage and/or necrosis. Microscopically,

STOs constitute highly cellular, cytologically pleomorphic, mitotically active sarcomas, spindle cell to epithelioid in appearance. The defining feature is the presence of neoplastic osteoid and/or bone. The latter usually presents in a 'lace like' manner, although solid sheets of amorphous osteoid can also be found. When the bone/osteoid matrix is found only focally in the tumour, largely demonstrates a nonspecific, undifferentiated, spindle cell sarcomatous appearance. Lobules of highly cellular, atypical hyaline/fibrocartilage may also present. Osteoclast-like giant cells have also been described. Various histologic subtypes of bone osteosarcoma can be seen in extraskeletal osteosarcoma. Osteoblastic variant is the most common type, followed by fibroblastic, chondroid, telangiectatic, small cell and well-differentiated variants. Common to all variants is the production of osteoid, intimately associated with tumour cells, which may be deposited in a lacy, trabecular or sheet-like pattern. Neoplastic bone formation is more prominent in the centre of the tumour with the peripheral areas being more cellular, a reverse pattern of myositis ossificans. In essence, any of the microscopic patterns of high-grade intraosseous osteosarcoma may be seen in EO.

The differential diagnosis should always include spindle cell (sarcomatoid) carcinomas and the exclusion of metastasis from a primary osteosarcoma, as well as carcinosarcomas, malignant tumours with osseous metaplasia and sarcomas. Metaplastic ossification, ranging from osteoid to woven bone formation can be seen in synovial sarcoma, epithelioid sarcoma, liposarcoma and carcinosarcoma. Osteogenic differentiation can also be seen as a phenomenon of dedifferentiation in various soft tissue sarcomas. In the above tumours, other histologic lineages or histologic characteristics of original tumours are usually present. The key to diagnosis, is the identification of the matrix surrounding the tumour cells and lack of epithelial differentiation. Furthermore, except osteoblastic, chondroblastic and fibroblastic differentiation, no other lineages of histologic differentiation should be detectable in EOs. Diagnostic confirmation using immunohistochemical markers is necessary to ensure the absence of an epithelial component and exclude the neoplasms of biphasic origin.

Immunohistochemical studies indicate that the EOs' immunophenotype is similar to bone osteosarcoma. EOs are uniformly positive for vimentin, they express smooth muscle actin (68%), desmin (25%), S-100 protein (20%), including non-cartilaginous areas, EMA (52%), Keratin (8%) and are negative for PLAP.

Differential diagnosis from recurrent or metastatic osteosarcoma is based on clinical history.

3. The use of cytology in the preoperative investigation of bone tumours with emphasis in osteosarcoma

Fine needle aspiration (FNA) of bone lesions has been performed ever since the technique was introduced (Coley et al, 1931). It has certain advantages over open biopsy, as it is less disruptive to bone and permits multiple sampling without complications. Its main use is to confirm malignancy. Although, cytomorphology of primary bone tumours has been extensively described in correlation with histology (Hajdu, 1975; Stormby & Akerman, 1973Walaas &Kindblom, 1990; White et al, 1988), FNA is not as good for diagnosing primary bone tumours.

There are two main indications of FNA of soft tissue and bone lesions: preoperative diagnosis before definitive treatment and the investigation of lesions suspicious of tumour recurrence or metastasis. Eventhough, the first use has limitations, however, at present, the use of FNA as the diagnostic, pre-treatment tool for musculoskeletal tumours is accepted in many orthopaedic centres, provided that certain requirements are fulfilled and that the final cytologic diagnosis is based on the combined evaluation of clinical data, radiographic findings and cytomorphology (Domansky et al, 2010). One important reason, why FNA is preferred upon open biopsy, is when the preoperative evaluation of a lesion as malignant is of most importance, rather the subtype of the lesion. On the other hand, in the use of neo-adjuvant treatment (radio- or chemotherapy), before surgery, the FNA diagnosis is of major importance, analogous to histopathologic examination, in regard to subtype and tumour grade. This is mostly the case with small round cell sarcomas. Regarding bone lesions, FNA may also replace open biopsy in the primary diagnosis. It is the task of the pathologist to distinguish benign and malignant primary bone tumours from metastatic deposits and from the wide range of benign and inflammatory reactive lesions of the bone. Furthermore, the pathologist should give a confident diagnosis of the various benign bone tumours and sarcomas, if open biopsy is to be avoided. Skeletal aspiration is not different from other aspirations, but it is important to remember that intact cortical bone cannot be penetrated by regularly used (22 gauge) needles, something that can be easily done with partly destroyed or eroded bone. A 18-gauge needle can be used in intact bone, under anaesthesia and multiple passes can be performed. Many malignant bone tumours have palpable soft tissue involvement, which can be much easier penetrated by the needle. In any case, it is strongly recommended that the pathologist is familiar with the radiological findings, discuss the best approach to the tumour with the radiologist and that non-palpable lesions are aspirated under image-guided techniques. Essentially, when the aspirated material is technically satisfactory, it is suitable for use of specialized techniques, likewise biopsy material, to assist in the diagnosis.

The FNA cytological findings of osteosarcoma have thoroughly been described (Mertens et al, 1982; Walaas &Kindblom, 1990; White et al, 1988). They include mixture of cell clusters and dispersed cells, pleomorphic, spindle and rounded cells with frequent mitoses, including atypical forms, intercellular tumour matrix of osteoid, benign osteoclast-like giant cells, epithelioid tumour cells, which may be of osteoblastic type, or resemble chondroblasts, in osteoblastic and chondroblastic variants respectively, atypical spindle-shaped cells in fibroblastic subtypes. The presence of osteoid-like material can be 'prominent, or scarce, dissociated, or in association with cell clusters, either as moderate-sized fragments, or not easily discernible globule-like particles'. This material could be associated either with the predominat histologic pattern or with the sampled area represented in the smears. Osteoid-like matrix material has been originally described as 'homogeneous or vacuolated eosinophilic plaques' or pink-purple acellular material in May Grunwald Giemsa (MGG) smears and green-blue in Papanicolaou-stained (PAP) smears. Another cause of difficulty in accurately assessing the presence of osteoid in the smears is that osteoid, cartilage and dense collagen fibers appear very similar in both Diff-Quick and PAP stains. Furthermore, osteoid resists the suction, during aspiration, and when aspirated, the small, disrupted fragments lack the characteristic lattice-like pattern observed in histological sections (Mertens & Langnickel, 1982; Nikol et al, 1998).

FNA has proven to be of value in the preoperative diagnosis of breast EOs (Trihia et al, 2007). Its diagnosis is often delayed because of a desceptively benign clinical and radiologic appearance (Watt et al, 1984). Although differential diagnosis from metaplastic carcinoma may not be possible on cytological grounds alone, FNA has proven to be of value in preoperative diagnosis of malignancy and prompt surgical intervention, as clinically and mammographically these lesions can be underdiagnosed as a benign tumour (Trihia et al, 2007).

4. The role of immunohistochemistry in the diagnosis of osteosarcoma

The diagnostic algorithm of primary bone tumors is, and always has been, a collaborative effort in which clinical, radiologic, and pathologic findings have to be considered. In the majority of cases, the pathologist can rely exclusively on histopathologic examination to provide an accurate diagnosis. In some cases, however, ancillary studies have to be employed to distinguish entities that share morphologic characteristics.

When evaluating a bone tumor, the pathologist is confronted with several difficulties. Bone tumors are rare entities, and not all pathologists are exposed to bone pathology with the frequency needed to gain the necessary level of diagnostic expertise. Also, certain osseous tumors share histopathologic features and, in many cases, important diagnostic features may not be readily evident in small specimens. Finally, intramedullary lesions often must be decalcified, a process that may be associated with loss in cellular morphologic detail. All of these factors complicate the diagnostic process. Diagnosis for many entities can be reached by the evaluation of histopathologic features alone, or can be interpretated in the context of clinico-radiologic findings, but for others, only a differential diagnosis can be reached without ancillary studies.

Several studies have shown that gentle decalcification methods preserve antigenicity relatively well for the most commonly used markers.

One of the greatest challenges in bone and soft tissue pathology is the reliable recognition of osseous matrix production in malignant lesions. Although several antigens have been explored, unfortunately, little is known about the antigenic specificity of normal bone tissue and bone neoplasms and currently there is no specific marker to distinguish the bone matrix from its collagenous mimics.

Since late 1990's, due to their central function in the process of mineralization, a group of proteins have been proposed for tumor diagnosis: alkaline phosphatase, osteonectin, and osteocalcin. Osteocalcin (OCN) and osteonectin (ONN) have been applied to paraffin sections and been used to highlight osteoid. OCN is one of the most prevalent intraosseous proteins and is produced exclusively by bone-forming cells-osteoblasts and therefore has received special attention as a specific marker (Fanburg et al, 1997, 1999; Takada et al, 1992). In the detection of bone-forming tumors, osteocalcin has been associated with 70% sensitivity and 100% specificity, compared with the 90% sensitivity and 54% specificity reported for ONN. Nevertheless, OCN is rarely used in clinical practice. ONN is a protein that is implicated in regulating the adhesion of osteoblasts and platelets to their extracellular matrix, as well as early mineralization and should only be used as part of a panel of reagents, directed at several lineage-related proteins (Serra et al, 1992; Wuisman et al, 1992).

Strong labeling of the osseous isozyme of alkaline phosphatase has been used to distinguish EO from other pleomorphic sarcomas. The major drawback of this marker is that it can only be used on cryostat sections and imprint smears.

Ancillary techniques have a limited role in diagnosing osteosarcoma, as the tumour is largely recognized by its morphologic features. Because of the many varieties of osteosarcoma, diverse tumours are considered in its differential diagnosis.

Currently, immunohistochemistry has limited application in the differential diagnosis of primary bone tumors. In general, osteosarcoma has a broad immunoprofile that lacks diagnostic specificity. Vimentin, OCN, ONN, S-100 protein, muscle protein smooth muscle actin (SMA), neuron specific enolase (NSE) and CD99 are some of the antigens that are commonly expressed. Importantly, some tumours also stain with antibodies to keratin and epithelial membrane antigen (EMA). Also, it's worth noticing, that osteosarcoma usually does not stain with antibodies to factor VIII and CD31.

Osteosarcoma is distinguished from benign tumours and fibro-osseous lesions, by virtue of its infiltrative growth pattern, with the tumour replacing the marrow space and surrounding bony trabeculae, which may also serve as scaffolding for the deposition of neoplastic bone.

Telangiectatic osteosarcoma differs from aneurysmal bone cyst because it contains cytologically malignant cells within the cyst walls, whereas the cells in aneurysmal bone cyst are banal in appearance.

Biopsies of osteosarcoma that lack neoplastic bone can be problematic because its immunophenotype can generate a broad list of differential diagnoses that include Ewing's sarcoma/Primitive Neuroectodermal Tumour-PNET, metastatic carcinoma and melanoma, leiomyosarcoma and malignant peripheral nerve sheath tumour.

The subtype of osteosarcoma that most likely will benefit from the application of an immunohistochemistry panel is the "small-cell" type. The diagnosis of this entity is difficult due to the paucity of osteoid and the similarity to other small round-cell tumors. Although the antigenic profile of small-cell osteosarcoma is unknown, expression of markers specific for other small-cell tumors, help in ruling out this diagnosis.

In these circumstances, immunohistochemical analysis, electron microscopic evaluation and molecular studies may be helpful. Small cell osteosarcoma is distinguished from Ewing's sarcoma by the presence of neoplastic bone and dilated rough endoplasmic reticulum by electron microscopy, as osteosarcoma cells have the features of mesenchymal cells with abundant endoplasmic reticulum and the matrix contains collagen fibres, which may show calcium hydroapatite crystal deposition and the absence of t(11;22) translocation, or its variants, which is diagnostic of Ewing's sarcoma.

MIC-2 gene product (CD99), which is located in the short arm of the sex chromosome, encodes a surface protein, first described in T-cell and null-cell acute lymphoblastic leukemia. Osteosarcoma usually has a diffuse moderate to strong intracytoplasmic staining for CD99. Tumour cells of the small cell variant of osteosarcoma may be positive for CD99, vimentin, osteocalcin, osteonectin, smooth muscle actin, Leu-7 and KP1.

The differential diagnosis of osteosarcoma from other sarcomas (e.g., malignant fibrous histiocytoma, fibrosarcoma) is important because of the specific therapy available for osteosarcoma patients. Most osteosarcomas express vimentin and, according to some authors, some tumors focally express cytokeratin and desmin, although these findings have not been widely confirmed. Bone matrix proteins, such as OCN, alkaline phosphatase, and ONN, are expressed in osteosarcomas. However, their presence has also been detected in chondrosarcomas, Ewing's sarcoma, fibrosarcomas, and malignant fibrous histiocytomas. Caution should also be used in the interpretation of focal expression of a variety of markers (e.g., S-100, actin, epithelial membrane antigen) found occasionally in otherwise typical osteosarcomas. Extraskeletal osteosarcomas of the fibroblastic subtype often have sparse amounts of osteoid and can be differentiated from malignant fibrous histiocytoma on the basis of strong expression of alkaline phosphatase. Chondroblastic osteosarcoma and chondrosarcoma, however, cannot be distinguished immunohistochemically.

The different types of collagen present in the bone matrix are also produced by other tumors and therefore have no application in differential diagnosis. The basic calponin gene, a smooth muscle differentiation-specific gene that encodes an actin-binding protein involved in the regulation of smooth muscle contractility, is expressed in osteosarcomas (Yamamura, et al, 1998).

The list of entities included in the differential diagnosis of MFH is extensive. Immunohistochemistry helps in the distinction of MFH (CD68+, OCN-, alkaline phosphatase-) from leiomyosarcoma (CD68-), malignant neurilemmoma (S-100+) and from fibroblastic osteosarcoma (occasionally positive for both OCN, alkaline phosphatase). The distinction of cytokeratin-positive MFH from sarcomatoid carcinoma may be impossible by immunohistochemistry and is best accomplished by electron microscopy.

Finally, stress fracture and accompanying callus can sometimes be confused with osteosarcoma because the reactive bone and cartilage are deposited around pre-existing bony trabeculae, mimicking an infiltrative pattern of growth. However, the cells in reactive tissues are banal and osteoblastic rimming is usually present.

In conclusion, although immunohistochemistry does not currently play an important diagnostic role in primary bone tumors as it does in soft-tissue counterparts, research efforts to characterize the histogenesis of many of these neoplasias may offer new alternatives for diagnosis in the near future. For the distinction of primary tumors versus metastases of non-osseous origin and for the characterization of a small subset of neoplasias, such as those with small round-cell morphology, immunohistochemistry remains the technique of choice.

5. Molecular pathology of osteosarcoma

Traditionally, our understanding of osteosarcoma has been largely based on anatomic and histologic features. However, recent studies in the molecular pathology of osteosarcoma have provided new insight into its pathogenesis. Through the identification of molecular pathways of osteosarcoma development and progression, the roles played by mutated tumor suppressor genes, oncogenes, and cell cycle regulatory molecules in bone oncogenesis, differentiation, cell death and cell migration have been explored. Furthermore, numerous cytogenetic abnormalities have been associated with osteosarcoma, including chromosomal amplifications, deletions, rearrangements, and translocations.

Thus, the diagnostic and prognostic significance of molecular aberrations are beginning to be evaluated and novel approaches for therapeutic interventions of osteosarcoma are being developed.

5.1 Bone growth, differentiation and osteosarcoma tumorigenesis

It is well known that osteosarcoma has a propensity for developing in bone growth plates characterized by rapid bone turnover during childhood and adolescence (Broadhead et al., 2011; Gelberg et al., 1997)

Additionally, patients affected by Paget's disease, a disorder characterized by both excessive bone formation and breakdown, also have a higher incidence of osteosarcoma (Vigorita, 2008). These observations, along with the knowledge that normal bone differentiation process occurs in the epiphyseal growth plates, strongly suggest that osteosarcoma is caused by genetic and epigenetic disturbances in the osteoblast proliferation and differentiation pathways (Tang et al., 2008; Thomas et al., 2006).

Osteogenesis results from a regulated sequence of events involving epithelial mesenchymal interactions, condensation, and terminal differentiation. Several major signal transduction pathways, such as Wnt, BMP, FGF, and hedgehog signaling, play an important role in regulating osteogenic differentiation (Glass & Karsenty, 2007; Luu et al., 2007; Reya &Clevers, 2005). Bone lineage commitment and terminal differentiation are regulated by several osteogenic transcriptional factors such as, Runx2, Osterix, ATF4, and TAZ (Chien & Karsenty, 2005; Deng et al., 2008; Kansara & Thomas, 2007; Karsenty, 2000; Karsenty, 2002; Karsenty, 2003; Hong et al., 2005; Yang & Karsenty, 2004) in coordination with their activators, like Rb which transactivates Runx2 (Ogasawara et al., 2004; Thomas et al., 2001) and their repressors, like WWOX which suppresses RUNX2 transcriptional activity (Del Mare et al., 2011).

Among these factors, Runx2 is the most important regulator of bone development and serves as a hub to direct progenitors to osteogenic lineage through BMP-induced osteogenesis, synergistically inducing many terminal differentiation markers (Lian et al., 2006; Nakashima et al., 2002; Thomas et al., 2004; Yamaguchi et al., 2000). Additionally, Runx2 associates with p27KIP1 protein and through interaction with the hypophosphorylated form of Rb and transactivation of Osterix transcription factor, promotes terminal cell cycle exit and the formation of a differentiated osteoblastic phenotype (Nakashima et al., 2002; Nishio et al., 2006; Thomas et al., 2004).

Furthermore, the canonical Wnt pathway has been identified to play a crucial role in osteoblast differentiation, as evidenced by the fact that Wnt3a expression leads to cell proliferation and suppression of osteogenic differentiation in adult mesenchymal stem cells (Boland et al., 2004), and that multiple aberrations in the Wnt signaling pathway have been associated with osteosarcoma tumorigenesis (Haydon et al., 2002, Reya & Clevers, 2005, Clevers, 2006).

Disruption of the well-coordinated balance between osteogenic progenitors proliferation and differentiation may lead to osteosarcoma development. The defects caused by genetic (eg, activation of oncogenes or inactivation of p53 and RB tumor suppressor genes) and epigenetic alterations may occur at different stages of osteogenic differentiation leading to more or less aggressive tumorigenic phenotypes (Kansara and Thomas, 2007).

Moreover, osteosarcoma cells utilize an alternative lengthening of telomere (ALT) pathway that prevents telomere shortening, allowing the tumor cells to evade senescence and resemble their stem cell progenitors (Wang, 2005).

5.2 Osteosarcoma invasion and metastasis

Osteosarcoma is an aggressive tumor with high metastatic potential. Osteosarcoma invasion of bone and metastasis to other organs relies on complex cell-cell and cell-matrix interactions. The invasion and metastatic sequence involves the detachment of osteosarcoma cells from the primary site, lysis of bone matrix, local migration, invasion through stromal tissue, intravasation, and extravasation. In this process, interactions between osteosarcoma cells, osteoblasts and osteoclasts are the main events leading to the substantial osteolysis exhibited by some osteosarcomas as a result of increased osteoclastic activity.

During the initial stages of osteosarcoma invasion, TGF-β is released from the degraded bone matrix and acts on osteosarcoma cells, stimulating the release of PTHrP, interleukin-6 (IL-6) and interleukin-11 (IL-11) (Quinn et al., 2001). These cytokines then stimulate osteoclasts, facilitating further invasion and release of proresorptive cytokines. Osteoblasts function as mediators in this process of bone resorption. Osteosarcoma cells release endothelin-1 (ET-1), VEGF, and PDGF in response to the hypoxic and acidotic conditions leading to angiogenesis and stimulation of osteoblastic function (Kingsley et al., 2007; Chirgwin et al., 2007). PTHrP and IL-11 also act on osteoblasts, stimulating increased expression of receptor activator of nuclear factor κB ligand (RANKL). RANKL is a main mediator of osteoclast differentiation and activity, and osteosarcoma cells produce RANKL independently (Kinpara, 2000). RANKL activates osteoclasts through binding to RANK on the osteoclast surface. RANK expression is regulated by cytokines IL-1, IL-6, IL-8, tumour necrosis factor-α (TNF-α), PTHrP, and TGF-α (Hofbauer & Heufelder, 1998).

Receptor-ligand binding leads to activation of both NFκB and MAPK pathways, with a resulting increase in nuclear factor of activated T cells (NFATc1) activity. RANK/RANKL also activates the c-Fos component of AP-1, resulting in additional NFATc1 upregulation. NFATc1 then activates the transcription of genes involved in osteoclast activity and maturation (Takayanagi, 2007).

Activated osteoclasts release proteases such as cathepsin K (Cat K) necessary for breakdown of collagen I, osteopontin, and osteonectin (Stoch & Wagner, 2008) aiding the invasion process (LeGall et al., 2007). This protease is essential for osteoclast function in normal bone remodelling and also in pathological states of osteolysis. For patients with high-grade metastatic osteosarcoma, low Cat K levels at the time of diagnosis confers a better prognosis (Husmann et al., 2008).

Invasion of the surrounding tissues by osteosarcoma also involves degradation of the extracellular matrix. Matrix metalloproteinases (MMPs) are principally involved in the breakdown of the extracellular matrix and are regulated by natural inhibitors such as tissue inhibitors of MMPs (TIMPs), RECK, and α2 macroglobulin (Birkedal-Hansen et al., 1993; Chakraborti et al., 2003). In the setting of osteosarcoma, MMPs break down extracellular collagens, facilitating both tumour and endothelial cell invasion. MMPs play also a role in angiogenesis aiding further the metastatic process.

The urokinase plasminogen activator (uPA) and its receptor (uPAR) system is another key regulator of osteosarcoma invasion, which acts as an activator of pro-MMPs. An inverse relationship between uPA levels and overall survival has been demonstrated in osteosarcoma cases (Choong et al., 1996).

5.3 Syndromes associated with osteosarcoma

A variety of genetically based diseases and syndromes show a susceptibility to the development of osteosarcoma, such as Paget's disease, Rothmund-Thomson, Bloom,Werner and Li-Fraumeni syndromes, as well as Hereditary Retinoblastoma.

In patients affected by Paget's, a hereditary disorder characterized by rapid bone remodelling leading to dysregulated bone turnover, about 1 % of them will develop osteosarcoma. This percentage accounts for a substantial fraction of the osteosarcoma cases diagnosed over 60 years of age (McNairm et al., 2001). Although the complete pattern of genetic aberrations leading to Paget's disease remains unclear, LOH18CRI located at 18q21-q22 locus has been identified as the major underlying genetic abnormality linked to Paget osteosarcoma (Cody et al., 1997; Good et al., 2002; Hansen et al.,1999; Nelissery et al., 1998). Furthermore, the genes SQSTMI at 5q31 and MAPK8 at 5q35qter, which are implicated in IL-1/TNF and RANK signalling pathways, respectively, seem to be involved in Paget osteosarcoma pathogenesis (Kansara & Thomas, 2007).

Rothmund-Thomson, Bloom and Werner syndromes are characterized by germline mutations in RecQ helicases genes whose products are responsible for separation of double-stranded DNA prior to replication (German, 1993; Goto et al., 1996; Hickson, 2003). Among them Rothmund-Thomson syndrome, an autosomal recessive disorder, is related to the highest osteosarcoma incidence (32 %) with a tendency to occur at a younger age (Tang et al., 2008; Wang, 2001; Wang et al, 2003; Wang et al., 2005).

Li-Fraumeni syndrome patients are characterized by germline mutations in p53 gene and have an increasesd risk in developing osteosarcomas among other malignancies (Malkin et al., 1990).

Hereditary Retinoblastoma patients have germline mutations in Rb1 tumor suppressor gene and are predisposed to develop osteosarcoma (Araki et al., 1991). Such bone sarcomas are likely to show LOH at 13q and molecular alterations of the Rb1 gene (Andreassen et al., 1993; Wadayama et al., 1994; Wunder et al., 1991).

5.4 Cytogenetic aberrations

5.4.1 Conventional osteosarcoma

5.4.1.1 Cytogenetics

Although the germline mutations explain part of the osteosarcoma cases, most osteosarcomas are sporadic. Sporadic osteosarcomas have a wide range of genetic abnormalities and display extensive genetic heterogeneity. However involvement of certain chromosomal loci is recurrent and chromosomal regions 1p11-13, 1q11-12, 1q21-22, 11p14-15, 14p11-13, 15p11-13, 17p and 19q13 are most frequently affected (Mertens et al., 1993; Tarkkanen et al., 1993). Numerical chromosomal abnormalities associated with conventional osteosarcoma include loss of chromosomes 6q, 9, 10, 13, and 17 as well as gain of chromosome 1 (Boehm et al., 2000; Bridge et al., 1997; Stock et al., 2000).

Recent studies have identified amplifications of chromosomes 6p21, 8q24, and 12q14, as well as loss of heterozygosity of 10q21.1, as being among the most common genomic alterations in osteosarcoma. Furthermore, patients carrying these aberrations had a poorer prognosis (Smida et al., 2010).

Cytogenetic features of gene amplification, such as ring chromosomes, double minutes, and homogeneously staining regions are frequently identified in conventional osteosarcomas (Menghi-Sartorio et al., 2001).

Despite intensive research, no consensus specific chromosomal aberrations that could be used diagnostically in osteosarcoma tumors have been identified.

5.4.1.2 DNA copy numbers

Osteosarcoma tumors contain multiple random chromosomal aberrations and only a few deletions and amplifications appear common to comparative genomic hybridization (CGH) studies (Atiye et al., 2005; Selvarajah et al., 2008).

Comparative genomic hybridization analysis reveals that chromosomal regions 3q26, 4q12-13, 5p13-14, 7q31-32, 8q21-23, 12q12-13, 12q14-15, and 17p11-12 are most frequently gained (Menghi-sartorio et al., 2001; Stock et al., 2000; Tarkannen et al., 1995). Gain of 8q23 is detected in 50% of tumors (Stock et al., 2000) and is correlated with poor prognosis (Tarkkanen et al., 1989). Increased copy number of the MYC gene localized to 8q24 was detected by in situ hybridization in 44% of cases (Stock et al., 2000). The most frequent losses are found at 2q, 6q, 8p, and 10p (Knutila et al., 2000; Tarkannen et al., 1995).

In a recent study with 10 osteosarcomas, CGH whole-genome analysis showed changes including: hypomethylation, gain, and overexpression of histone cluster 2 genes at chromosome 1q21.1-q21.3; loss of chromosome 8p21.2-p21.3 and underexpression of DOCK5 and TNFRSF10A/D genes; and amplification-related overexpression of RUNX2 at chromosome 6p12.3-p21.1. Amplification and overexpression of RUNX2 could disrupt G2/M cell cycle checkpoints and bone differentiation leading to genomic instability. Disruption of DOCK5-signaling, together with p53 and TNFRSF10A/D related cell cycle and death pathways, may play a critical role in abrogating apoptosis (Sadicovic et al., 2009)

Diploid ploidy pattern by DNA fluocytometry has been reported to be a poor prognostic sign (Kusuzaki et al., 1999).

5.4.1.3 Loss of heterozygosity (LOH)

Loss of heterozygocity are detected more frequently at the long arms of chromosomes 3, 13 and 18 and at the short arm of chromosome 17 (Kruzelock et al., 1997). As the incidence of LOH is high at 3q26.6-26.3, this area has been suggested to harbour a putative suppressor gene (Kruzelock et al., 1997).

5.4.2 Telangiectatic osteosarcoma

A limited number of cases show highly complex chromosomal changes, and only one case is characterized by trisomy 3 (Bridge et al., 1997; Fletcher et al., 1994; Hoogerwerf et al., 1994). Mutations in the TP53 and RAS genes, LOH at the TP53, CDKN2A and RB1 loci, and amplification of the MDM2 and MYC genes are rare in telangiectatic osteosarcomas (Radig et al., 1998).

Telangiectatic osteosarcoma can be distinguished from aneurysmal bone cyst by the balanced tranlocations between the short arm of chromosome 17 and the long arm of chromosome 16 (Panoutsakopoulos et al., 1999). This rearrangement is characteristic of aneurysmal bone cyst. However, there are many variations on this theme, and at least five different chromosomes can serve as translocation partners with chromosome 17 (Dal Cin et al., 2000; Herens et al., 2001; Wyatt-Ashmead et al., 2001).

5.4.3 Small cell osteosarcoma

No specific cytogenetic abnormalities have been detected in small cell osteosarcoma.

Small cell osteosarcoma can be distinguished from Ewing sarcoma by the presence of neoplastic bone and the absence of the t(11:22) translocation or one of its variants.

5.4.4 Low grade central osteosarcoma

Low grade central (intramedullary) osteosarcoma show minimal chromosomal imbalances compared with the complex cytogenetic aberrations identified in high grade osteosarcoma. Cytogenetic studies revealed ring chromosomes of amplified regions 12q13-15, as well as abnormalities in chromosome 6p, 14 and 15 (Werner et al., 1998).

Comparative genomic hybridization demonstrate recurrent gains in chromosomal regions at 12q13-14, 12p, and 6p21 (Tarkkanen et al., 1998). MDM2, CDK4, and SAS at the 12q13-15 amplicon have been reported to be amplified at frequencies of 35%, 65% and 15%, respectively (Ragazzini et al., 1999).

5.4.5 Postradiation osteosarcoma

Cytogenetic and DNA copy number changes are complex and similar to those in conventional osteosarcomas (Mertens et al.; 2000). Postradiation osteosarcomas frequently exhibit 3p and 1p chromosomal losses compared to sporadic osteosarcoma which show more gains than losses (Mertens et al., 2000; Tarkkanen et al;, 2001).

In one study, a high (58%) incidence of TP53 mutations was found (Nakanishi et al., 1998).

5.4.6 Parosteal osteosarcoma

Chromosomal alterations in parosteal osteosarcomas (low grade surface osteosarcomas) are characterized by one or more supernumerary ring chromosomes, often as the sole alteration (Mertens et al., 1993; Örndal et al., 1993; Sinovic et al., 1992).

Comparative genomic hybridization studies indicate 12q13-15 amplified region in the chromosomal rings (Szymanska et al., 1996). The SAS, CDK4, and MDM2 genes are coamplified and overexpressed in the majority of cases (Wunder et al., 1999).

Mutations in RB1 (Wadayama et al., 1994) or microsatellite instability (Tarkkanen et al., 1996) have not been found to be present in parosteal osteosarcoma.

5.4.7 Periosteal osteosarcoma

Most of the periosteal osteosarcomas show complex karyotypic aberrations (Gisselsson et al., 1998; Hoogerwerf et al., 1994; Tarkkanen et al., 1993).

5.4.8 Extraskeletal osteosarcomas

Clonal chromosomal aberrations with complex patterns have been reported (Mandahl et al., 1989; Mertens et al. 1998). So far, no genetic differences between osteosarcomas of bone and extraskeletal origin have been identified.

5.5 Molecular genetic alterations

A number of molecular defects in tumor suppressor genes, oncogenes, bone differentiation genes and genes involved in cell migration have been observed in osteosarcomas.

5.5.1 Tumor suppressor genes

The p53 and retinoblastoma (Rb) genes are the major tumor-suppressor genes affected in osteosarcoma (Marina et al., 2004).The p53 gene is mutated in 22% of osteosarcomas (Ta et al., 2009) and its expression seems to be higher in low grade osteosarcomas and correlate with reduced metastatic disease and improved survival (Hu et al., 2010). p53 mutation has also been shown to be more common in high-grade conventional osteosarcomas versus low grade central osteosarcomas (Park et al., 2004). However, other studies showed no correlation between survival and the p53 protein, while coexpression of p53 and P-glycoprotein was associated with a poorer prognosis (Lonardo et al., 1997; Park et al., 2001).

In addition to p53, the Rb tumour suppressor has also been implicated in the tumorigenesis of osteosarcoma. Both germ-line and somatic mutations of Rb confer an increased risk of osteosarcoma (Benassi et al., 1999). Loss of heterozygosity for Rb has been reported to confer both an improved and poorer prognosis for patients (Heinsohn et al., 2007; Wadayama et al., 1994; Feugeas et al., 1996).

5.5.2 Oncogenes

Transcription factors c-Fos and c-Jun are significantly upregulated in high-grade osteosarcomas compared with benign osteogenic lesions and low-grade osteosarcomas (Wu et al., 1990; Franchi et al., 1998) and are associated with the propensity to develop metastases (Gamberi et al., 1998).

Another transcription factor involved in cell proliferation, is c-Myc, whose amplification has been implicated in osteosarcoma pathogenesis and resistance to chemotherapeutic drugs. Overexpression of Myc in bone marrow stromal cells leads to osteosarcoma development and loss of adipogenesis (Shimizu et al., 2010).

Overexpression of MET (Ferracini et al., 1995; Rong et al., 1993) and c-Fos (Wu et al., 1990) has been reported in more than 50% of osteosarcoma cases, whereas c-Myc is overexpressed in less than 15% of cases (Barrios et al., 1993; Ladanyi et al., 1993). c-Myc, c-Fos, and cathepsin L have been shown to be overexpressed in a high proportion of relapsed tumours and metastases (Gamberi et al., 1998; Park et al., 1996).

Transforming growth factor beta (TGF-β) family proteins are also implicated in osteosarcomagenesis through impairment of osteoblast proliferation, differentiation and cell death. High-grade osteosarcomas are found to express TGF-β1 in significantly higher amounts than low-grade osteosarcomas (Franchi et al., 1998).

IGF (insulin-like growth factor)-I and IGF-II are growth factors that are often overexpressed by osteosarcomas (Rikkof et al., 2009).

Connective tissue growth factor (CTGF) is related to a number of proteins in the CCN family (CTGF/Cyr61/ Cef10/NOVH). This protein family act via integrin signalling pathways (Lau et al., 1999) and, is involved in a diverse range of functions including adhesion, migration, proliferation, survival, angiogenesis, and differentiation. A related protein, CCN3, was found to be overexpressed in osteosarcoma and associated with a worse prognosis (Perbal et al., 2008).

In one study, a substantial percentage (42.6%) of osteosarcomas displayed high levels of HER2/neu (c-erbB2,ERBB2) expression, relative to adjacent normal tissues (Gorlick et al., 1999).

5.5.3 Genes amplifications

Amplifications at 1q21-23 and at 17p are frequent findings in conventional osteosarcoma (Knuutila et al., 2000). Several genes have been reported to be involved in the 1q21-23 amplicon (Forus et al., 1998; Meza-Zepeda et al., 2002). Similarly, a variety of genes in the 12q13-15 region are co-amplified (Berner et al., 1997; Forus et al., 1994; Khatib et al., 1993; Momand et al., 1992; Oliner et al., 1992; Roberts et al., 1989; Smith et al., 1992; Yotov et al., 1999).

FISH analysis has revealed that genes, including CCND2, ETV6, and KRAS2, at 12p and MDM2 at 12q were differently amplified in low grade osteosarcomas (parosteal osteosarcoma) and high grade osteosarcomas (Gisselson et al., 2002).

MDM2 (Ladanyi et al., 1993; Oliner et al., 1992) and PRIM1 (Yotov et al., 1999) amplifications have been detected in 14-27% and 41% of osteosarcoma cases, respectively. In aggressive osteosarcomas CDK4 is most consistently amplified, alone or together with MDM2 (Berneret al., 1996; Forus et al., 1994; Maelandsmoet al., 1995).

Recently, it was shown that APEX1 gene was amplified in osteosarcomas and that APEX1 expression was an independent predictor of the osteosarcoma local recurrence and/or metastasis (Yang et al., 2010).

5.5.4 Gene expression

Osteosarcoma cells share many similar features to undifferentiated osteoprogenitors, including a high proliferative capacity, resistance to anoikis, and expression of many osteogenic markers, such as CTGF, Runx2, ALP, Osterix, Osteocalcin and Osteopontin (Tang et al., 2008; Haydon et al., 2007; Luu et al., 2007). Furthermore, the more aggressive osteosarcoma phenotypes often have features of early osteogenic progenitors, while less aggressive tumors seem to be more similar to osteogenic mesenchymal stem cells that have progressed further along the differentiation cascade (Broadhead et al., 2011; He et al., 2010).

Osteogenic differentiation of mesenchymal stem cells can be monitored by using bone morphogenetic proteins (BMPs) and their downstream mediators, such as Id proteins and connective tissue growth factor (CTGF), as early markers, alkaline phosphatase and Osterix as early/middle markers and osteocalcin and osteopontin as late markers of bone formation (Tang et al., 2008).

Analysis of the expression of these osteogenic markers in osteosarcoma cells demonstrates a much lower alkaline phosphatase expression in tumor cells when compared to committed osteoblastic cell lines (Harris et al., 1995; Luo et al., 2008). Similarly, the late osteogenic markers osteopontin and osteocalcin are highly expressed in mature, differentiated osteoblasts, but are minimally expressed in both primary OS tumors and OS cell lines (Cheng et al., 2003; Luu et al., 2007). CTGF, a multifunctional growth factor that is normally upregulated at the earliest stages of osteogenic differentiation, also shows elevated basal expression in human osteosarcoma cells (Luo et al., 2004).

Recent studies have revealed that *WWOX*, a gene involved in bone differentiation, is deleted in 30% of osteosarcoma cases and WWOX protein is absent or reduced in ~60% of osteosarcoma tumors (Del Mare et al., 2011). WWOX associates with Runx2, a key regulator of bone differentiation. Interestingly, Runx2 has a very low expression in osteosarcoma cell lines. Runx2 also associates with BMPs, Rb, and p27KIP1 playing a crucial role in cell cycle and bone differentiation regulatory pathways. Thus, it is natural that any alterations would lead to uncontrolled proliferation and loss of differentiation. Accordingly, high-grade osteosarcomas show decreased expression of p27KIP1, while lower-grade tumors have detectable p27KIP1 levels (Thomas et al., 2004).

Bone morphogenetic proteins (BMPs) such as bone morphogenetic protein-6 and bone morphogenetic protein receptor 2 are expressed in more than 50% of osteosarcomas and related to poor prognosis (Gobbi et al., 2002; Guo et al., 1999; Yoshikawa et al., 2004).

As above mentioned, Wnt pathway plays a crucial role in osteoblast differentiation and elevated levels of β-Catenin, an important regulator of the Wnt pathway, are correlated with osteoprogenitor proliferation and osteosarcoma metastasis (Iwaya et al., 2003). In addition, osteosarcoma tumors overexpressing LRP5, a Wnt co-receptor, are associated with a poorer prognosis and decreased patient survival (Hoang et al., 2004). Furthermore, Wnt mutations causing excessive Wnt (Wingless and int) signalling are associated to decreased survival and increased metastatic capacity (Hoang et al., 2004; Iwaya et al., 2003; Kansara and Thomas, 2007).

Other genes with altered expression associated to osteosarcoma include overexpression of MAGE genes (Sudo et al., 1997), p19INK4D (a cyclin dependent kinase inhibitor involved in cell cycle regulation, found in 7 % of osteosarcomas) (Miller et al., 1997), transforming growth factor-beta (TGFβ) isoforms, of which TGFβ3 is strongly related to disease progression (Kloen et al., 1997) and vascular endothelial growth factor (VEGF, expression correlated with survival) (Jung et al., 2005). Antiangiogenic proteins such as thrombospondin 1, TGF-β , troponin I, pigment epithelial-derived factor (PEDF), and reversion-inducing cysteine rich protein with Kazal motifs (RECK) are downregulated in osteosarcoma (Ren et al., 2006; Cai et al., 2006; Clark et al., 2007).

Overexpression of Ezrin, a protein involved in cell movement, correlates with poor outcome in paediatric osteosarcoma (Khanna et al., 2004) and according to animal studies, is overexpressed in highly metastatic osteosarcoma compared to tumors with lower metastatic potential (Khanna et al., 2000).

MMP2 and MMP9 were overexpressed in osteosarcoma cells and associated with the ability of the cells to metastasize (Bjornland et al., 2005). Increased expression of membrane-type MMP1 has been correlated with poor prognosis (Ushibori et al., 2006) and upregulation of TIMP1 is associated with poor clinical outcome (Ferrari et al., 2004).

5.6 Epigenetics

Compared to large number of studies describing genetic alterations in osteosarcoma, relatively few studies investigating epigenetic alterations have been reported so far (Benassi et al., 2001; Benassi et al., 1999; Harada et al., 2002; Hou et al., 2006; Thomas and Kansara, 2006; Tsuchiya et al., 2000).

Recent studies have identified a close association between the aberrant methylation of histone cluster 2 genes, p14ARF/CDKN2A, p16 and Ras effector homologue (RASSF1A) genes and osteosarcoma tumorigenesis (Hou et al., 2006; Rao-Bindal & Kleinerman, 2011**).** It is believed that hypermethylation and subsequent transcriptional silencing of tumor suppressor genes contributes to the neoplastic process by increasing the mutation rate (Jones & Baylin, 2002; Wajed et al., 2001).

5.7 Epilogue

Understanding of the molecular pathogenesis of osteosarcoma has advanced considerably over recent decades. The processes involved in osteosarcoma oncogenesis have been outlined above with emphasis on the disruption of bone differentiation machinery.

However, the study of pathogenic mechanisms is in itself not enough. Translational studies are critical if an effective treatment for osteosarcoma is to arise from this understanding of osteosarcoma molecular pathology. If osteosarcoma results from bone differentiation defects, future research should focus on identifying relevant biomarkers and therapies targeting cellular differentiation thereby avoiding complications associated with conventional chemotherapy and be most effective in treatment of this debilitating tumor.

6. References

Acchiapati G, Randelli G, & Randelli M (1965). Observations on osteogenous- osteogenic sarcoma. *Arch Orthop*, 78:57-156

Ackerman A.J (1948). Multiple osteogenic sarcoma. Report of two cases. *Am J Roentgenol Radium Ther Nucl Med*, 60:623-632

Adler C.P (1980). Case report 111. *Skeletal Radiol*, 5(1):56-60

Amstutz H.C (1969). Multiple osteogenic osteosarcomata-metastatic or multicentric? Review of two cases and review of the literature. *Cancer*, 24:923-931

Allan C.J, Soule E.H (1971). Osteogenic sarcoma of the somatic soft tissues. Clinicopathologic study of 26 cases and review of the literature. *Cancer*, 27:1121-1133

Andreassen A, Oyjord T, Hovig E, Holm R, Florenes VA, Nesland JM, Myklebost O, Hoie J, Bruland OS & Borresen AL. (1993). p53 abnormalities in different subtypes of human sarcomas. *Cancer Res*, 53: 468-471.

Araki N, Uchida A, Kimura T, Yoshikawa H, Aoki Y, Ueda T, Takai S, Miki T & Ono K (1991). Involvement of the retinoblastoma gene in primary osteosarcomas and other bone and soft-tissue tumors. *Clin Orthop*, 270:271-277.

Atiye J, Wolf M, Kaur S, Monni O, Bohling T, Kivioja A, Tas E, Serra M, Tarkkanen M & Knuutila S. (2005).Gene amplifications in osteosarcoma-CGH microarray analysis. *Genes Chromosomes Cancer*, 42:158–163.

Bane B.L, Evans H.L, Ro J.Y, et al (1990). Extraskeletal osteosarcoma. A clinicopathologic review of 26 cases. *Cancer*, 65:2762-2770

Barrios C, Castresana JS, Ruiz J, Kreicbergs A (1993). Amplification of c-myc oncogene and absence of c-Ha-ras point mutation in human bone sarcoma. *J Orthop Res*, 11: 556-563

Bartkowski S & Kleczynski A (1974). A case of sarcoma developing in the course of chronic non specific osteitis. *Pol Przegl Chir*, 46:783-785

Baydar D.E, Himmetoglu C.,Yazici S., et al. (2009). Primary osteosarcoma of the urinary bladder following cyclophosphamide therapy for systemic lupus erythematosus: a case report. *Journal of Medical Case Reports*, 3(39):1-5

Benassi, M. S., Molendini, L., Gamberi, G., Magagnoli, G., Ragazzini, P., Gobbi, G. A., Sangiorgi, L., Pazzaglia, L., Asp, J., Brantsing, C., & Picci, P. (2001). Involvement of INK4A gene products in the pathogenesis and development of human osteosarcoma. *Cancer* 92: 3062-3067

Benassi, M. S., Molendini, L., Gamberi, G., Ragazzini, P., Sollazzo, M. R., Merli, M., Asp, J., Magagnoli, G., Balladelli, A., Bertoni, F., & Picci, P. (1999). Alteration of pRb/p16/cdk4 regulation in human osteosarcoma. *Int J Cancer*, 84: 489-493

Benson J.E, Goske M, Han J.S, et al (1984). Primary osteogenic sarcoma of the calvaria. *Am J Neuroradiol*, 5:810-813

Berner JM, Forus A, Elkahloun A, Meltzer PS, Fodstad O & Myklebost O (1996). Separate amplified regions encompassing CDK4 and MDM2 in human sarcomas. *Genes Chromosomes Cancer* 17: 254-259

Berner JM, Meza-Zepeda LA, Kools PF, Forus A, Schoenmakers EF, Van de Ven WJ, Fodstad O & Myklebost O (1997). HMGIC, the gene for an architectural transcription factor, is amplified and rearranged in a subset of human sarcomas. *Oncogene*, 14: 2935-2941

Bjornland K, Flatmark K, Pettersen S, Aaasen AO, Fodstad O & Maelandsmo GM. (2005). Matrix metalloproteinases participate in osteosarcoma invasion. *J Surg Res.*, 127:151-156

Birkedal-Hansen H., W. G. I. Moore, M. K. Bodden et al. (1993). Matrix metalloproteinases: a review. *Critical Reviews in Oral Biology and Medicine*, 4(2):197–250

Boehm AK, Neff JR, Squire JA, Bayani J, Nelson M & Bridge JA (2000). Cytogenetic findings in 36 osteosarcoma specimens and a review of the literature. *Ped Pathol Mol Med*, 19: 359-376

Boland G. M., G. Perkins, D. J. Hall, and R. S. Tuan (2004). Wnt 3a promotes proliferation and suppresses osteogenic differentiation of adult human mesenchymal stem cells. *Journal of Cellular Biochemistry*, 93(6):1210–1230

Brien W.W, Salvati E.A, Healey J.H, et al (1990). Osteogenic sarcoma arising in the area of a total hip replacement. A case report. *J Bone Joint Surg Am*, 72:1097-1099

Bridge JA, Nelson M, McComb E, McGuire MH, Rosenthal H, Vergara G, Maale GE, Spanier S & Neff JR (1997). Cytogenetic findings in 73 osteosarcoma specimens and a review of the literature. *Cancer Genet Cytogenet*, 95:74-87.

Broadhead M. L., Clark J. C. M., Myers D. E., Dass C. R., & Choong P. F. M. (2011). The Molecular Pathogenesis of Osteosarcoma: A Review. *Sarcoma*, 2011: Article ID 959248, 12 pp

Broders A.C (1920). Squamous cell epithelioma of the lip: A study of 537 cases. *JAMA*, 74:659-664

Burke A. P, Virmani R. (1991). Osteosarcoma of the heart. *Am J Surg Path*, 15:289-295

Cahan W.G., Woodard H.Q., Higinbothan N.L., & al. (1948). Sarcoma arising in irradiated bone. Report of eleven cases. *Cancer, 1 :3-29*

Cai J., Parr C., Watkins G., Jiang W. G., & Boulton M.(2006). Decreased pigment epithelium-derived factor expression in human breast cancer progression. *Clinical Cancer Research,* 12(11): 3510–3517

Coley B.L, Sharp G.S & Ellis E.B (1931). Diagnosis of bone tumours by aspiration. *Am J Surg Pathol,* 13:215-224

Chakraborti S, Mandal M., Das S., Mandal A, & Chakraborti T. (2003). Regulation of matrix metalloproteinases. An overview. *Molecular and Cellular Biochemistry,* 253(1-2):269–285

Cheng H., W. Jiang, F. M. Phillips et al. (2003). Osteogenic activity of the fourteen types of human bone morphogenetic proteins (BMPs). *Journal of Bone and Joint Surgery A,* 85(8):1544–1552

Chien KR & Karsenty G.(2005). Longevity and lineages: toward the integrative biology of degenerative diseases in heart, muscle and bone. *Cell,*120:533–544

Chirgwin J. M. & T. A. Guise (2007). Skeletal metastases: decreasing tumor burden by targeting the bone microenvironment. *Journal of Cellular Biochemistry,* 102(6):1333–1342

Choong P. M., Ferno M., Akermans M. et al. (1996). Urokinaseplasminogen-activator levels and prognosis in 69 soft-tissue sarcomas. *International Journal of Cancer,* 69(4):268–272

Chung E.B, Enzinger F.M (1987). Extraskeletal osteosarcoma. *Cancer,* 60:1132-1142

Clark J. C. M., D. M. Thomas, P. F. M. Choong, & C.R. Dass (2007). RECK—a newly discovered inhibitor of metastasis with prognostic significance in multiple forms of cancer. *Cancer and Metastasis Reviews,* 26(3-4):675–683

Clevers H. (2006). Wnt/β-catenin signaling in development and disease. *Cell,* 127(3):469–480

Cody JD, Singer FR, Roodman GD, Otterund B, Lewis TB, Leppert M & Leach RJ (1997). Genetic linkage of Paget disease of the bone to chromosome 18q. *Am J Hum Genet,* 61: 1117-1122

Dal Cin P, Kozakewich HP, Goumnerova L, Mankin HJ, Rosenberg AE, & Fletcher JA (2000). Variant translocations involving 16q22 and 17p13 in solid variant and extraosseous forms of aneurysmal bone cyst. *Genes Chromosomes Cancer,* 28: 233-234.

Dass C. R., Nadesapillai A. P. W., Robin D. et al. (2005). Downregulation of uPAR confirms link in growth and metastasis of osteosarcoma. *Clinical and Experimental Metastasis,* 22(8):643–652

Del Mare S., Kurek K.C., Stein G.S, Lian J.B., & Aqeilan R.I. (2011). Role of the WWOX tumor suppressor gene in bone homeostasis and the pathogenesis of osteosarcoma. *Am J Cancer Res.,* 1(5): 585–594

Deng ZL, Sharff KA, Tang N, Song WX, Luo JXL, Chen J, Bennett E & Reid R. Manning D, Xue A, Montag AG, Luu HH, Haydon RC, He T-C. (2008). Regulation of osteogenic differentiation during skeletal development. *Frontiers in Biosci.,* 13:2001–2021

De Santos L.A, Rosengren J-E, Wooten W.B, et al (1978). Osteogenic sarcoma after the age of 50: a radiographic evaluation. *Am J Roentgenol,* 131:481-484

Dick D.C, Morley W.N & Watson J.J (1982). Rothmund-Thompson syndrome and osteogenic sarcoma. *Clin Exp Dermatol,* 7:119-123

Dix D., McDonald M., & Cohen P. (1983). Adolescent bone cancer: is the growth spurt implicated? (Letter to the Editor) *Eur J Cancer Clin Oncol,* 19:859-860

Domanski H., Akerman M. & Silverman J. (2010). Soft tissue and musculoskeletal system In: *Diagnostic Cytopathology* by W. Gray and G. Kocjan, Elsevier editions

Dorfman H.D & Czerniak B. (1005). Bone cancers. *Cancer*, 75:201-210,

Dorfman H.D & Czerniak B. (1998). Osteosarcoma In: *Bone Tumors*. Mosby, pp.128-252, St.Louis, USA

Dorfman H.D, Czerniak B. & Kotz R. (2002). WHO classification of tumors of bone: Introduction In: *Pathology and Genetics. Tumors of soft tissue and bone*, IARCPress, 226-232, Lyon, France

Edge S.B, Byrd D.R, Carducci M.A, et al: eds (2009). *AJCC Cancer Staging Manual 7th ed.*, Springer, New York,USA

Ewing J (1922). A review and classification of bone sarcomas. *Arch Surg*, 4:483-533

Ewing J. (1939). A review of the classification of bone tumors. *Bull Am Coll Surg*, 24:290-295

Fanburg J.C, Rosenberg A.E, Weaner D.L, et al (1997). Osteocalcin and osteonectin immunoreactivity in the diagnosis of osteosarcoma. *Am J Clin Pathol*, 108:464-473

Fanburg-Smith J.C, Bratthauer G.L & Miettinen M. (1999). Osteocalcin and osteonectin immunoreactivity in extraskeletal osteosarcoma: A study of 28 cases. *Hum Pathol*, 30:32-38

Ferracini R, Di Renzo MF, Scotlandi K, Baldini N, Olivero M, Lollini P, Cremona O, Campanacci M & Comoglio PM (1995). The Met/HGF receptor is over-expressed in human osteosarcomas and is activated by either a paracrine or an autocrine circuit. *Oncogene*, 10: 739-749.

Ferrari C, Benassi S, Ponticelli F, Gamberi G, Ragazzini P, Pazzaglia L, Balladelli A, Bertoni F & Picci P. (2004). Role of MMP-9 and its tissue inhibitor TIMP-1 in human osteosarcoma: findings in 42 patients followed for 1–16 years. *Acta Orthop Scand.*, 75:487–491

Feugeas O., N. Guriec, A. Babin-Boilletot et al. (1996). Loss of heterozygosity of the RB gene is a poor prognostic factor in patients with osteosarcoma. *Journal of Clinical Oncology*, 14(2):467–472

Fletcher JA, Gebhardt MC & Kozakewich HP (1994). Cytogenetic aberrations in osteosarcomas. Nonrandom deletions, rings, and double-minute chromosomes. *Cancer Genet Cytogenet*, 77: 81-88.

Fornasier V.L: Osteoid: An ultrastructural study(1997). Hum Pathol 8:243-254

Forus A, Berner JM, Meza-Zepeda LA, Saeter G, Mischke D, Fodstad O, & Myklebost O (1998). Molecular characterization of a novel amplicon at 1q21-q22 frequently observed in human sarcomas. *Br J Cancer*, 78: 495-503

Forus A, Florenes VA, Maelandsmo GM, Fodstad O & Myklebost O (1994). The protooncogene CHOP/GADD153, involved in growth arrest and DNA damage response, is amplified in a subset of human sarcomas. *Cancer Genet Cytogenet*, 78:165-171.

Forus A, Flørenes VA, Maelandsmo GM, Meltzer PS, Fodstad O & Myklebost O. (1993). Mapping of amplification units in the q13-14 region of chromosome 12 in human sarcomas: some amplica do not include MDM2. *Cell Growth Differ.*, 4(12):1065-70

Franchi A., L. Arganini, G. Baroni et al. (1998). Expression of transforming growth factor β isoforms in osteosarcoma variants: association of TGFβ1 with high-grade osteosarcomas. *Journal of Pathology*, 185(3):284–289

Franchi A., A. Calzolari & G. Zampi (1998). Immunohistochemical detection of c-fos and c-jun expression in osseous and cartilaginous tumours of the skeleton. *Virchows Archiv*, 432(6):515–519

Gamberi G, Benassi MS, Böhling T, Ragazzini P, Molendini L, Sollazzo MR, Pompetti F, Merli M, Magagnoli G, Balladelli A & Picci P (1998). C-myc and c-fos in human osteosarcoma: prognostic value of mRNA and protein expression. *Oncology*, 55: 556-563.

Gaylord H.R (1903). On the pathology of so-called bone aneurism. *Ann Surg*, 37:834-847

Gelberg K. H., E. F. Fitzgerald, S. A. Hwang & R. Dubrow (1997). Growth and development and other risk factors for osteosarcoma in children and young adults. *International Journal of Epidemiology*, 26(2):272–278.

German, J. (1993). Bloom syndrome: a mendelian prototype of somatic mutational disease. *Medicine (Baltimore)*, 72: 393-406.

Gisselsson D, Höglund M, Mertens F, Mitelman F & Mandahl N (1998). Chromosomal organization of amplified chromosome 12 sequences in mesenchymal tumors detected by fluorescence in situ hybridization. *Genes Chromosomes Cancer*, 23: 203-212

Gisselsson D, Pålsson E, Höglund M, Domanski H, Mertens F, Pandis N, Sciot R, Dal Cin P, Bridge JA & Mandahl N (2002). Differentially amplified chromosome 12 sequences in low- and high-grade osteosarcoma. *Genes Chromosomes Cancer*, 33: 133-140

Glass DA 2nd & Karsenty G. (2007). In vivo analysis of Wnt signaling in bone. *Endocrinology*, 148:2630–2634

Gobbi, G., Sangiorgi, L., Lenzi, L., Casadei, R., Canaider, S., Strippoli, P., Lucarelli, E., Ghedini, I., Donati, D., Fabbri, N., et al. (2002). Seven BMPs and all their receptors are simultaneously expressed in osteosarcoma cells. *Int J Oncol*, 20:143-147

Goes M., (1952) Knochenwachstum und osteogenes sarckom. *Strahlentherapie*, 89:194-210

Good DA, Busfield F, Fletcher BH, Duffy DL, Kesting JB, Andersen J & Shaw JT (2002). Linkage of Paget disease of bone to a novel region on human chromosome 18q23. *Am J Hum Genet*, 70: 517-525.

Gorlick R, Huvos AG, Heller G, Aledo A, Beardsley GP, Healey JH & Meyers PA. (1999). Expression of HER2/c-erbB-2 correlates with survival in osteosarcoma. *J Clin Oncol.*, 17:2781–2788

Goto, M., Miller, R. W., Ishikawa, Y. & Sugano, H. (1996). Excess of rare cancers in Werner syndrome (adult progeria). *Cancer Epidemiol Biomarkers Prev*, 5:239-246

Gradt van Roggen J.F, Zonderland H.M, Welvaart K., et al (1998). Local recurrence of a phylloedes tumour of the breast presenting with widespread differentiation to a telangiectatic osteosarcoma. *J Clin Pathol*, 51(9):706-708

Greenwood S.M, & Meschter S.C (1989). Extraskeletal osteogenic sarcoma of the mediastinum. *Arch Pathol Lab Med*, 1113:430-433

Guo W, Gorlick R, Ladanyi M, Meyers PA, Huvos AG, Bertino JR & Healey JH (1999). Expression of bone morphogenetic proteins and receptors in sarcomas. *Clin Orthop Relat Res.*, 365: 175-183.

Haibach H., Farrell C. & Dittrich F.J (1985). Neoplasms arising in Paget's disease of bone. A study of 82 cases. *Am J Clin Pathol*, 83:594-600

Hansen M.F, Koufos A., Gallie B.L, et al (1985). Osteosarcoma and retinoblastoma: a shared chromosomal mechanism revealing recessive predisposition. *Proc Natl Acad Sci USA*, 82:6216-6220

Hajdu S.I (1975). Aspiration biopsy of primary malignant bone tumours. *Front Radiat Ther Oncol*, 10:73-81

Hansen MF, Nellissery MJ & Bhatia P (1999). Common mechanisms of osteosarcoma and Paget's disease. *J Bone Miner Res*, 14 (Suppl 2): 39-44.

Harada, K., Toyooka, S., Maitra, A., Maruyama, R., Toyooka, K. O., Timmons, C. F., Tomlinson, G. E., Mastrangelo, D., Hay, R. J., Minna, J. D. & Gazdar, A. F. (2002). Aberrant promoter methylation and silencing of the RASSF1A gene in pediatric tumors and cell lines. *Oncogene* 21, 4345-4349

Harris S. A., R. J. Enger, B. L. Riggs & T. C. Spelsberg (1995). Development and characterization of a conditionally immortalized human fetal osteoblastic cell line. *Journal of Bone and Mineral Research*, 10(2):178–186

Haydon R. C., A. Deyrup, A. Ishikawa et al. (2002). Cytoplasmic and/or nuclear accumulation of the β-catenin protein is a frequent event in human osteosarcoma. *International Journal of Cancer*, 102(4): 338–342

Haydon R. C., Luu H. H. & He T. C. (2007). Osteosarcoma and osteoblastic differentiation: a new perspective on oncogenesis. *Clinical Orthopaedics and Related Research*, 454:237–246

He B. C., L. Chen, G. W. Zuo et al. (2010). Synergistic antitumor effect of the activated PPARγ and retinoid receptors on human osteosarcoma. *Clinical Cancer Research*, 16(8):2235–2245

Heinsohn S., U. Evermann, U. Zur Stadt, S. Bielack, and H. Kabisch, (2007). Determination of the prognostic value of loss of heterozygosity at the retinoblastoma gene in osteosarcoma. *International Journal of Oncology*, 30(5):1205–1214

Herens C, Thiry A, Dresse MF, Born J, Flagothier C, Vanstraelen G, Allington N & Bex V (2001). Translocation (16;17)(q22;p13) is a recurrent anomaly of aneurysmal bone cysts. *Cancer Genet Cytogenet*, 127: 83-84.

Hickson, I. D. (2003). RecQ helicases: caretakers of the genome. *Nat Rev Cancer*, 3:169-178

Hirakawa T., Tsuneyoshi M, Enjoji M., et al (1998). Ovarian stroma with histologic features of telangiectatic osteosarcoma of the bone. *Am J Surg Pathol*, 12(7):567-572

Hoang, B. H., Kubo, T., Healey, J. H., Sowers, R., Mazza, B., Yang, R., Huvos, A. G., Meyers, P.A. & Gorlick, R. (2004). Expression of LDL receptor-related protein 5 (LRP5) as a novel marker for disease progression in high-grade osteosarcoma. *Int J Cancer*, 109:106-111.

Hofbauer L. C. & A. E. Heufelder (1998). Osteoprotegerin and its cognate ligand: a new paradigm of osteoclastogenesis. *European Journal of Endocrinology*, 139(2):152–154

Hong JH, Hwang ES, McManus MT, Amsterdam A, Tian Y, Kalmukova R, Mueller E, Benjamin T, Spiegelman BM, Sharp PA, Hopkins N & Yaffe MB.(2005). TAZ, a transcriptional modulator of mesenchymal stem cell differentiation. *Science*, 309:1074–1078

Hoogerwerf WA, Hawkins AL, Perlman EJ & Griffin CA (1994). Chromosome analysis of nine osteosarcomas. *Genes Chromosomes Cancer*, 9: 88-92.

Hou, P., Ji, M., Yang, B., Chen, Z., Qiu, J., Shi, X. & Lu, Z. (2006). Quantitative analysis of promoter hypermethylation in multiple genes in osteosarcoma. *Cancer* 106:1602-1609

Hu X., A. X. Yu, B. W. Qi et al. (2010). The expression and significance of IDH1 and p53 in osteosarcom. *Journal of Experimental & Clinical Cancer Research*, 29: 43

Husmann K., R. Muff, M. E. Bolander, G. Sarkar, W. Born & B. Fuchs (2008). Cathepsins and osteosarcoma: expression analysis identifies cathepsin K as an indicator of metastasis. *Molecular Carcinogenesis*, 47(1):66–73

Huvos A.G (1986). Osteogenic sarcoma of bones and soft tissues in older persons. A clinicopathologic analysis of 117 patients older than 60 years. *Cancer*, 57:1442-1449

Huvos A.G, Butler A. & Bretsky S.S (1983). Osteogenic sarcoma in the American black. *Cancer*, 52:1959-1965

Huvos A.G, Butler A. & Bretsky S.S (1983). Osteogenic sarcoma associated with Paget's disease of bone. A clinicopathologic study of 65 cases. *Cancer*, 52:1489-1495

Huvos A.G, Woodard H.Q, Cahan W.G, et al (1985). Postirradiation osteogenic sarcoma of bone and soft tissues. A clinicopathologic study of 66 patients. *Cancer*, 55:1244-1255

Inwards C.Y & Unni K. (1995). Classification and grading of bone sarcomas. *Haematol Oncol Clin North Am*, 9(3):545-569

Iwaya, K., Ogawa, H., Kuroda, M., Izumi, M., Ishida, T. & Mukai, K. (2003). Cytoplasmic and/or nuclear staining of beta-catenin is associated with lung metastasis. *Clin Exp Metastasis*, 20:525-529.

Johnson L.C, Vetter H. & Putschar W.G.J (1962). Sarcoma arising in bone cysts. *Virchows Arch (Pathol. Anat.)*, 335:428-451

Jones, P. A., and Baylin, S. B. (2002). The fundamental role of epigenetic events in cancer. Nat Rev Genet, 3:415-428

Jung, S. T., Moon, E. S., Seo, H. Y., Kim, J. S., Kim, G. J. & Kim, Y. K. (2005). Expression and significance of TGF-beta isoform and VEGF in osteosarcoma. *Orthopedics* 28: 755-760

Kansara, M. & Thomas, D. M. (2007). Molecular pathogenesis of osteosarcoma. *DNA Cell Biol*, 26:1-18

Karsenty G. (2000). Bone formation and factors affecting this process. *Matrix Biol.* ,19:85–89

Karsenty G. (2003). The complexities of skeletal biology. *Nature*, 423: 316–318

Karsenty G & Wagner EF. (2002). Reaching a genetic and molecular understanding of skeletal development. *Dev Cell*, 2:389–406

Kemmer H., Grass C., Siemer S., et al (2008). First case of a primary osteosarcoma of the ureter: diagnostic findings, course of disease and treatment. *Q J Med*, 101:663-665

Khanna, C., Wan, X., Bose, S., Cassaday, R., Olomu, O., Mendoza, A., Yeung, C., Gorlick, R., Hewitt, S. M. & Helman, L. J. (2004). The membrane-cytoskeleton linker ezrin is necessary for osteosarcoma metastasis. *Nat Med* 10: 182-186

Khanna, C., Prehn, J., Yeung, C., Caylor, J., Tsokos, M. & Helman, L. (2000). An orthotopic model of murine osteosarcoma with clonally related variants differing in pulmonary metastatic potential. *Clin Exp Metastasis*, 18:261-271

Khatib ZA, Matsushime H, Valentine M, Shapiro DN, Sherr CJ & Look AT (1993). Coamplification of the CDK4 gene with MDM2 and GLI in human sarcomas. *Cancer Res.*, 53: 5535-5541.

Kingsley L. A., P. G. J. Fournier, J. M. Chirgwin & T.A. Guise (2007). Molecular biology of bone metastasis. *Molecular Cancer Therapeutics*, 6(10):2609–2617

Kinpara K. (2000). Osteoclast differentiation factor in human osteosarcoma cell line. *Journal of Immunoassay*, 21(4):327–340

Kloen, P., Gebhardt, M. C., Perez-Atayde, A., Rosenberg, A. E., Springfield, D. S., Gold, L. I. & Mankin, H. J. (1997). Expression of transforming growth factor-beta (TGF-beta) isoforms in osteosarcomas: TGF-beta3 is related to disease progression. *Cancer,* 80: 2230-2239.

Knuutila S, Autio K & Aalto Y (2000). Online access to CGH data of DNA sequence copy number changes. *Am J Pathol,* 157: 689

Koppers B., Rakow D. & Schmidt L. (1977). Osteogenic sarcoma combined with non-ossifying fibroma in one bone. *Roentgenblaetter,* 30:261-266

Kozlowski K., Scougall J.S & Oates R.K (1980). Osteosarcoma in a boy with Rothmund-Thomson syndrome. *Pediatr,* 10:42-45

Kruzelock RP, Murphy EC, Strong LC, Naylor SL & Hansen MF (1997). Localization of a novel tumor suppressor locus on human chromosome 3q important in osteosarcoma tumorigenesis. *Cancer Res,* 57: 106-109.

Kurt A.M, Unni K.K, McLeod R.A, et al (1990). Low-grade intraosseous osteosarcoma. *Cancer,* 65:1418-1428

Kusuzaki K, Takeshita H, Murata H, Hirata M, Hashiguchi S, Ashihara T & Hirasawa Y (1999). Prognostic significance of DNA ploidy pattern in osteosarcomas in association with chemotherapy. *Cancer Lett,* 137: 27-33.

Kyriakos M. & Hardy D. (1991). Malignant transformation of aneurismal bone cyst, with an analysis of the literature. *Cancer,* 68(8):1770-1780

Ladanyi M, Cha C, Lewis R, Jhanwar SC, Huvos AG & Healey JH (1993). MDM2 gene amplification in metastatic osteosarcoma. *Cancer Res,* 53: 16-18

Ladanyi M, Park CK, Lewis R, Jhanwar SC, Healey JH & Huvos AG (1993). Sporadic amplification of the MYC gene in human osteosarcomas. *Diagn Mol Pathol,* 2: 163-167

Lau L. F. & S. C. T. Lam (1999). The CCN family of angiogenic regulators: the integrin connection. *Experimental Cell Research,* 248(1):44–57

Laurent H-R, Rebonl J., Picot A, et al (1973). Multicentric osteogenic sarcoma. *Bordeaux Med,* 17: 2685-2694

Lee J.S, Fetsch J.F, Wasdhal D.A, et al (1995). A review of 40 patients with extraskeletal osteosarcoma. *Cancer,* 76: 2253-2259

Le Gall C., A. Bellahcene, E. Bonnelye et al. (2007). A cathepsin K inhibitor reduces breast cancer-induced osteolysis and skeletal tumor burden. *Cancer Research,* 67(20) : 9894–9902

Lian JB, Stein GS, Javed A, van Wijnen AJ, Stein JL, Montecino M, Hassan MQ, Gaur T, Lengner CJ & Young DW. (2006). Networks and hubs for the transcriptional control of osteoblastogenesis. *Rev Endocr Metab Disord.,* 7:1–16

Lidang J.M, Schumacher B., Myhre J.O, et al (1998). Extraskeletal osteosarcomas: a clinicopathologic study of 25 cases. *Am J Surg Pathol,* 22:588-594

Logue J.P & Cairnduff F. (1991). Radiation induced extraskeletal osteosarcoma. *Br J Radiol,* 64:171-172

Lonardo F., T. Ueda, A. G. Huvos, J. Healey & M. Ladanyi (1997). p53 and MDM2 alterations in osteosarcomas: correlation with clinicopathologic features and proliferative rate. *Cancer,* 79(8):1541–1547

Loose J.H, El-Naggar A.K, Ro J.Y, et al (1990). Primary osteosarcoma of the lung: Report of two cases and review of the literature. *J Thorac Cardiovasc Surg,* 100:867-873

Luo X., J. Chen, W. X. Song et al. (2008). Osteogenic BMPs promote tumor growth of human osteosarcomas that harbor differentiation defects. *Laboratory Investigation,* 88(12):1264–1277

Luo Q., Q. Kang, W. Si et al. (2004). Connective tissue growth factor (CTGF) is regulated by Wnt and bone morphogenetic proteins signaling in osteoblast differentiation of mesenchymal stem cells. *Journal of Biological Chemistry*, 279(53):55958–55968

Luu HH, Song WX, Luo X, Manning D, Luo J, Deng ZL, Sharff KA, Montag AG, Haydon RC & He TC. (2007). Distinct roles of bone morphogenetic proteins in osteogenic differentiation of mesenchymal stem cells. *J Orthop Res.*, 25:665–677

Maelandsmo GM, Berner JM, Florenes VA, Forus A, Hovig E, Fodstad O & Myklebost O (1995). Homozygous deletion frequency and expression levels of the CDKN2 gene in human sarcomas - relationship to amplification and mRNA levels of CDK4 and CCND1. *Br J Cancer*, 72: 393-398

Malkin, D., Li, F. P., Strong, L. C., Fraumeni, J. F., Jr., Nelson, C. E., Kim, D. H., Kassel, J., Gryka, M. A., Bischoff, F. Z., Tainsky, M. A., et al. (1990). Germ line p53 mutations in a familial syndrome of breast cancer, sarcomas, and other neoplasms. *Science*, 250: 1233-1238

Mandahl N, Heim S, Willén H, Rydholm A, Eneroth M, Nilbert M, Kreicbergs A & Mitelman F (1989). Characteristic karyotypic anomalies identify subtypes of malignant fibrous histiocytoma. *Genes Chromosomes Cancer*, 1: 9-14

Marina N., M. Gebhardt, L. Teot & R. Gorlick (2004). Biology and therapeutic advances for pediatric osteosarcoma. *Oncologist*, 9(4):422–441

Mark R.J, Poen J., Tran L.M, et al (1994). Postirradiation sarcomas. A single-institution study and review of the literature. *Cancer*, 73:2653-2662

McDonald J. & Budd J.W (1943). Osteogenic sarcoma: I. A modified nomenclature and a review of 118 five-year cures. *Surg Gynecol Obstet*, 76:413-421

McNairm J. D. K., T. A. Damron, S. K. Landas, J. L. Ambrose & A. E. Shrimpton (2001). Inheritance of osteosarcoma and Paget's disease of bone: a familial loss of heterozygosity study. *Journal of Molecular Diagnostics*, 3(4):171–177

Menghi-Sartorio S, Mandahl N, Mertens F, Picci P & Knuutila S (2001). DNA copy number amplifications in sarcomas with homogeneously staining regions and double minutes. *Cytometry*, 46: 79-84

Mertens F, Fletcher CD, Dal Cin P, de Wever I, Mandahl N, Mitelman F, Rosai J, Rydholm A, Sciot R, Tallini G, van den Berghe H, Vanni R & Willén H (1998). Cytogenetic analysis of 46 pleomorphic soft tissue sarcomas and correlation with morphologic and clinical features: a report of the CHAMP study group. *Genes Chromosomes Cancer*, 22: 16-25.

Mertens H.H, Langnickel D. & Staedtler F. (1982). Primary osteogenic sarcoma of the breast. *Acta Cytol*, 26:512-516

Mertens F, Larramendy M, Gustavsson A, Gisselsson D, Rydholm A, Brosjö O, Mitelman F, Knuutila S & Mandahl N (2000). Radiation-associated sarcomas are characterized by complex karyotypes with frequent rearrangements of chromosome arm 3p. *Cancer Genet Cytogenet*, 116: 89-96.

Mertens F, Mandahl N, Örndal C, Baldetorp B, Bauer HC, Rydholm A, Wiebe T, Willén H, Åkerman M, Heim S & Mitelman F (1993). Cytogenetic findings in 33 osteosarcomas. *Int J Cancer*, 55: 44-50

Meza-Zepeda LA, Forus A, Lygren B, Dahlberg AB, Godager LH, South A, Serra M, Nezetic D, Tarkkanen M, Knuutila S & Myklebost O (2002). Positional cloning identifies a novel cyclophilin as a candidate amplified oncogene in 1q21. *Oncogene*, 21: 2261-2269

Micolonghi T.S, Liang D. & Schwarz S. (1984). Primary osteosarcoma of the kidney. *J Urol*, 131:1164-1166

Miller,C. W., Yeon, C., Aslo, A., Mendoza, S., Aytac, U. & Koeffler, H. P. (1997). The p19INK4D cyclin dependent kinase inhibitor gene is altered in osteosarcoma. *Oncogene*, 15:231-235

Mirra J.M, Bullough P.G, Marcove R.C, et al (1974). Malignant fibrous histiocytoma and osteosarcoma in association with bone infarcts. Report of four cases, two in caisson workers. *J Bone Joint Surg (Am)*, 56:932-940

Mohamed AN, Zalupski MM, Ryan JR, Koppitch F, Balcerzak S, Kempf R & Wolman SR (1997). Cytogenetic aberrations and DNA ploidy in soft tissue sarcoma. A Southwest Oncology Group Study. *Cancer Genet Cytogenet*, 99: 45-53

Momand J, Zambetti GP, Olson DC, George D & Levine AJ (1992). The mdm-2 oncogene product forms a complex with the p53 protein and inhibits p53-mediated transactivation. *Cell*, 69: 1237-1245

Nakanishi H, Tomita Y, Myoui A, Yoshikawa H, Sakai K, Kato Y, Ochi T & Aozasa K (1998). Mutation of the p53 gene in postradiation sarcoma. *Lab Invest*, 78: 727-733.

Nakashima K, Zhou X, Kunkel G, Zhang Z, Deng JM, Behringer RR & de Crombrugghe B. (2002). The novel zinc finger-containing transcription factor osterix is required for osteoblast differentiation and bone formation. *Cell*, 108:17–29

Nellissery MJ, Padalecki SS, Brkanac Z, Singer FR, Roodman GD, Unni KK, Leach RJ & Hansen MF (1998). Evidence for a novel osteosarcoma tumor-suppressor gene in the chromosome 18 region genetically linked with Paget disease of bone. *Am J Hum Genet*, 63: 817-824

Nikol K.K, Ward W.G, Savage P.D, et al (1998). Fine-needle aspiration biopsy of skeletal versus extraskeletal osteosarcoma. *Cancer (Cancer Cytopathol)*, 84:176-185

Nishio, Y., Dong, Y., Paris, M., O'Keefe, R. J., Schwarz, E. M. & Drissi, H. (2006). Runx2-mediated regulation of the zinc finger Osterix/Sp7 gene. *Gene*, 372: 62-70

Nitzsche E.U, Seeger L.L, Klosa B., et al (1992). Primary osteosarcoma of the thyroid gland. *J Nucl Med*, 33:1399-1401

Ogasawara, T., Kawaguchi, H., Jinno, S., Hoshi, K., Itaka, K., Takato, T., Nakamura, K. & Okayama, H. (2004). Bone morphogenetic protein 2-induced osteoblast differentiation requires Smad-mediated down-regulation of Cdk6. *Mol Cell Biol*, 24: 6560-6568

Okada K., Frassica F.J, Sim F.H, et al (1994). Parosteal osteosarcoma. A clinicopathological study. *J Bone Joint Surg Am*, 76:366-378

Oliner JD, Kinzler KW, Meltzer PS, George DL & Vogelstein B (1992). Amplification of a gene encoding a p53-associated protein in human sarcomas. *Nature* ,358: 80-83

Örndal C, Mandahl N, Rydholm A, Willén H, Brosjö O & Mitelman F (1993). Chromosome aberrations and cytogenetic intratumor heterogeneity in chondrosarcomas. *J Cancer Res Clin Oncol*, 120: 51-56

Panoutsakopoulos G, Pandis N, Kyriazoglou I, Gustafson P, Mertens F & Mandahl N (1999). Recurrent t(16;17)(q22;p13) in aneurysmal bone cysts. *Genes Chromosomes Cancer*, 26: 265-266

Park IC, Lee SY, Jeon DG, Lee JS, Hwang CS, Hwang BG, Lee SH, Hong WS, Hong SI (1996). Enhanced expression of cathepsin L in metastatic bone tumors. J Korean Med Sci, 11: 144-148

Park Y. B., H. S. Kim, J. H. Oh & S. H. Lee (2001). The co-expression of p53 protein and P-glycoprotein is correlated to a poor prognosis in osteosarcoma. *International Orthopaedics*, 24(6):307–310

Park H. R., W. Won Jung, F. Bertoni et al. (2004). Molecular analysis of p53, MDM2 and H-ras genes in low-grade central osteosarcoma. *Pathology Research and Practice*, 200(6):439–445

Perbal B., M. Zuntini, D. Zambelli et al. (2008). Prognostic value of CCN3 in osteosarcoma. *Clinical Cancer Research*, 14(3):701–709

Piscioli F., Govoni E., Polla E., et al (1985). Primary osteosarcoma of the uterine corpus: Report of a case and a critical review of the literature. *Int J Gynaecol Obstet*, 23:377-385

Quinn J. M. W., Itoh K., Udagawa N. et al. (2001).Transforming growth factor β affects osteoclast differentiation via direct and indirect actions. *Journal of Bone and Mineral Research*, 16(10):1787–1794

Radhi J.M, Loewy J. (1999). Dedifferentiated chondrosarcoma with features of telangiectatic osteosarcoma. *Pathology*, 31(4):428-430

Radig K, Schneider-Stock R, Mittler U, Neumann HW & Roessner A (1998). Genetic instability in osteoblastic tumors of the skeletal system. *Pathol Res Pract*, 194: 669-677

Ragazzini P, Gamberi G, Benassi MS, Orlando C, Sestini R, Ferrari C, Molendini L, Sollazzo MR, Merli M, Magagnoli G, Bertoni F, Böhling T, Pazzagli M & Picci P (1999). Analysis of SAS gene and CDK4 and MDM2 proteins in low-grade osteosarcoma. *Cancer Detect Prev*, 23: 129-136

Rao-Bindal K. & Kleinerman E.S. (2011). Epigenetic Regulation of Apoptosis and Cell Cycle in Osteosarcoma. *Sarcoma*, 2011, ID article 679457, 5 pages

Reya T & Clevers H. (2005). Wnt signalling in stem cells and cancer. *Nature*, 434:843–850

Ren B., K. O. Yee, J. Lawler & R. Khosravi-Far (2006). Regulation of tumor angiogenesis by thrombospondin-1. *Biochimica et Biophysica Acta*, 1765(2):178–188

Rikhof B., S. De Jong, A. J.H. Suurmeijer, C.Meijer & W. T. A. van der Graaf (2009). The insulin-like growth factor system and sarcomas. *Journal of Pathology*, 217(4):469–482

Roberts WM, Douglass EC, Peiper SC, Houghton PJ & Look AT (1989). Amplification of the gli gene in childhood sarcomas. *Cancer Res*, 49: 5407-5413

Rong S, Jeffers M, Resau JH, Tsarfaty I, Oskarsson M & Vande Woude GF (1993). Met expression and sarcoma tumorigenicity. *Cancer Res*, 53: 5355-5360

Ruggieri P., Sim F.H, Band J.R, et al (1995). Osteosarcoma in a patient with polyostotic fibrous dysplasia and Albright's syndrome. *Orthopedics*, 18:71-75

Sadikovic B., M. Yoshimoto, S. Chilton-MacNeill, P. Thorner, J. A. Squire & M. Zielenska (2009). Identification of interactive networks of gene expression associated with osteosarcoma oncogenesis by integrated molecular profiling. *Human Molecular Genetics*, 18(11):1962–1975

Schajowicz F., Santini A.E & Berenstein M. (1983). Sarcoma complicating Paget's disease of bone. A clinicopathological study of 62 cases. *J Bone Joint Surg Br*, 65:299-307

Schweitzer G. & Gand Pirie D. (1971). Osteosarcoma arising in a solitary osteochondroma. *S Afr Med J*, 45:810-811

Selvarajah S, Yoshimoto M, Ludkovski O, Park PC, Bayani J, Thorner P, Maire G, Squire JA & Zielenska M. (2008). Genomic signatures of chromosomal instability and osteosarcoma progression detected by high resolution array CGH and interphase FISH. *Cytogenet Genome Res.*, 122:5–15

Serra M., Morini M.C, Scotlandi K., et al (1992). Evaluation of osteonectin as a diagnostic marker of osteogenic bone tumours. *Hum Pathol*, 23:1326-1331

Shimizu T., T. Ishikawa, E. Sugihara et al. (2010). c-MYC overexpression with loss of Ink4a/Arf transforms bone marrow stromal cells into osteosarcoma accompanied by loss of adipogenesis. *Oncogene*, 29(42):5687–5699

Shui-Xiang Tao, Guo-Quin Tian, Meng-Hua Ge, et al (2011). Primary extraskeletal osteosarcoma of omentum majus. *World J of Surg Oncol*, 9:25-27

Silver SA & Tavassolli FA (1980). Primary osteogenic sarcoma of the breast: A clinicopathologic analysis of 50 cases. *Am J Surg Pathol*, 22:925-933

Sinovic JF, Bridge Jab & Neff JR (1992). Ring chromosome in parosteal osteosarcoma. Clinical and diagnostic significance. *Cancer Genet Cytogenet*, 62: 50-52

Siu F.H, Unni K.K, Beabout J.W, et al (1979). Osteosarcoma with small cells simulating Ewing's tumor. *J Bone Joint Surg (Am)*, 61:201-215

Smida J., Baumhoer D., Rosemann M. et al. (2010). Genomic alterations and allelic imbalances are strong prognostic predictors in osteosarcoma. *Clinical Cancer Research*, 16(16):4256–4267

Smith G.D, Chalmer J. & McQeen M.M (1986). Osteosarcoma arising in relation to an echondroma. A report of three cases. *J Bone Joint Surg (Br)*, 68:315-319

Smith SH, Weiss SW, Jankowski SA, Coccia MA & Meltzer PS (1992). SAS amplification in soft tissue sarcomas. *Cancer Res*, 52: 3746-3749

Stoch S. A. & Wagner J. A (2008). Cathepsin K inhibitors: a novel target for osteoporosis therapy. *Clinical Pharmacology and Therapeutics*, 83(1):172–176

Stock C, Kager L, Fink FM, Gadner H & Ambros PF (2000). Chromosomal regions involved in the pathogenesis of osteosarcomas. *Genes Chromosomes Cancer*, 28:329-336

Soloviev, Yu. N (1969). On the relationship between the rate of skeleton growth and occurrence of primary osteogenic sarcoma. *Vopr Onkol*, 15(5):3-7

Sordillo P.P, Hadju S.I, Magill G.B, et al (1983). Extraosseous osteogenic sarcoma. A review of 48 patients. *Cancer*, 51:727-734

Spyra S. (1976). Osteogenic sarcoma in chronic osteitis. *Chir Narzadow Ruchu Ortop Pol*, 41:99-100

Stormby N. & Akermanm M (1973). Cytodiagnosis of bone lesions by means of fine needle aspiration biopsy. *Acta Cytol*, 17:166-172

Sudo T, Kuramoto T, Komiya S, Inoue A & Itoh K (1997). Expression of MAGE genes in osteosarcoma. *J Orthop Res* ,15: 128-132

Szymanska J, Mandahl N, Mertens F, Tarkkanen M, Karaharju E & Knuutila S (1996). Ring chromosomes in parosteal osteosarcoma contain sequences from 12q13-15: a combined cytogenetic and comparative genomic hybridization study. *Genes Chromosomes Cancer*, 16: 31-34

Ta H. T., Dass C. R., Choong P. F. M. & Dunstan D. E. (2009). Osteosarcoma treatment: state of the art. *Cancer and Metastasis Reviews*, 28(1-2):247–263

Takada J., Ishii S., Ohta T., et al (1992). Usefulness of a novel monoclonal antibody against human osteocalcin in immunohistochemical diagnosis. *Virchows Arch A*, 420:507-511

Takayanagi H. (2007). The role of NFAT in osteoclast formation. *Annals of the New York Academy of Sciences*, 1116: 227–237

Tang, N., Song, W. X., Luo, J., Haydon, R. C. & He, T. C. (2008). Osteosarcoma development and stem cell differentiation. *Clin Orthop Relat Res*, 466: 2114-2130

Tarkkanen M, Aaltonen LA, Böhling T, Kivioja A, Karaharju E, Elomaa I & Knuutila S (1996). No evidence of microsatellite instability in bone tumours. *Br J Cancer* , 74: 453-455

Tarkkanen M, Böhling T, Gamberi G, Ragazzini P, Benassi MS, Kivioja A, Kallio P, Elomaa I, Picci P & Knuutila S (1998). Comparative genomic hybridization of low grade central osteosarcoma. *Mod Pathol* , 11: 421-426

Tarkkanen M, Elomaa I, Blomqvist C, Kivioja AH, Kellokumpu-Lehtinen P, Böhling T, Valle J & Knuutila S (1999). DNA sequence copy number increase at 8q: a potential new prognostic marker in high grade osteosarcoma. *Int J Cancer*, 84: 114-121

Tarkkanen M, Kaipainen A, Karaharju E, Böhling T, Szymanska J, Helio H, Kivioja A, Elomaa I & Knuutila S (1993). Cytogenetic study of 249 consecutive patients examined for a bone tumor. *Cancer Genet Cytogenet,* 68:1-21

Tarkkanen M, Karhu R, Kallioniemi A, Elomaa I, Kivioja AH, Nevalainen J, Böhling T, Karaharju E, Hyytinen E, Knuutila S & Kalioniemi OP (1995). Gains and losses of DNA sequences in osteosarcomas by comparative genomic hybridization. *Cancer Res,* 55: 1334-1338

Tarkkanen M, Wiklund TA, Virolainen MJ, Larramendy M, Mandahl N, Mertens F, Blomqvist C, Tukiainen E, Miettinen M, Elomaa I & Knuutila S (2001). Comparative genomic hybridization of postirradiation sarcomas. *Cancer,* 92: 1992-1998

Thomas, D. M., Carty, S. A., Piscopo, D. M., Lee, J. S., Wang, W. F., Forrester, W. C. & Hinds, P. W. (2001). The retinoblastoma protein acts as a transcriptional coactivator required for osteogenic differentiation. *Mol Cell,* 8: 303-316.

Thomas D. M., Johnson S. A., Sims N. A. et al. (2004). Terminal osteoblast differentiation, mediated by runx2 and p27, is disrupted in osteosarcoma. *Journal of Cell Biology,* 167(5):925–934

Thomas, D. & Kansara, M. (2006). Epigenetic modifications in osteogenic differentiation and transformation. *J Cell Biochem,* 98: 757-769

Trihia H., Valavanis C., Markidou S., et al (2007). Primary osteogenic sarcoma of the breast. Cytomorphologic study of three cases and histologic correlation. *Acta Cytologica,* 51(3): 443-450

Trowell J.E & Arkell D.G (1976). Osteosarcoma of the thyroid gland. Case report. *J Pathol,* 119:123-127

Tsuchiya, T., Sekine, K., Hinohara, S., Namiki, T., Nobori, T. & Kaneko, Y. (2000). Analysis of the p16INK4, p14ARF, p15, TP53, and MDM2 genes and their prognostic implications in osteosarcoma and Ewing sarcoma. *Cancer Genet Cytogenet*, 120:91-98.

Tsuneyoshi M. & Dorfman H.D (1987). Epiphyseal osteosarcoma: distinguishing features from clear cell chondrosarcoma, chondroblastoma and epiphyseal echondroma. *Hum Pathol,* 18:664-651

Uchibori M, Nishida Y, Nagasaka T, Yamada Y, Nakanishi K & Ishiguro N. (2006). Increased expression of membrane-type matrix metalloproteinase-1 is correlated with poor prognosis in patients with osteosarcoma. *Int J Oncol.* 28:33–42.

Unni K.K, Dahlin D.C & Beabout J.W (1976). Periosteal osteosarcoma. *Cancer,* 37:2476-2485

Unni K.K, Dahlin D.C, McLeod R.A, et al (1977). Intra-osseous well-differentiated osteosarcoma. *Cancer,* 40:1337-1347

Vigorita V. J. (2008).*Orthopaedic Pathology,* Lippincott, Williams & Wilkins, Philadelphia, Pa, USA

Wadayama B, Toguchida J, Shimizu T, Ishizaki K, Sasaki MS, Kotoura Y, & Yamamuro T (1994). Mutation spectrum of the retinoblastoma gene in osteosarcomas. *Cancer Res,* 54: 3042-3048

Wajed, S. A., Laird, P. W. & DeMeester, T. R. (2001). DNA methylation: an alternative pathway to cancer. *Ann Surg,* 234:10-20

Walaas L. & Kindblom L-G (1990). Light and electron microscopic examinations of fine needle aspirates in the preoperative diagnosis of osteogenic tumours. *Diagn Cytopath,* 6:27-38

Wang, L. L. (2005). Biology of osteogenic sarcoma. *Cancer J,* 11:294-305

Wang, L.L., Gannavarapu, A., Kozinetz, C.A., Levy, M.L., Lewis, R.A., Chintagumpala, M. M.,Ruiz-Maldanado, R., Contreras-Ruiz, J., Cunniff, C., Erickson, R. P., et al. (2003). Association between osteosarcoma and deleterious mutations in the RECQL4 gene in Rothmund-Thomson syndrome. *J Natl Cancer Inst,* 95:669-674

Wang, L. L., Levy M. L., Lewis, R. A., Chintagumpala, M. M., Lev, D., Rogers, M. & Plon, S.E. (2001). Clinical manifestations in a cohort of 41 Rothmund-Thomson syndrome patients. *Am J Med Genet,* 102:11-17

Watt A.C, Haggar A.M & Krasicky G.A (1984). Extraosseous osteogenic sarcoma of the breast. Mammographic and pathologic findings. *Radiology,* 150:34

Wegner R.E, McGrath K.M, Luketoch J.D, et al (2010). Extraosseous osteosarcoma of the esophagus: a case report. *Sarcoma,* vol 2010, article ID 907127, 3 pages

Werner M, Rieck J & Delling G. (1998). Cytogenetic changes in low grade central osteosarcomas. *Verh Dtsch Ges Pathol.,* 82:189-94

White V.A, Fanning C.V, Ayala A, et al (1988). Osteosarcoma and the role of fine-needle aspiration: a study of 51 cases.Cancer, 62:1238-1246

Wick M.R, Siegal G.P, Unni K.K, et al (1981). Sarcoma of bone complicating osteitis deformans (Paget' disease): fifty years' experience. *Am J Surg Pathol,* 5:47-59

Wilimas J., Barrett G. & Pratt C. (1977). Osteosarcoma in two very young children. *Clin Pediatr,* 16:548-551

Wines A., Bonar F. & Lam P. (2000). Telangiectatic differentiation of a parosteal osteosarcoma. *Skeletal Radiol.,* 29(10):597-600

Wold L.E, Unni K.K & Beabout J.W, et al (1984). Dedifferentiated parosteal osteosarcoma. *J Bone Joint Surg Am,* 66:53-59

World Health Organization Classification of Tumours. *Pathology and Genetics of Tumours of Soft Tissue and Bone.* Lyon: IARC Press: 2002

Wu J. X., Carpenter P. M., Gresens C. et al. (1990). The protooncogene c-fos is over-expressed in the majority of human osteosarcomas. *Oncogene,* 5(7):989–1000

Wuisman P., Roessner A., Bosse A., et al (1992). Osteonectin in osteosarcomas: A marker of differential diagnosis and/or prognosis? *Ann Oncol,* 3(2):533-535

Wunder JS, Czitrom AA, Kandel R & Andrulis IL (1991). Analysis of alterations in the retinoblastoma gene and tumor grade in bone and soft-tissue sarcomas. *J Natl Cancer Inst,* 83: 194-200

Wunder JS, Eppert K, Burrow SR, Gokgoz N, Bell RS, Andrulis IL & Gogkoz N (1999). Co-amplification and overexpression of CDK4, SAS and MDM2 occurs frequently in human parosteal osteosarcomas. *Oncogene,* 18: 783-788

Wyatt-Ashmead J, Bao L, Eilert RE, Gibbs P, Glancy G & McGavran L (2001). Primary aneurysmal bone cysts: 16q22 and/or 17p13 chromosome abnormalities. *Pediatr Dev Pathol,* 4: 418-419

Yamaguchi A, Komori T & Suda T. (2000). Regulation of osteoblast differentiation mediated by bone morphogenetic proteins, hedgehogs, and Cbfa1. *Endocr Rev.*, 21:393–411

Yamamura H., Yashikawa H., Tatsuta M., et al (1998). Expression of the smooth muscle calponin gene in human osteosarcoma and its possible association with prognosis. *Int J Cancer*, 79:245-250

Yang X & Karsenty G. (2004). ATF4, the osteoblast accumulation of which is determined post-translationally, can induce osteoblast specific gene expression in non-osteoblastic cells. *J Biol Chem.* , 279:47109–47114

Yang J, Yang D, Cogdell D, Du X, Li H, Pang Y, Sun Y, Hu L, Sun B, Trent J, Chen K & Zhang W. (2010). APEX1 gene amplification and its protein overexpression in osteosarcoma: correlation with recurrence, metastasis, and survival. *Technol Cancer Res Treat.*, 9(2):161-9.

Yoshikawa, H., Nakase, T., Myoui, A., & Ueda, T. (2004). Bone morphogenetic proteins in bone tumors. *J Orthop Sci* 9:334-340

Yotov WV, Hamel H, Rivard GE, Champagne MA, Russo PA, Leclerc JM, Bernstein ML & Levy E (1999). Amplifications of DNA primase 1 (PRIM1) in human osteosarcoma. *Genes Chromosomes Cancer*, 26: 62-69

Young R.H & Rosenberg A.E (1987). Osteosarcoma of the urinary bladder: Report of a case and review of the literature. *Cancer*, 59:174-178

2

Imaging Osteosarcoma

Ali Nawaz Khan[1], Durr-e-Sabih[2],
Klaus L. Irion[3], Hamdan AL-Jahdali[4] and
Koteyar Shyam Sunder Radha Krishna[1]
[1]North Manchester General Hospital Manchester,
[2]Multan Institute of Nuclear Medicine & Radiotherapy,
Nishtar Medical College & Hospital, Multan,
[3]Cardiothoracic Centre, Liverpool NHS Trust,
The Royal Liverpool University Hospitals, Liverpool,
[4]Division of Pulmonology, Dept. of Medicine,
Head of Pulmonary Division, Sleep Disorders Center,
King Saud University for Health Science,
King Abdulaziz Medical City, Riyadh,
[1,3]UK
[2]Pakistan
[4]Saudi Arabia

1. Introduction

The World Health Organization subdivides the histologic appearance of OS into central and surface tumors, and recognises a number of subtypes within each group [1]. OS frequently originate in the metaphysis of the distal femur, proximal tibia and proximal humerus. OSs are subdivided into the classic form (75%) and osteosarcoma variants (25%) [2, 3 & 4]. The variants form a heterogeneous group with a range of different imaging and behavioral features (Figures 1-7).

The long-term survival has improved thanks to more accurate diagnosis and better staging by imaging. The classic OS grows in a radial manner, which invades the bony cortex forming a ball-like area of new bone formation/destruction that compresses the surrounding soft tissues/muscles effectively forming a pseudocapsule termed as the "reactive zone." Satellite nodules invade the reactive zone. To ensure effective surgical therapy the entire abnormal bone including the reactive zone containing the satellites is resected with wide surgical margins. OS may metastasize regionally or systemically. The presence of metastasis worsens the prognosis dramatically. Tumor nodules that grow outside the reactive zone but within the same bone or across a neighbouring joint are called "skip lesions" and represent regional metastases. Lungs are the commonest site of systemic metastases. The skeleton forms the second most common site of metastatic disease but generally occur after pulmonary metastases.

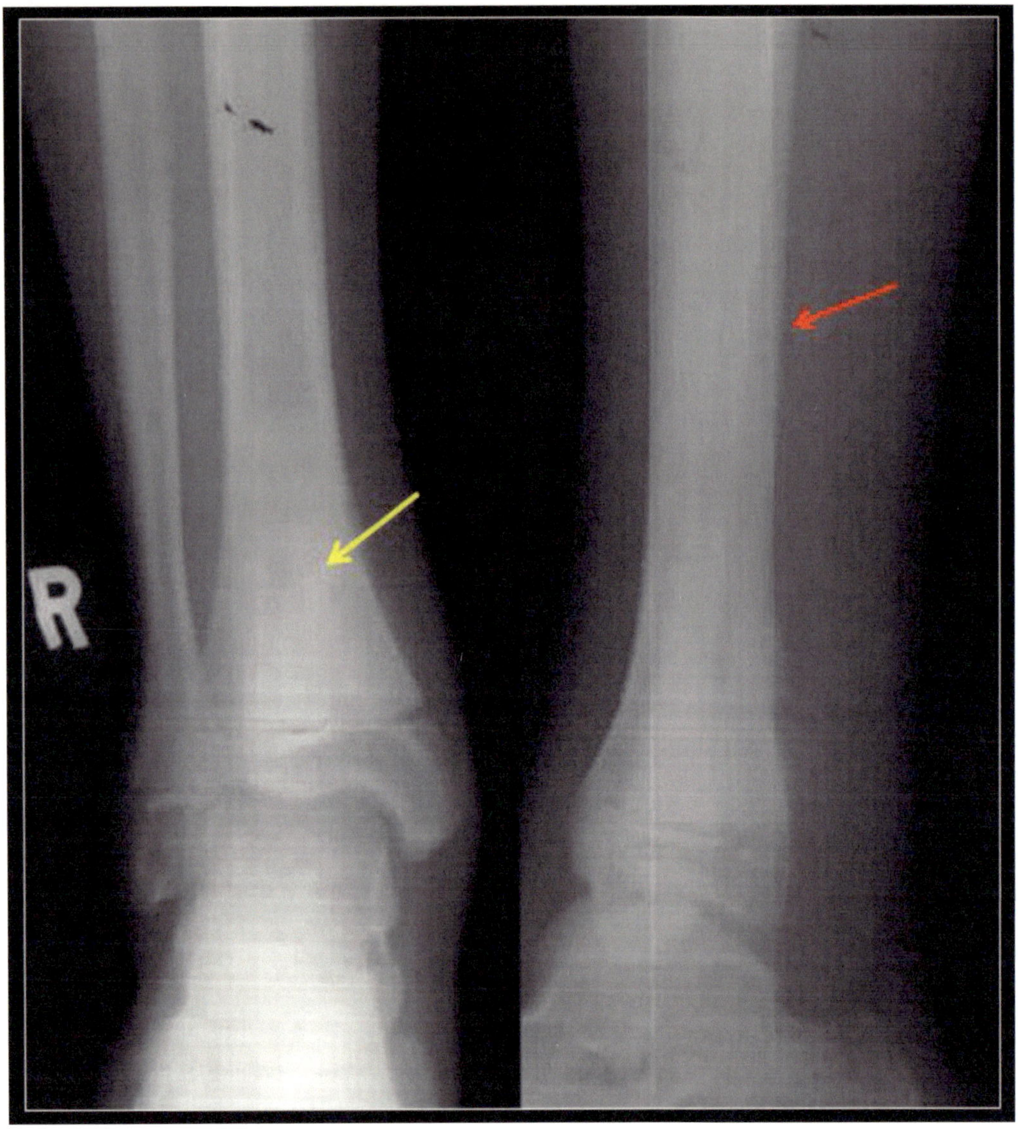

Fig. 1. The illustration shows a radiograph of a right ankle in a 12-year old. He presented with vague ankle pain and a slight limp. The radiograph shows mixed lytic and osteosclerotic lower tibial metaphyseal lesion (yellow arrow). Note the subtle laminated periosteal reaction (red arrow). A surgical biopsy confirmed a classical osteogenic sarcoma.

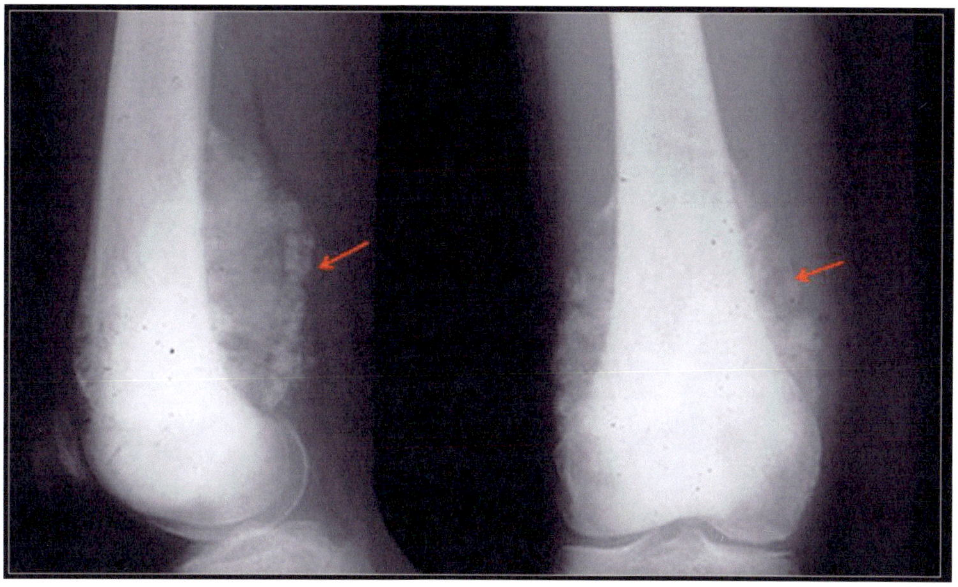

Fig. 2. Radiograph of the lower femur shows a sclerotic lesion of the lower femoral metaphysis. An associated exuberant "sun ray" periosteal reaction (red arrows) is seen. A biopsy revealed an osteosarcoma. Note the area of sclerosis is extending into the epiphysis.

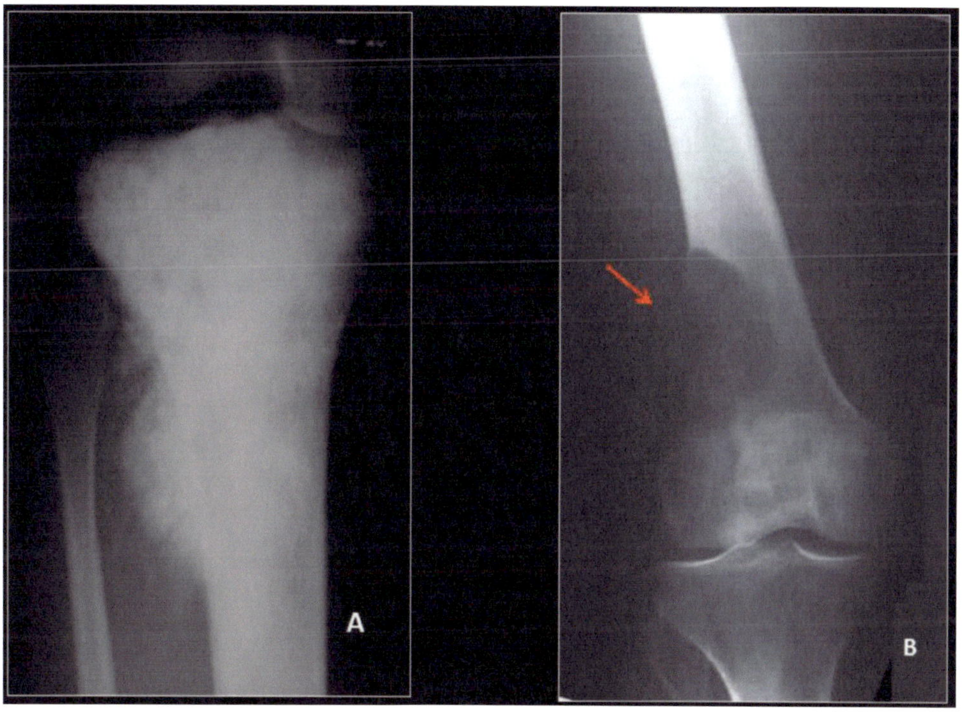

Fig. 3. The figure show radiographs from two different patients depicting a markedly osteosclerotic lesion of the upper tibia (A) and radiograph (B) from a more skeletally mature case that shows an entirely osteolytic lesions. Both lesions proved osteosarcomas on biopsy.

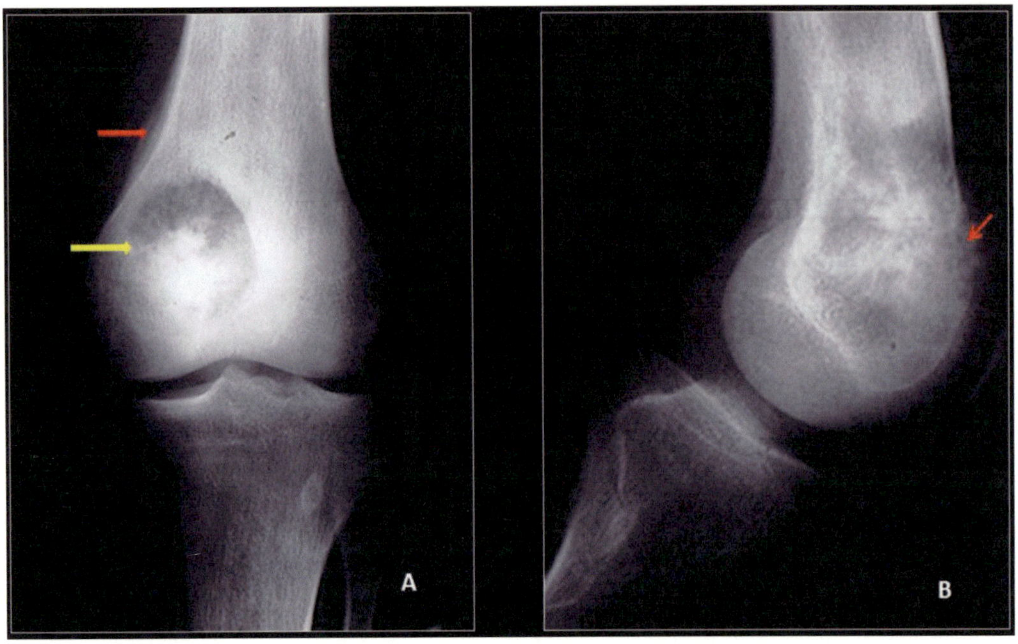

Fig. 4. The figure shows another mixed lytic and sclerotic metaphyseal tumor (yellow arrow). The tumor is crossing the epiphyseal line. Both 'sun ray' and onionskin periosteal reactions (red arrows) are shown.

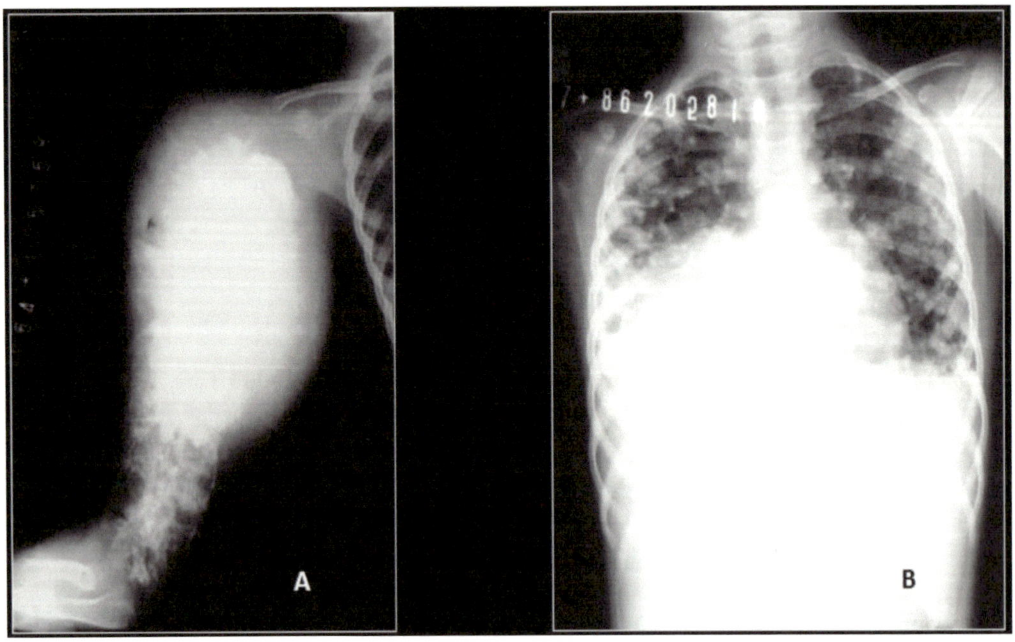

Fig. 5. Image A shows, biopsy proved osteosarcoma involving the whole shaft of the humerus. Image B depicts multiple lung metastases from the same patient. Note bilateral pleural effusions due to histologically proved pleural metastatic disease.

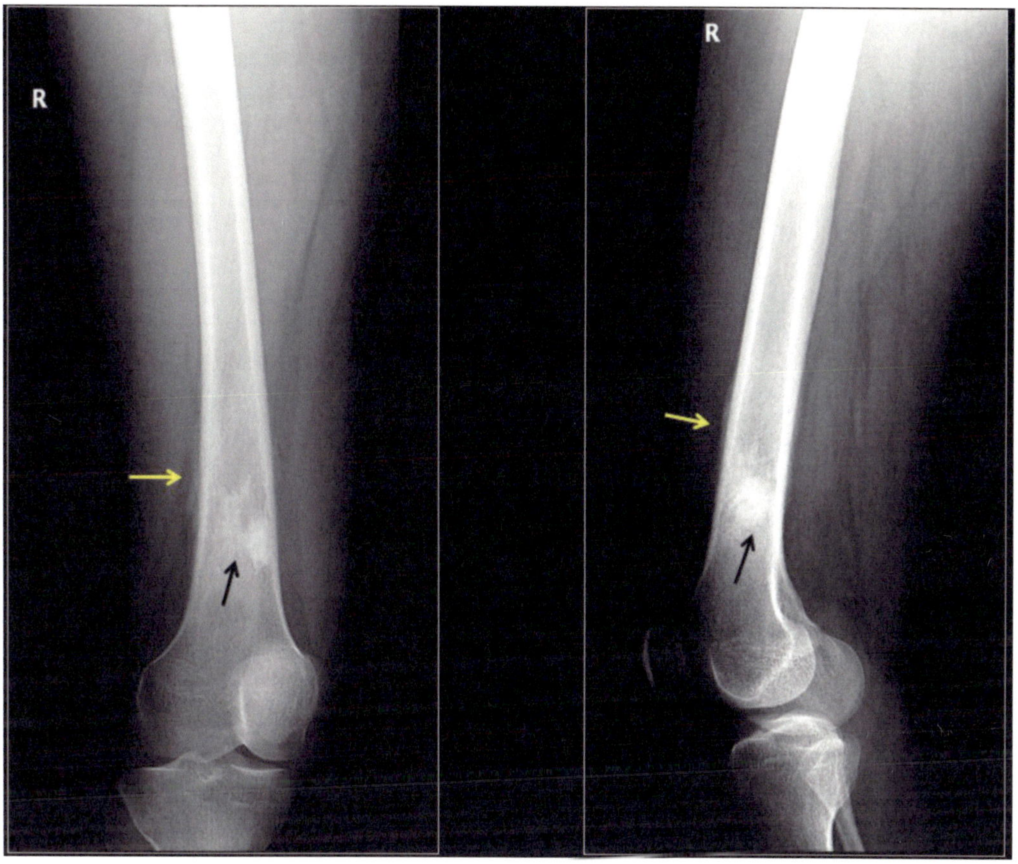

Fig. 6. AP and lateral radiographs of the lower femur shows a biopsy proved diaphyseal variant of OS. Note the mixed lytic/sclerotic lesion (black arrow) and the laminated periosteal new bone formation (yellow arrow).

2. Discussion

OS affects the age groups between 15-25 years in over 75% of cases with a gender ratio M: F=1.5:1. OS is uncommon in patients younger than 6 years or older than 60 years. OS in the older age group are usually secondary to Paget's disease, radiation or dedifferentiated chondrosarcomas. By far the highest percentage of OS (80% to 90%) occurs in the long tubular bones. The axial skeleton is rarely involved. Femur, tibia and humerus account for about 85% of extremity tumors. OS usually originate in the metaphysis of the long bones; tumors originating in the diaphysis and the epiphysis are rare Figures (1-7) [5 & 6].

The cause is not known but ionising radiation is implicated in 2% of OSs [7]. A genetic relationship exists with hereditary retinoblastoma. In patients with retinoblastoma, OS occurs 500 times more often than in the general population [8]. Three to four per cent children suffering from OS carry an inherent germline mutation in p539. The majority of children with germline p53 mutations have a family history suggestive of Li-Fraumeni syndrome Rarely OS is associated with single or multiple osteochondroma, solitary enchondroma or enchondromatosis, multiple hereditary exostoses, fibrous dysplasia, chronic osteomyelitis, sites of bone infarcts, sites of metallic prostheses and sites of previous internal fixation. Ionizing radiation is a well-documented etiologic factor. OS is also associated with the use of intravenous radium and Thorotrast and exposure to alkylating agents independent of the administration of radiotherapy (Figures 8-16) [9].

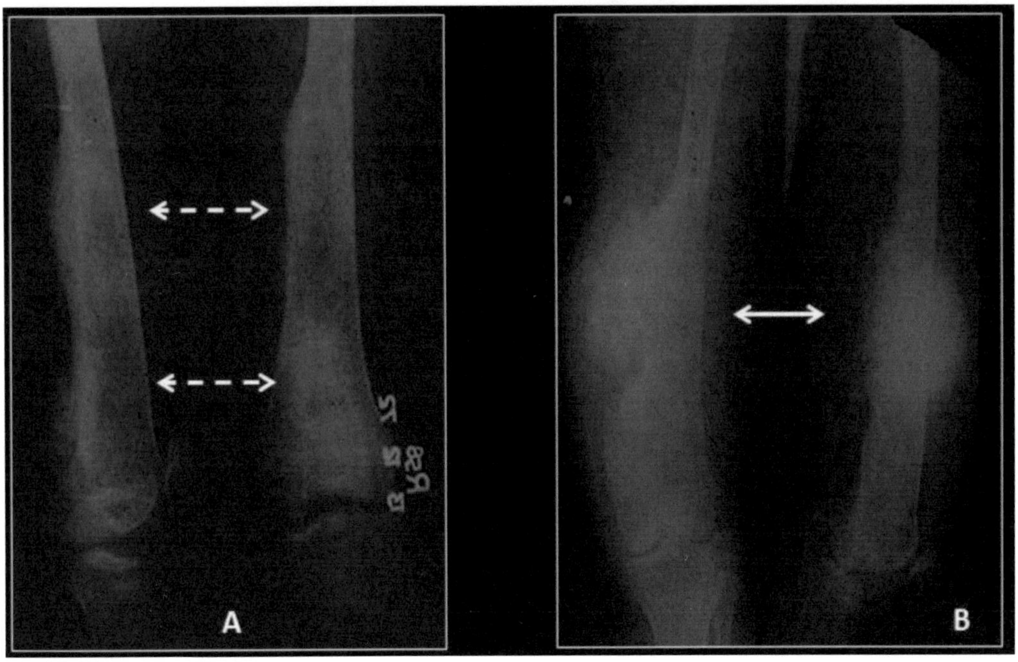

Fig. 7. Image A and B shows radiographs of the lower femur in two different patients. Both represent variants of OS. Image A shows a classic OS originating at the metaphysis and invading the diaphysis. Image B is from 18-year old female shows a tumor based at the lower femoral diaphysis sparing the metaphysis. Note the exuberant periosteal reaction. The diagnosis of image B was parosteal OS.

Patients typically present with pain and swelling, localized enlargement of the extremity and, occasionally, a pathologic fracture. Most patients have localized disease at presentation. Diagnosis and treatment of OS requires a multidisciplinary approach involving the primary health care physician, radiologist, pathologist, orthopedic surgeon/oncologist, and the medical oncologist. Imaging is crucial to early diagnosis. Imaging also can predict prognosis and allows separation from other focal bone pathology. Conventional radiography is usually the primary imaging used which often provides a clue to the diagnosis and often is a guide as to which modality should follow. Once the issue of an OS is raised, MRI is the critical next step in the local staging and the associated soft tissue involvement. CT scanning is less sensitive than MRI in local staging but is essential in depicting systemic metastases specifically to the lungs. Histologic confirmation is essential, and CT is often used as a guide to obtain tumor tissue. Conventional radiography generally depicts a combination of lytic and sclerotic areas within the tumor but purely lytic or sclerotic lesions may occur. The tumor appears moth eaten, with ill-defined margins, and may appear permeative with several small cortical erosions. The tumor near joints is often difficult to distinguish from joint effusions. Periosteal new bone formation usually occurs once the cortex is breached. Periosteal new bone formation may take a variety of shapes and forms including a Codman triangle, an onionskin appearance or hair on end/ and sunburst reactions, all indicate an aggressive process. Other imaging studies that contribute to the diagnosis and management include radionuclide studies, PET/CT and US. PET/CT holds a promise. Presently angiography is rarely used in the diagnosis of OSs except for specific indications. Bone OSs whatever the type are initially imaged by conventional radiography. Radiographs of the involved bone are obtained in various planes and often a chest radiograph is obtained in the same sitting. Once the diagnosis is suspected, MRI forms the next imaging modality of choice to assess the extent of the tumor distribution within the bone and associated soft tissue component if any. If MRI is not available, CT provides the same information though is not as sensitive. Nevertheless, CT is an essential part of a staging procedure especially in the staging of pulmonary metastases. Histological opinion is always required because of radiological mimics of OSs (Figure 17). Biopsy should always be performed before a base line MRI is obtained.

The various modalities are discussed in detail, and examples of different imaging are shown.

2.1 Stages of osteosarcoma

Staging of OSs is surgical based on Musculoskeletal Tumour Society staging system [10]:

Tumor grade (I = low grade; II = high grade);

Tumor extension (A = intraosseous involvement only; B = intra- and extraossseous extension);

Presence of distant metastases (III)

Nevertheless, imaging is required for correct staging including an isotope bone scan to rule out bone metastases and a chest radiograph and CT to rule out pulmonary metastases.

Differential diagnosis of OS includes many benign and malignant lesions and soft tissue tumors adjacent to bones particularly long tubular bones. Imaging studies alone, however, may be sometimes confusing and histological opinion is always required. Osteolytic osteosarcoma may mimic malignant fibrous histiocytoma, fibrosarcoma or giant cell tumors. The diaphyseal variant of OS may resemble Ewing's sarcoma or lymphoma [11].

Technetium-99m (99m Tc) methylene diphosphonate (MDP) radionuclide bone scans are extremely sensitive but has a low specificity for OS. Nevertheless, MDP scans are useful in depicting multifocal bone disease.

Other imaging studies that contribute to the diagnosis and management include radionuclide studies, PET/CT and ultrasound. PET/CT holds a promise. Angiography is no longer used in the diagnosis of osteosarcomas.

Although ultrasonography (US) is not considered when staging OS but it is a valuable modality in tissue sampling. US is also useful in patients with prosthetic implants in the detection of early local recurrence as MRI and CT may not be suitable, because of the artifact produced by the metal on CT scans or MRIs.

3. Conventional radiograph

Conventional radiography is a non-invasive, affordable and widely available means that often provides a clue to the initial diagnosis, aggressiveness of the tumor and hence prognosis and provides a summary differential diagnosis. It can evaluate the effects of chemotherapy and diagnose lung metastases. In a suspected bone lesion, conventional radiographs are usually the initial imaging procedure. Conventional radiography may confirm a bony lesion, suggest diagnosis and guide further imaging. The anatomical location of the bone lesion the age of the patient and the clinical presentation help to formulate the list of differential diagnosis.

In a review of 347 patients with extremity OS plain-film radiographic patterns of American Joint Committee on Cancer (AJCC) stage II OA were analysed and were found to be related with clinicopathological features. The study concluded that this finding has a potential use to provide valuable information for treatment decision-making in high-grade extremity OS [12].

OS present with a variety of radiographic findings. Most OSs presents as a combination of osteolytic and osteosclerotic areas but lesions may be entirely lytic or sclerotic. Most OSs appears aggressive tumors with a moth eaten appearance and indistinct edges. Some OSs appears permeative, associated with multiple small cortical holes. Periosteal new bone formation surrounding the tumor is a common occurrence and occurs when the tumor breaks through the cortex. A Codman triangle is created when a triangular area of new subperiosteal bone formation raises the periosteum away from the bone. The main causes for this sign are OS, Ewing's sarcoma, and a subperiosteal abscess. Other types of periosteal reactions are multilaminated ("onionskin"), spiculated, and sunburst appearance ("hair on end"), all of which represent an aggressive process. Extension of the tumor beyond the bone into the surrounding soft tissues is common. As most OSs are near joints, differentiation of soft tissue extension may sometimes be difficult to distinguish from a joint effusion on radiography. 'Cloudlike' areas of sclerosis, resulting from malignant osteoid production and calcification, may be seen within the mass. Lung metastases are depicted as cannon ball lesions, which may calcify/ossify (Figures 1-7).

Following chemotherapy, OSs becomes well defined often with a surrounding 'capsule'. Atypical features in OS present diagnostic problems. Most OSs present late with aggressive features highly suggestive of OSs. However, early detection may cause diagnostic issues and tumors may be mistaken for benign lesions [13]. In these circumstances cross sectional imaging may indicate aggressive features suggestive of OS [14]. Rarely an expanding type of tumor may be, confined to the intramedullary cavity with no apparent aggressive features. Osteosclerotic OS confined to the intramedullary cavity have been confused with avascular necrosis [14, 15]. An OS may resemble an osteoblastoma or osteoid osteoma as a lytic defect with calcification or ossification within the defect and surrounded by sclerosis [14, 16].

Intracortical OS is a rare variant, which, is contained within the cortex. Radiographs may indicate a fibrous cortical defect or a Brodie's abscess. A CT scan depicts the tumor in an intra-cortical location [14, 17].

A subchondral OS originates in the subchondral position extending across the epiphyseal plate into the metaphysis. This variant may resemble a giant cell tumor or a chondrosarcoma. These variants may be entirely lytic or sclerotic. The sclerotic type has a more malignant look [14, 18].

Diaphyseal OS located in the diaphysis are radiologically similar to classical OS. Rarely, diaphyseal OS may have a more sclerotic appearance resembling a benign process. A lytic tumor with or without multilaminated periosteal reaction may resemble Ewing's sarcoma [14, 19].

Cavarial OS are a rare variant that comprise less than 2% of all OSs [20]. The radiographic appearance is similar to classic OS. Lytic appearance is more common, but periosteal reaction is rare but a sclerotic hair on end appearance may indicate a poor prognosis. Most calvarial OS occur in young adults but a secondary type of OS occurs in the fifth decade or beyond and usually is associated with Paget's disease and radiation therapy [14].

Osteosarcoma of the calcaneus occurs in less than 1% of the cases. Radiographic findings are similar to the classic OS. There is a rare association with Rothmund-Thompson syndrome [14].

OS complicating Paget's is rare but well recognized with incidence of 0.95%. Paget's related OS primarily affect males in the seventh decade of life (Figure 8-11). The distribution of lesions is similar to that expected with uncomplicated Paget's disease. The sites most commonly affected sites are the pelvis, femur and humerus. The bones of the pelvis are most commonly involved; the humerus and the femur are next in frequency. No region of the skeleton is spared, with the exception of the forearms and hands. In 30 per cent of cases, these neoplasms are multifocal. The tumors are categorized radiographically as lytic, mixed, and sclerotic, in descending order of frequency. Diagnosis on plain radiographs may be quite difficult because of the underlying Paget's changes and osteolyic lesions that sometimes occur in Paget's disease. Histologically these tumors are typically highly polymorphic sarcomas. The prognosis is poor with only 3%-8% of patients surviving at five years. The main cause of death is pulmonary metastasis or local extension of tumor growth. A high index of suspicion should be maintained when evaluating radiographs of patients with Paget disease, especially of those who present with pain or a palpable mass [21, 22 & 23].

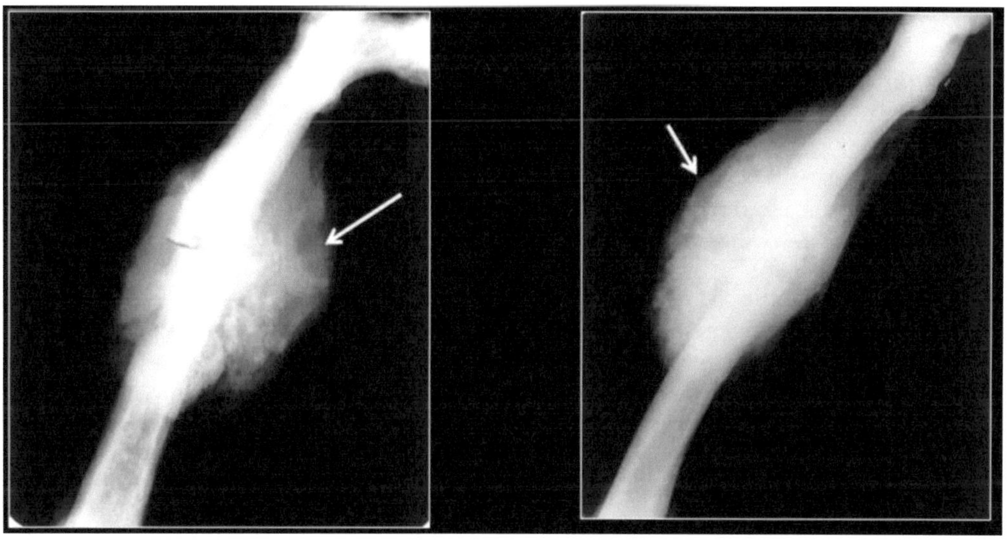

Fig. 8. Two images of the mid shaft of the femur that shows a pathological fracture. The fracture occurred in a Pagetic bone. Note the heavy periosteal reaction at the fracture site (arrows). The initial diagnosis was periosteal new bone formation around a fracture site. However, a biopsy was taken that revealed a sarcomatous transformation of Paget's disease.

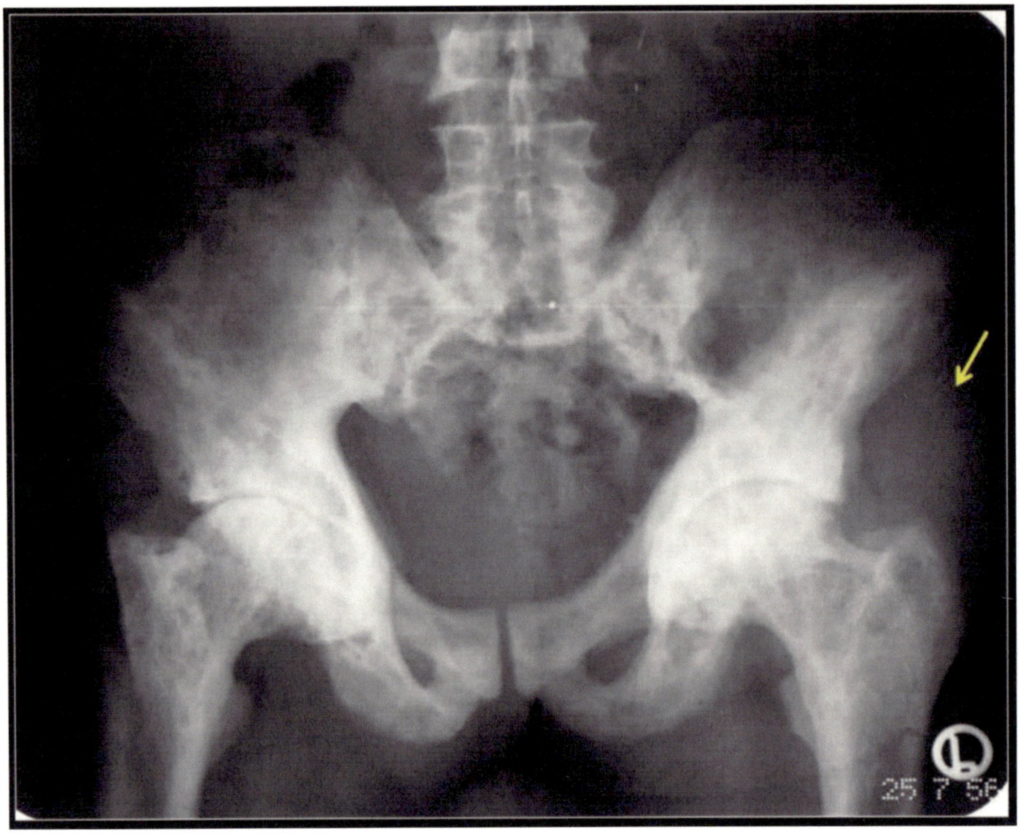

Fig. 9. Radiograph of a pelvis shows considerable sclerosis and coarsening of the trabecular pattern suggestive of Paget's disease. The diagnosis of Paget's disease was confirmed on previous imaging and blood biochemistry 10 years earlier. The patient had bone pain for some time but had recently worsened and had become more focal to the left hip. Note bilateral Paget's coxopathy and much more prominent sclerosis admixed with lysis in the left iliac bone. There is a soft tissue component superior to the left hip. Because of the atypical symptoms a radiographic changes a biopsy was taken. The biopsy confirmed sarcomatous transformation of Paget's disease.

There is a rare association of OS and a bone infarct. Imaging diagnosis may be difficult with such a relationship as changes seen suggest benign characteristics of a bone infarct. Diagnosis only become apparent with advanced OS. In a review of 50 cases of infarct associated OS, a disproportionate number of patients were black. In most patients, there was no known cause for the infarct, whereas in the remainder, the most common underlying disease was a earlier dysbaric event or alcoholism. Approximately 75% of the patients had multiple bone infarcts. Most infarct associated OS involved the femur, tibia, humerus and the radius in that border of frequency. The survival rate in patients with infarct-associated OS is poor [24, 25].

The main limitations of plain radiography in OS are underestimation of the tumor's extent within and outside of the bone and other bone lesions, such as Ewing sarcoma, chondrosarcoma, and fibrosarcoma, infections or Langerhans cell histiocytosis may resemble OS on plain radiographs [26].

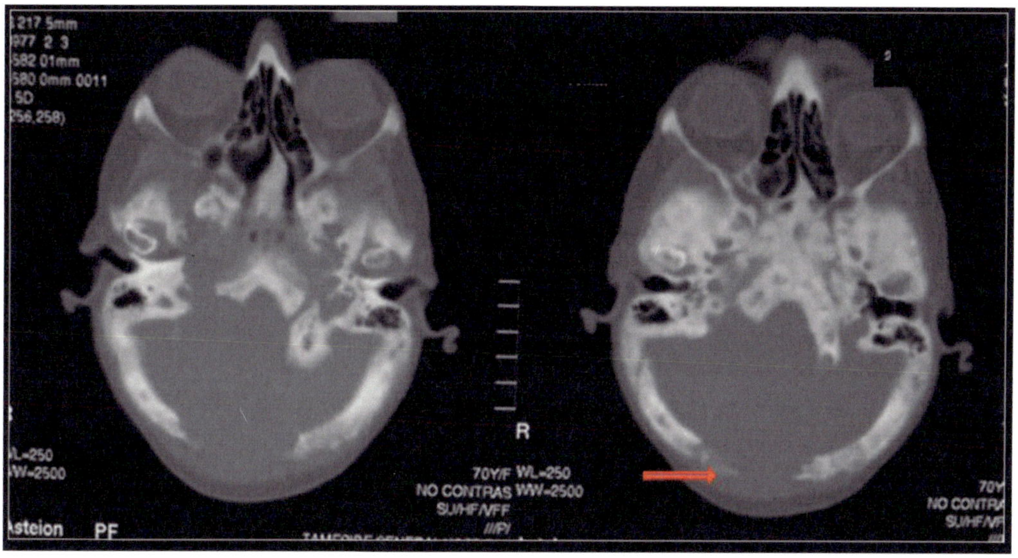

Fig. 10. Non-contrast CT scans performed on the skull of a 70-year old female known to have Paget's disease. The patient had recently presented with increasingly severe occipital headaches. The scans show dense sclerosis at the base of the skull in keeping with Paget's disease. Note the area of bone destruction of the occiput (arrow). The CT scans show the usefulness of the technique in the presence complex bone structure. A biopsy taken from the occipital bone revealed a sarcomatous transformation of Paget's disease.

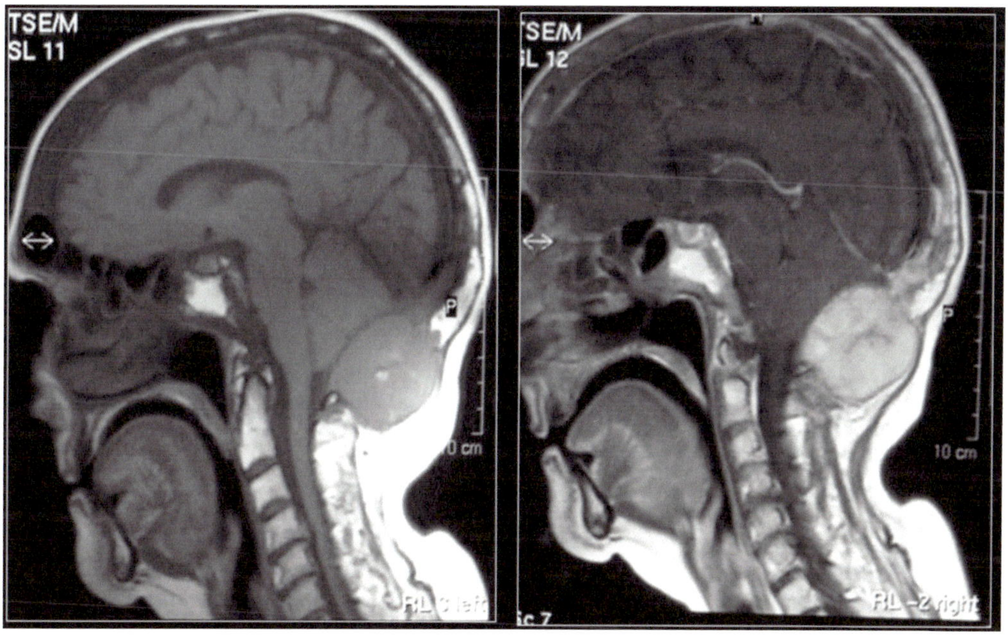

Fig. 11. MRI scans on the same patient as in Figure 10 depicted in T1W and Gadolinium enhanced axial, coronal and sagittal images. The images show an enhancing occipital skull diploic mass that is sparing the brain (see Figures 10).

4. Magnetic resonance imaging

MRI is the modality of choice in the evaluation of focal benign and malignant bone lesions. MRI has excellent capabilities in the local staging of malignant tumors because of its good bone marrow and soft tissue contrast and multiplanar facility. As calcium returns no signal, MRI is insensitive to small foci of calcification. Not only does MRI makes a significant contribution to correct local staging of OS it also assists in determining the most appropriate surgical management. The most fundamental purposes of local staging, is the assessment of tumor relationship of the anatomic domain from which it originates. MRI fulfills this job exceptionally well and defines individual bones, joints, and surrounding fascia and neurovascular bundles elegantly. Ultimate prognosis of OS depends on the number of compartments involved (Figures 13, 14 & 21-23, 25-26, 28) [27, 28, 29, 30 & 31].

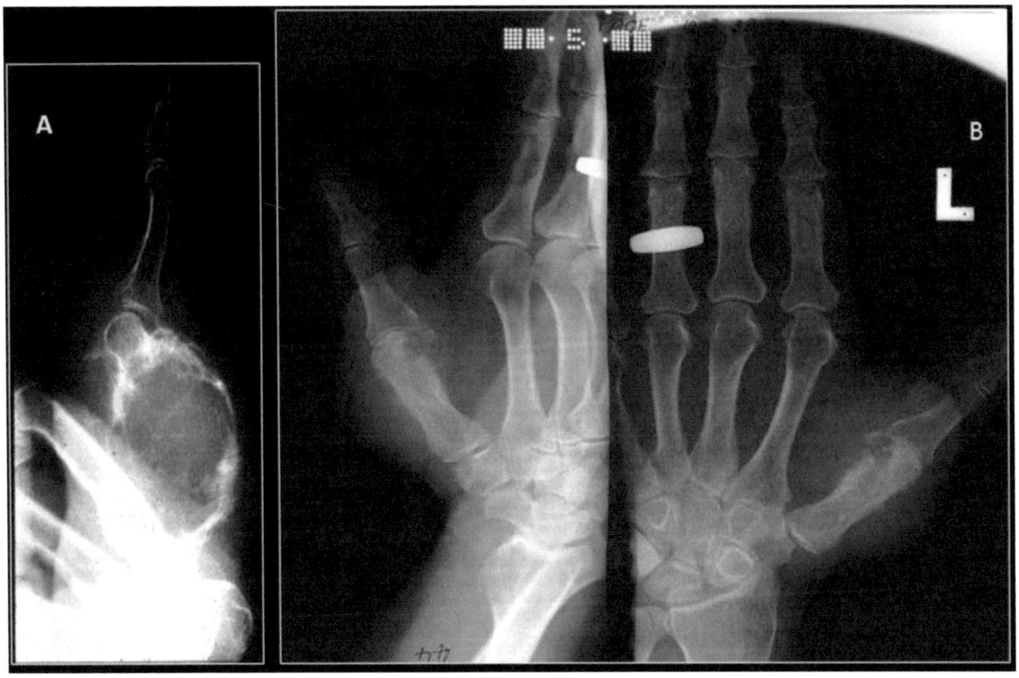

Fig. 12. Thumb and hand radiographs from the departmental archives of two unrelated patients. Patent A had suffered from a solitary enchondroma of the first metacarpal bone for some time. The radiograph shows an expansile lytic lesion in the first metacarpal bone. A histological diagnosis of OS was made. Image B is from a patient that had worked with radium watch dials 20 years earlier. The image shows a biopsy proved OS of the first metacarpal bone. Note the mixed lytic/sclerotic lesion of the first metacarpal bone, also note the periosteal reaction and surrounding soft tissue swelling.

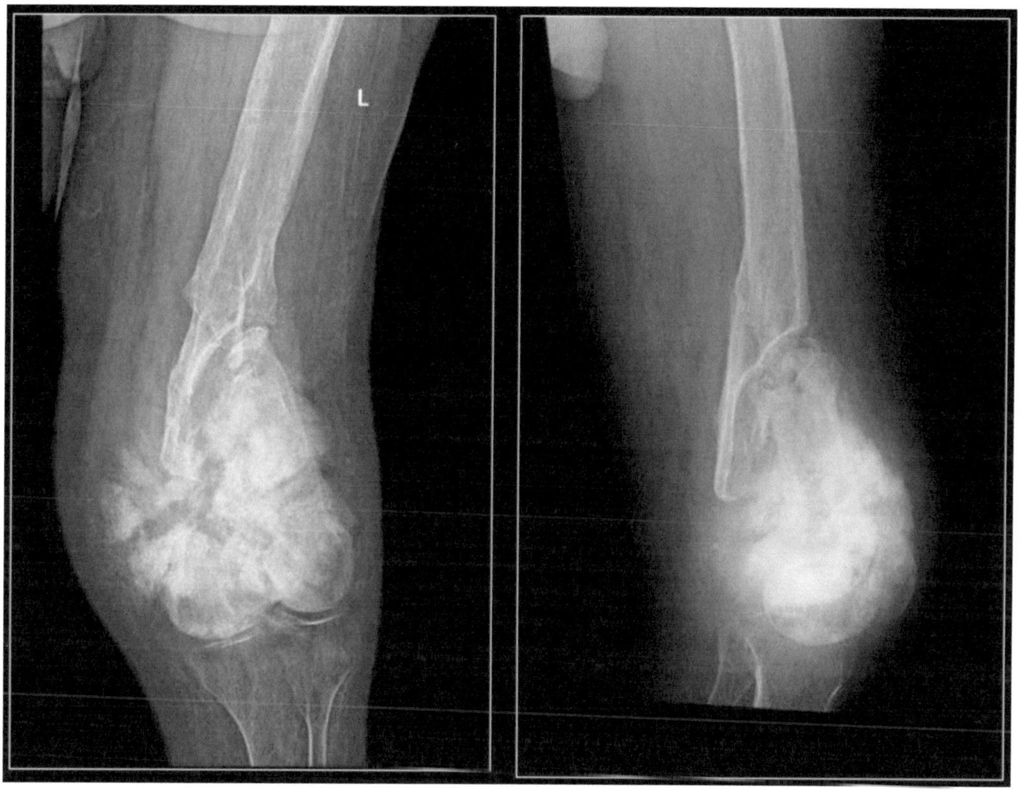

Fig. 13. AP and lateral radiographs of the lower femur of 76 year old man that had suffered from chronic osteomyelitis for some years. The patient recently presented with a change in the pattern of symptoms. The images show destruction of the lower femur associated with periosteal new bone formation. Some of the destroyed bone is well corticated indicative of a chronic process. Initial diagnosis was that of recrudesce of osteomyelitis. The patient was treated accordingly despite a negative aspiration. A repeat radiograph (see next image) show worsening "sun ray" periosteal that prompted a biopsy, which showed OS complicating chronic osteomyelitis.

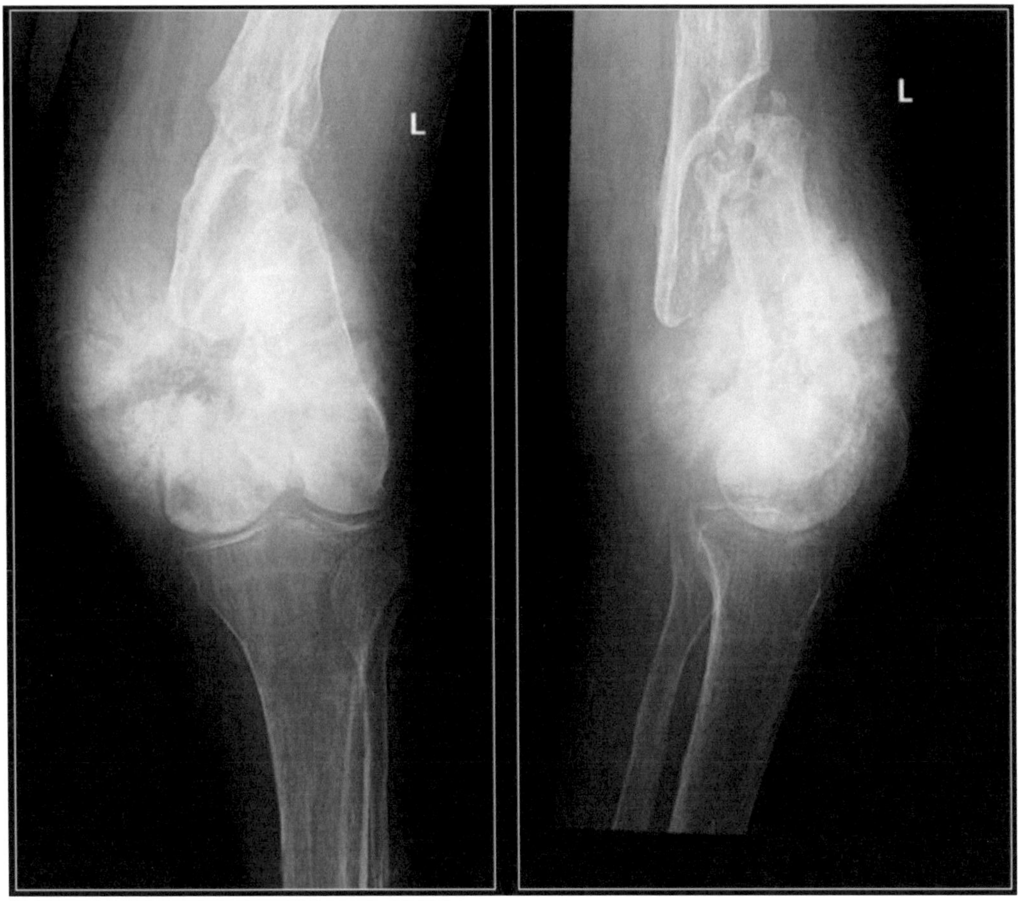

Fig. 14. AP and lateral radiographs of the lower femur of 76 year old man that had suffered from chronic osteomyelitis for some years. The patient recently presented with a change in the pattern of symptoms. The images show destruction of the lower femur associated with periosteal new bone formation. Some of the destroyed bone is well corticated indicative of a chronic process. Initial diagnosis was that of recrudesce of osteomyelitis. The patient was treated accordingly despite a negative aspiration. A repeat radiograph (see previous image) show worsening "sun ray" periosteal that prompted a biopsy, which showed OS complicating chronic osteomyelitis (also see Figure 13).

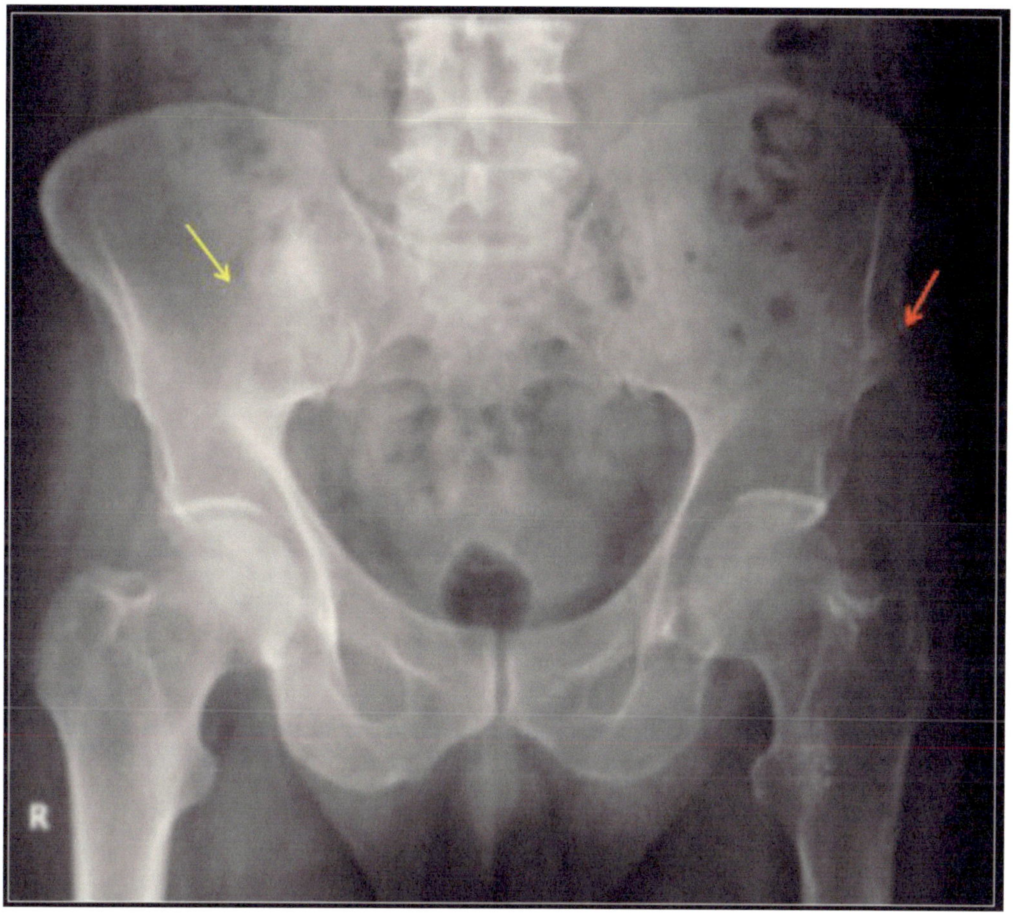

Fig. 15. An AP radiograph of pelvis from a patient with known multiple hereditary exostoses that presented with a 3 month history of increasing right buttock pain. There is a mixed lytic/osteosclerotic lesion in the right iliac bone adjacent to the right sacroiliac joint. A biopsy was taken, which showed a sarcomatous degeneration. An exostosis is noted arising from the region of the left anterior super iliac spine.

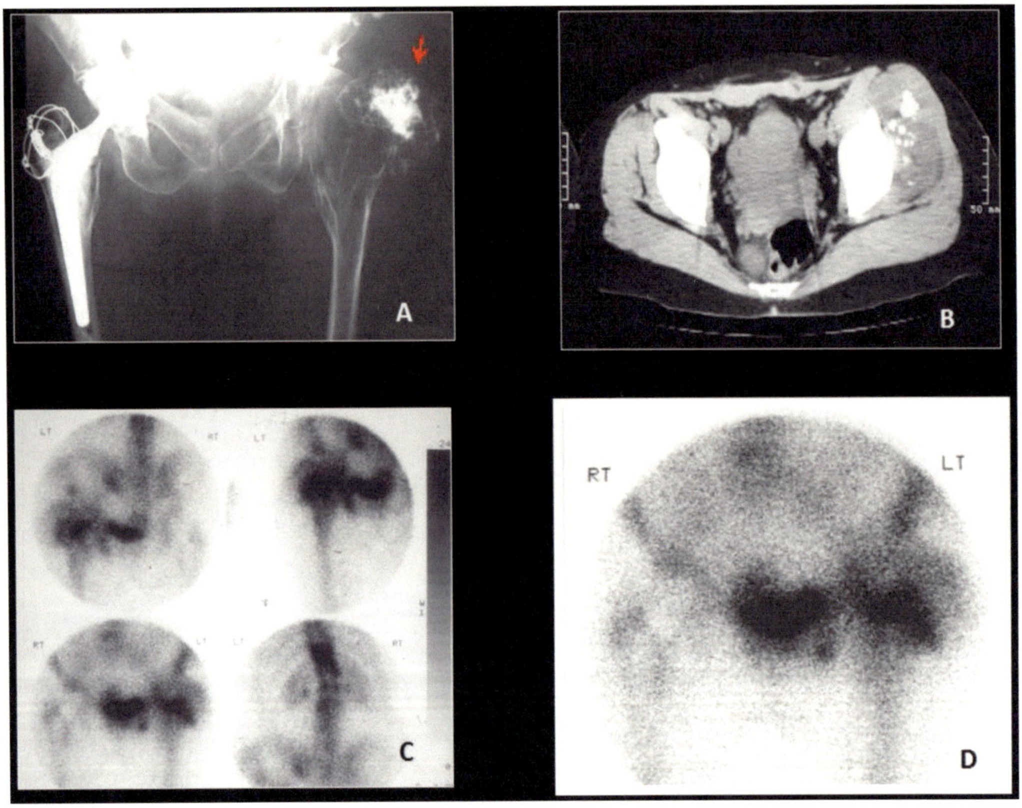

Fig. 16. Series of images from a patient with a long and family history of multiple hereditary exostoses are shown above. The patient presented with increasing pain over the left greater trochanter. An exostosis of the left greater trochanter was recorded 4 years earlier on radiograph taken prior to a right hip replacement. Image B is from an un-enhanced axial CT through the trochanter. The section shows calcification overlying the left greater trochanter associated with overlying prominent soft tissues. This finding by itself does not represent a malignant change. Images C and D show technetium-99m (99m Tc) methylene diphosphonate scans. The MDP scans show intense activity in the region of the left greater trochanter and L1/L2 vertebral bodies. A biopsy taken from the greater trochanter confirmed OS. The activity in L1/L2 were subsequently proved secondary to osteoporotic fractures.

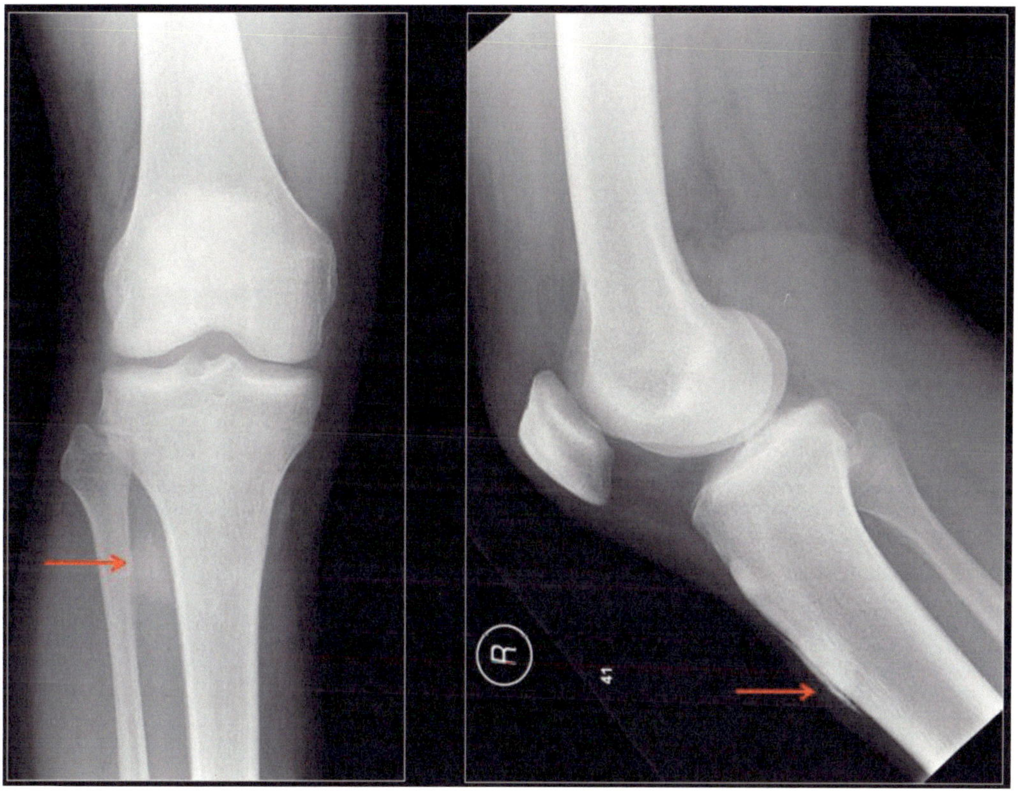

Fig. 17. Imaging studies may be sometimes confusing. Purely osteolytic osteosarcoma may mimic malignant fibrous histiocytoma, fibrosarcoma or giant cell tumours. Osteosarcoma with diaphyseal location may suggest Ewing's sarcoma or lymphoma. Occasionally traumatic periostitis/traumatic myositis ossificance may resemble OS as in this case.

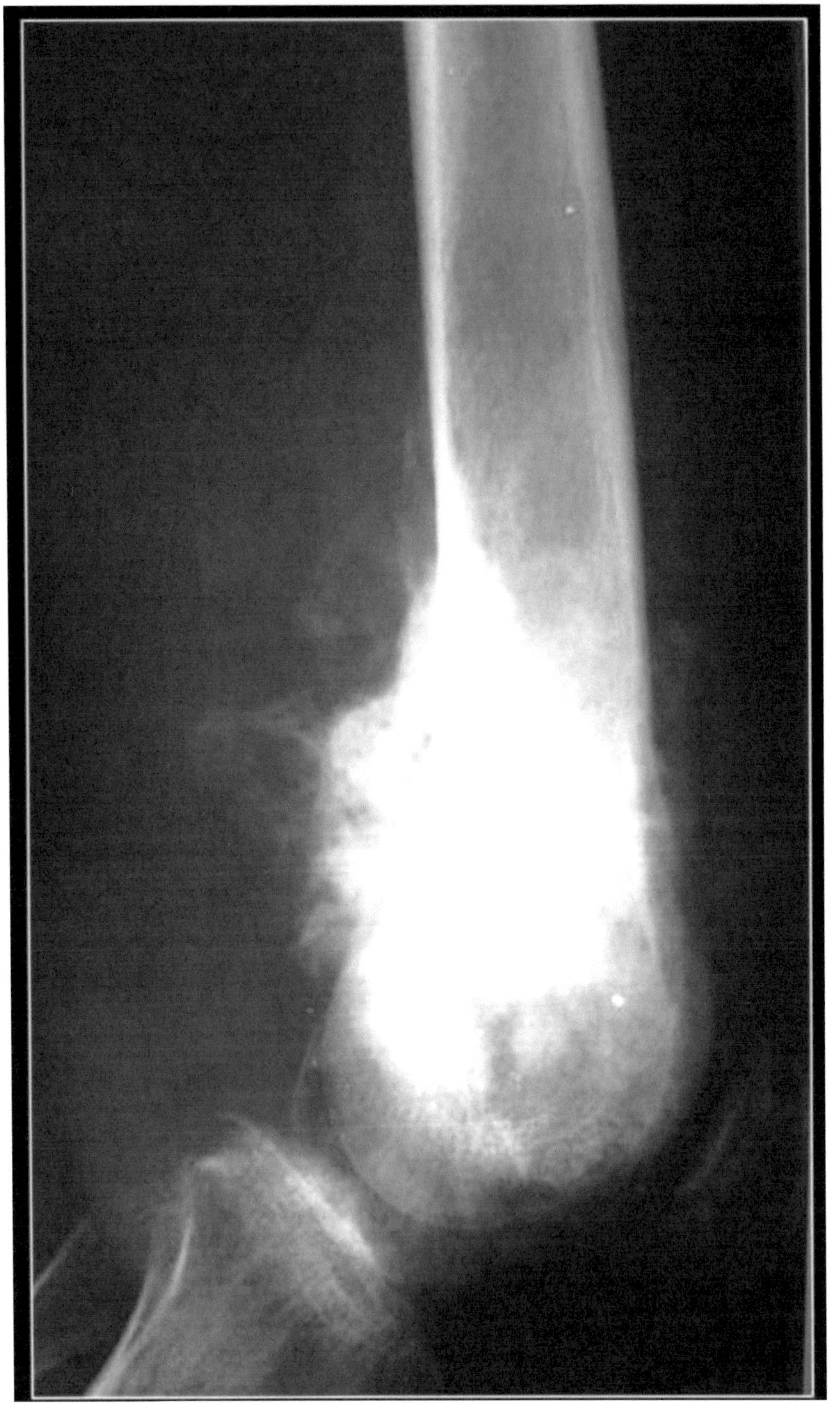

Fig. 18. A radiograph of the left knee of a 65-year old man is shown. The radiographic appearances are characteristically those of an OS. Figures 19-26 are images from the same patient showing the value of various modalities.

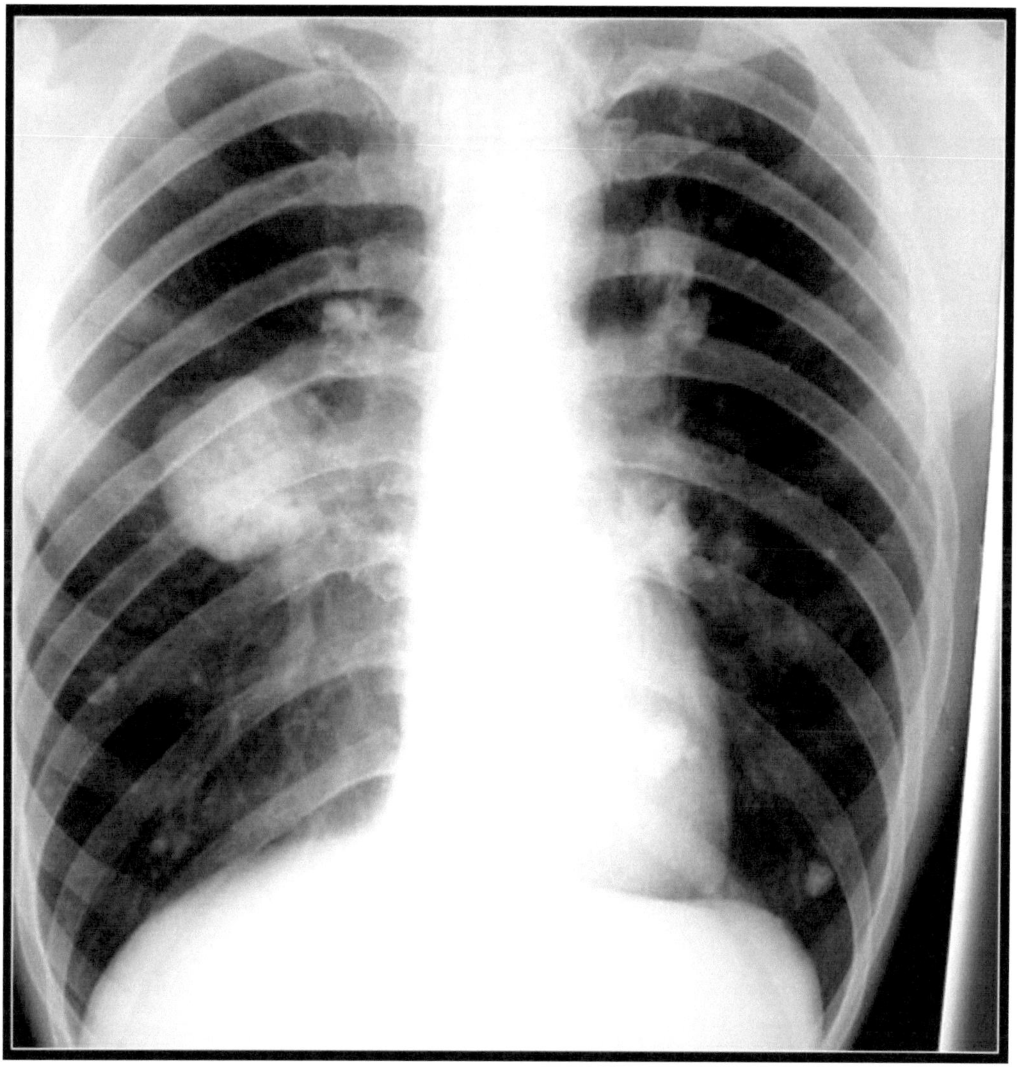

Fig. 19. A chest radiograph of the patient from figure 18 showing calcified cannon ball lung metastases.

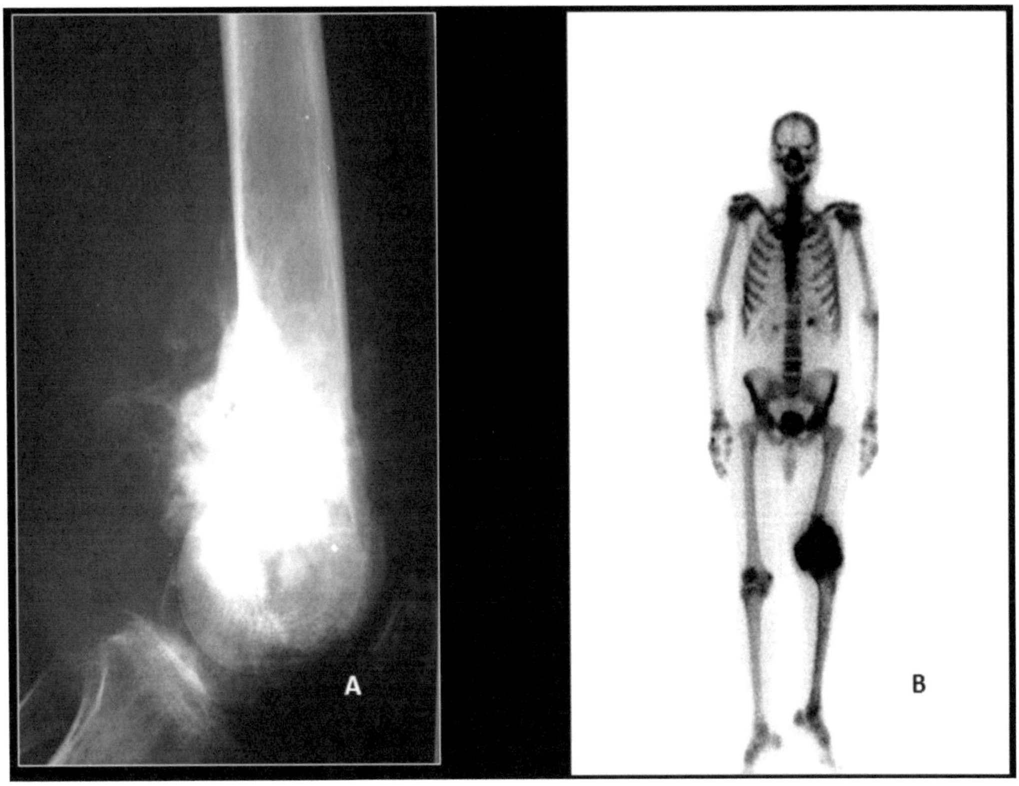

Fig. 20. A technetium-99m (99m Tc) methylene diphosphonate scan was performed on the same patient as in Figure 18 to look for other bone lesions. Activity is seen in the left lower femur associated intense hyperemic peritumoral isotope uptake.

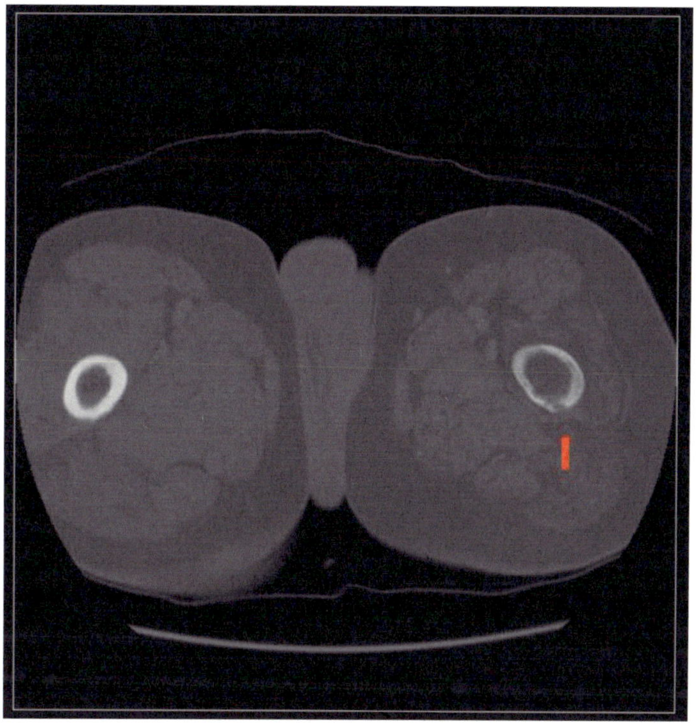

Fig. 21. Unenhanced CT scan through the upper left femur, which shows a break in the cortex (arrow) associated with cortical thinning and effacement of intramedullarly bone marrow. The described observations are at a much higher level than depicted by radiography and the MDP scan. It is difficult to be certain as to whether these findings are related to reactive bone changes or a skip lesion as no biopsy was taken from this focus. Nevertheless the CT scan demonstrate its potential.

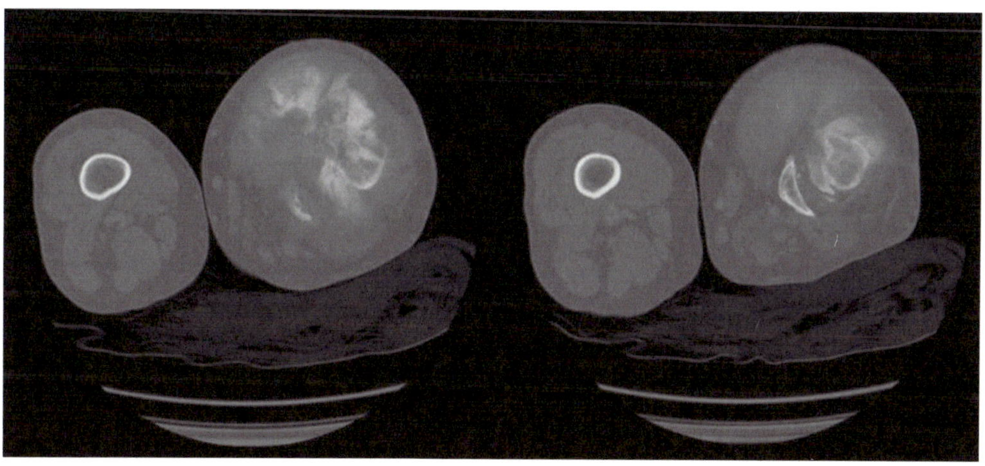

Fig. 22. Axial CT scans (the same patient as in Figure 18) through the lower left femoral tumor showing a mixture of osteosclerotic and lytic changes associated with 'sun ray' periosteal new bone formation. Also, seen are surrounding muscle and subcutaneous edema.

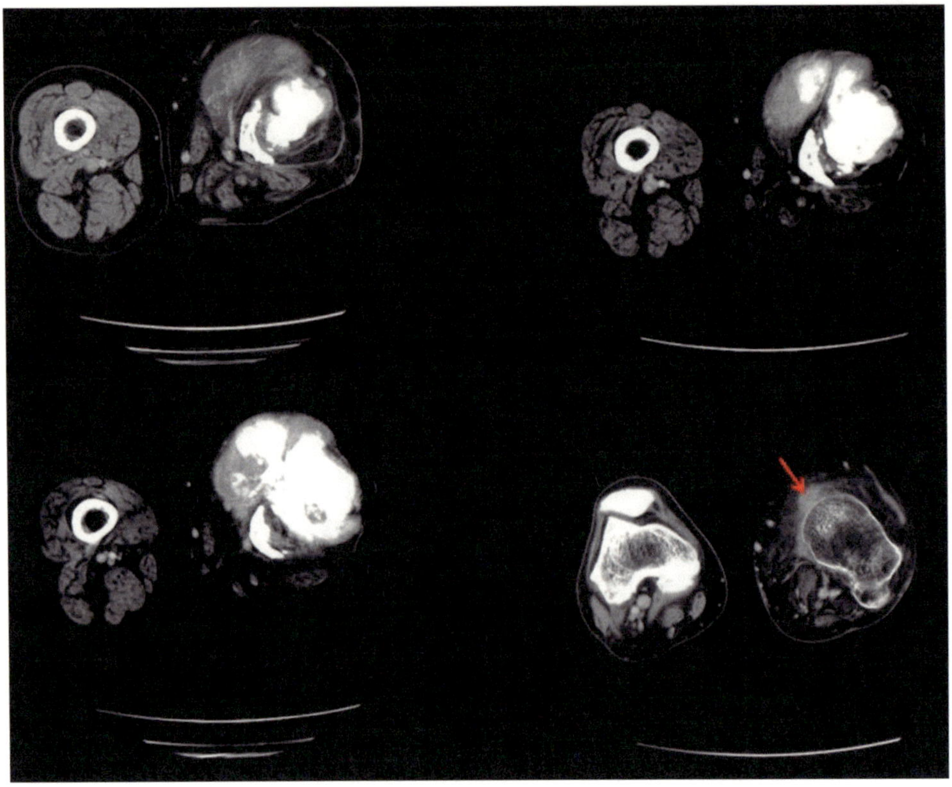

Fig. 23. Axial CT scans (the same patient as in Figure 18) through the lower left femoral tumor showing a mixture of osteosclerotic and lytic changes associated with 'sun ray' periosteal new bone formation. The images are interpreted on a soft tissue window. The images show growth of the tumor into the knee joint (arrow).

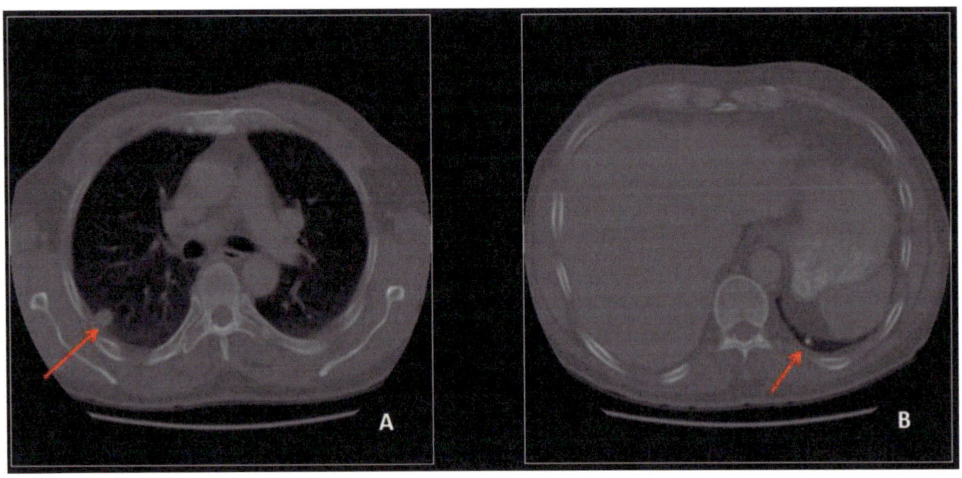

Fig. 24. Axial CT scans (same patient as in Figure 18) through the lungs interrogated on a bone window showing lung metastases. The lesion in the left costophrenic angle (image B) is calcified/ossified.

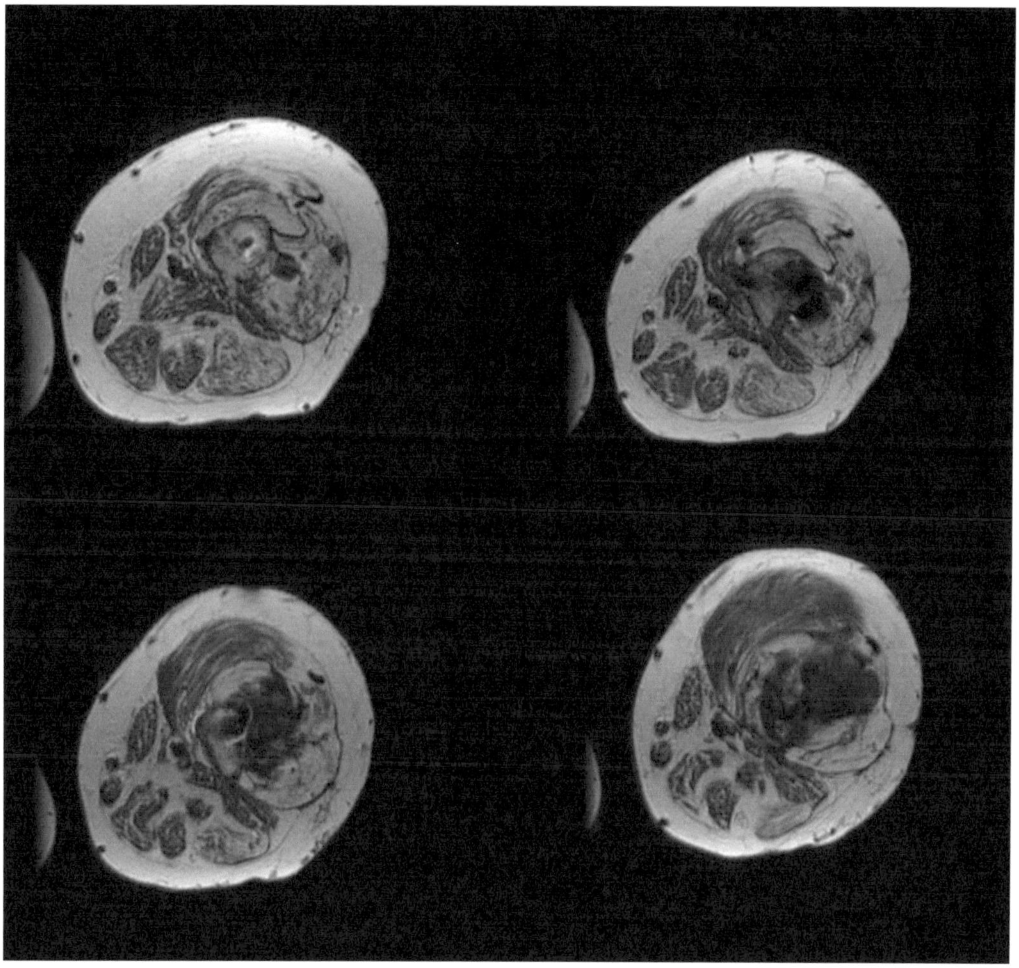

Fig. 25. Axial T1W MRI scans through the tumor (same patient as in Figure 18) showing low signal osteosclerotic bone lesion.

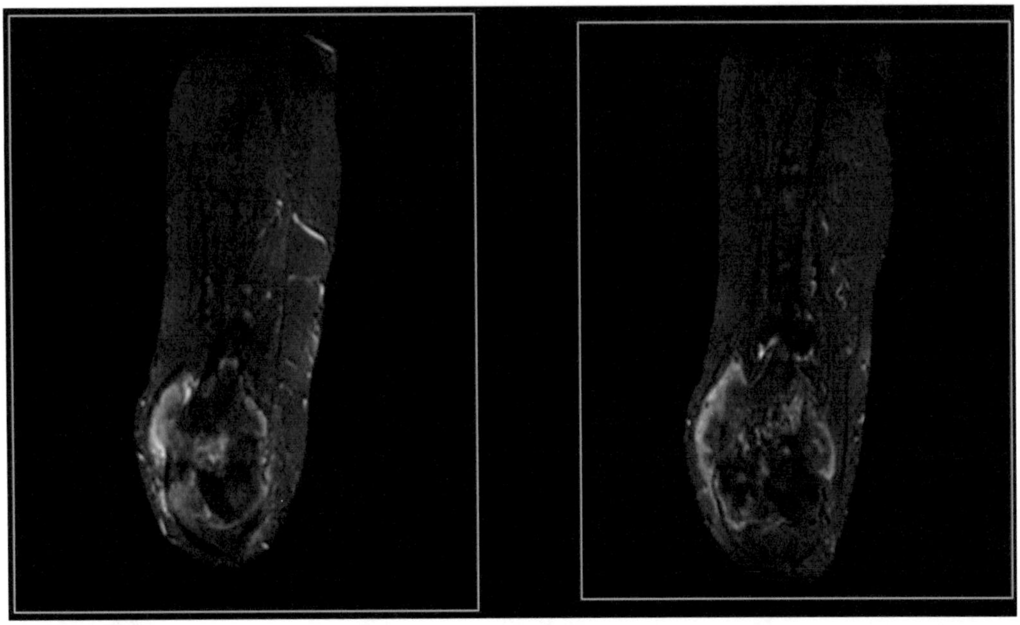

Fig. 26. STIR sequence coronal images (same patient as in Figure 18) show the extent of the tumor and tissue edema.

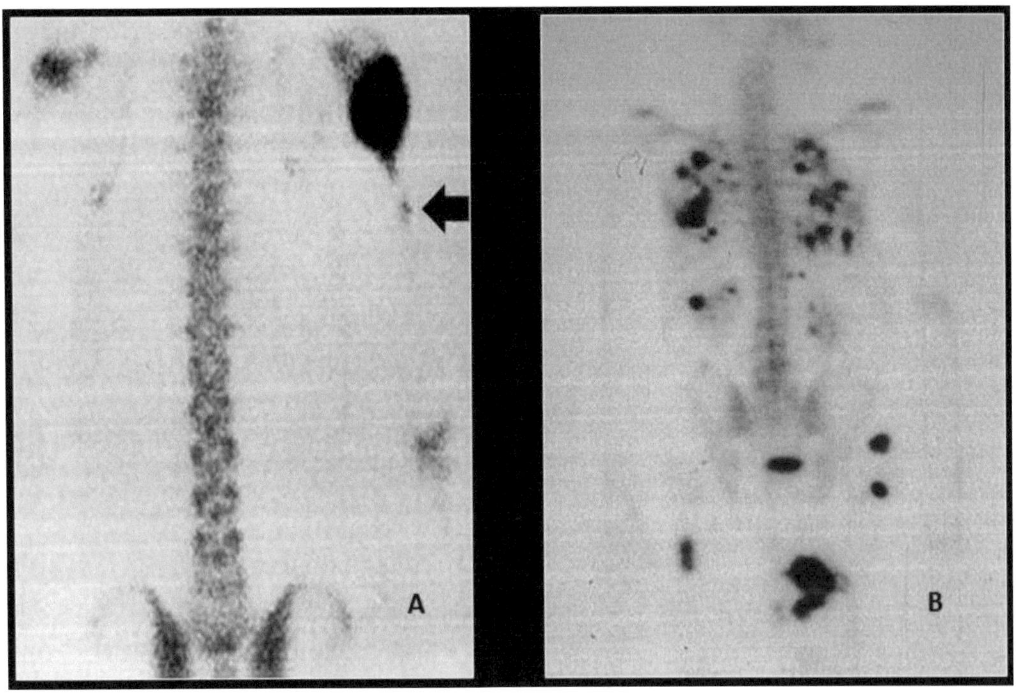

Fig. 27. Two images from technetium-99m (99m Tc) methylene diphosphonate bone scans are shown to demonstrate the importance of this technique in the diagnosis of OS. Image A show a skip lesion in OS (arrow). Image B shows extensive bony metastases from OS.

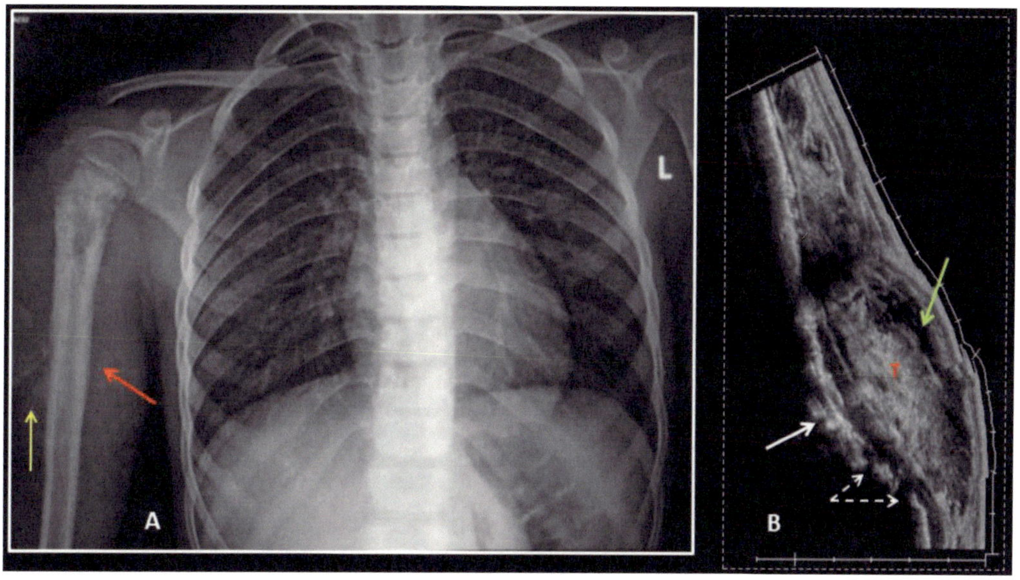

Fig. 28. A chest radiograph of a 13 year old boy showing a destructive lesion of the metaphysis and upper third of the shaft of the right humerus. The image shows a permeative lesion with surrounding periosteal reaction (red arrow) and a Codman triangle (yellow arrow). The child presented with pain in his right shoulder following minor trauma. Image B shows a longitudinal ultrasound examination of the right humerus. The image shows the tumor itself (T) periosteal new bone formation (white arrow) edema surrounding the tumor (green arrow) and a hole in the cortex (interrupted arrows). The areas pinpointed by the interrupted arrows would lend itself to a guided biopsy.

When assessing solitary bone lesions either a T1-weighted or a short-tau inversion recovery (STIR) sequence should be performed to include the entire bone.

The inclusion of the whole length of the bone is necessary to image skip lesions and evaluate the longitudinal distance of the tumor. The epiphysis is also included. Accurate assessment of the extent of intraosseous and extra osseous extension of the tumor is a crucial parameter that will ultimately affect the treatment and prognosis. Periosteal OS is of chondroblastic origin and present with high signal on T2W MRI [29, 32].

Histological opinion is required in suspected OS. Biopsy should be performed following MRI evaluation as hemorrhage occurring at the biopsy site alters the signal intensity characteristics of the tumor at subsequent MRI examinations [28].

T1W spin-echo MR images provide the most accurate estimate of the longitudinal extent of the tumor. STIR sequence overestimates the extent of the tumor because of edema and marrow hyperplasia, which may show signal changes similar to the tumor. It is necessary to determine the maximum longitudinal extent of the tumor, and its maximal distance from the articular surface of the nearest joint.

Epiphyseal tumor growth is associated with signal changes within the epiphysis similar to the tumor and may be seen in association with focal destruction of the growth plate. Both

STIR and T1-weighted sequences are correct in the diagnosis of epiphyseal tumor growth, and although T1W MR is more specific, STIR sequence images are slightly more sensitive.

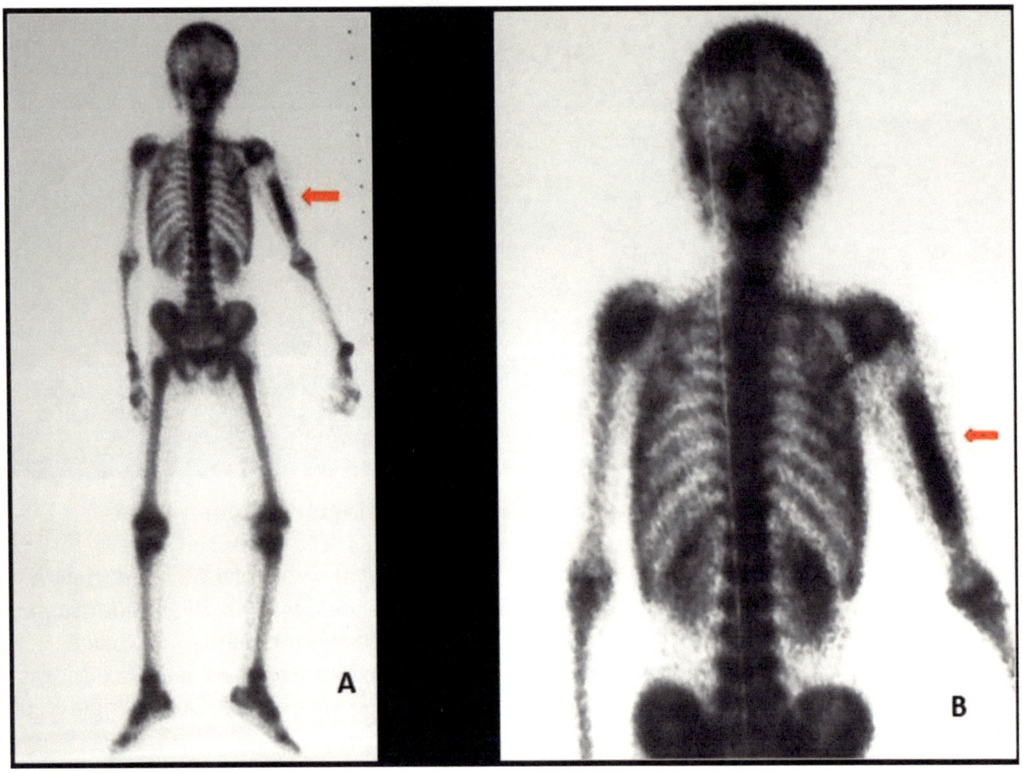

Fig. 29. An MDP bone scan on the same child as in Figure 28 shows a single lesion right humerus (arrow) B is a magnified of A. Note that the metaphysis is relatively photon deficient. Excessive osteoclastic activity may explain the reduced isotope uptake in the upper humerus.

Skip lesions associated with OS are foci of tumor quite distinct and at a distance from the primary tumor represent metastases. Tumor deposits across a joint but on the ipsilateral side are termed transarticular skip metastases. Patients with skip lesions have a more guarded prognosis and are more likely to have distant metastatic disease and shorter periods of disease-free survival.

The extent of extraosseous tumor element and its relationship to the muscle compartment and the neurovascular bundles and adjacent joints is well depicted on STIR and fat-suppressed, T2-weighted or proton density-weighted sequences. The neurovascular bundle is regarded as disease free when an intervening plane of muscle or fat is seen separating the tumor from the neurovascular bundle. When the tissue plane between the tumor and the neurovascular bundle is abolished, disease extension is presumed. Tumor extension to a joint is assumed when tumor tissue is seen within the joint breaching the subarticular bone and cartilage. Tumor infiltration along the cruciate ligaments is regarded diagnostic of tumor extension into the knee joint. MRI is more accurate in identifying tumor growth to the cruciate ligaments than to the intrasynovial joint space.

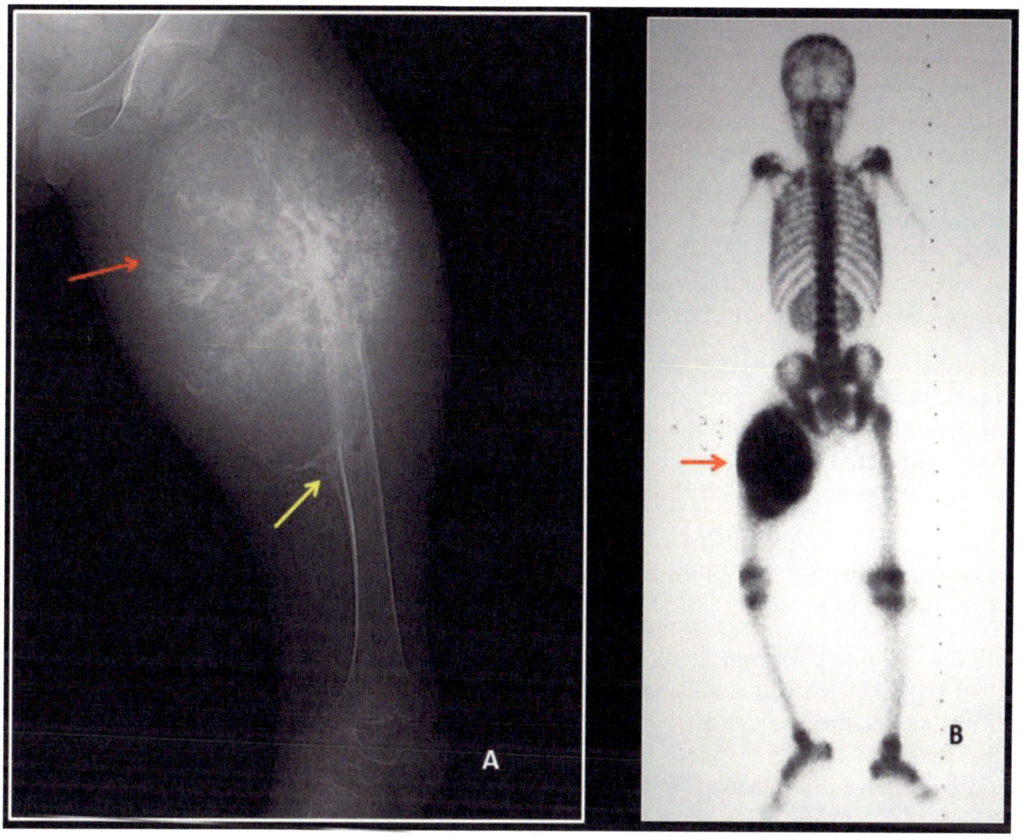

Fig. 30. This 12-year old boy presented with a painful swelling of the left upper thigh. A radiograph of the left, upper femur shows an aggressive bone lesion. There is destruction the femoral metaphysis and upper two third of the shaft of the femur. Note the exuberant periosteal 'sun ray' periosteal reaction (red arrow) and A Codman triangle (yellow arrow). Image B is an MDP scan showing intense activity at the tumor site.

Four patients with progressive pain associated with Paget's disease were evaluated with MRI. Conventional radiographs showed diffuse progressive osteolysis, cortical resorption, insufficiency fractures, bowing, and cortical and trabecular thickening. MRI showed preservation of fatty marrow signal in all phases of Paget's disease except in patients with an acute fracture and sarcoma. Small focal linear or oval areas of low signal were seen against a background of normal marrow signal on short or long TR/TE, which did not resemble a tumor. The findings suggest that unless an acute fracture or tumor is present fatty marrow signal is preserved in advanced Paget's disease [33].

MRI to confirm or exclude a sarcoma evaluated five symptomatic patients with Paget's disease. Two patients whose MRI showed a low signal' abnormality on the T1-weighted sequence corresponding to osteolysis on the radiograph were found to have malignant degeneration. Three patients with preservation of fat signal in areas of osteolysis were not biopsied and ultimately prove benign. In symptomatic patients, with Paget's disease with osteolysis but preserved marrow signal on T1-weighted MRI may be used in the basic decision-making process between conservative follow-up and biopsy [34].

Dynamic gadolinium contrast-enhanced MRI (DCE MRI) has been evaluated in a number of areas in the management of OS. The use of DCE MRI provides useful information as the characteristics of the enhancement pattern differ in viable tumor. DCE MRI has been found useful in high lighting the most appropriate location for a tissue biopsy. DCE MRI is useful in detecting joint involvement. Although MRI is highly sensitive for detecting joint invasion, false-positive diagnoses may lead to over staging of tumor and result in unnecessarily radical surgical procedures [35]. 'High signal' intensity on T2W MRI is not reliable in predicting the Grade of parosteal OS. Contrast enhanced T1-weighted images can be valuable to show the solid component in the heterogeneous areas on T2-weighted images, and can be useful in guiding a biopsy [36].

Gd-enhanced MR imaging could assist in obtaining diagnostic biopsy material of chondroblastic OS by identifying both osteoid and chondroid forming tissues. Geirnaerdt MJ et al found that septonodular and peripheral rim enhancement represented tumor with a pure chondroid matrix, whilst non-enhancing and heterogeneous enhancing areas represented tumor with both chondroid and osteoid matrix [36, 37].

Yakushiji et al found diffusion weighted MRI (DWI) more reliable than DCE MRI in differentiating between chondroblastic osteosarcoma and chondrosarcoma or other types of osteosarcoma [38].

In order to detect differences in MRI between chondroblastic osteosarcomas (CO) and the other types of osteosarcomas or chondrosarcomas (CS) using gadolinium-enhanced versus diffusion-weighted sequences Yakushiji T et al recruited 5 CO, 17 other types of OS and 18 CS. Both CO and CS showed a similar enhancement pattern; both showed septonodular and peripheral rim enhancement. The authors found DWI more useful for differentiating between CO, OS and CS or other types of osteosarcoma than Gd-enhanced MRI [38].

MRI can evaluate treatment response to chemotherapy. Oka et al evaluated the role of Diffusion-weighted MRI in 22 patients with OS, before and after chemotherapy, using the average and minimum apparent diffusion coefficient (ADC). The authors found the minimum ADC a better tool than the average apparent diffusion coefficient ADC for evaluating the chemotherapeutic response of patients with osteosarcoma. Conventional and diffusion-weighted MRI can predict chemotherapeutic response of OS early in the disease course, and it correlates well with necrosis. In addition, newly derived parameter diffusion per unit volume appears to be a sensitive substitute for response evaluation in OS [39, 40].

Gadolinium based contrast has been linked to nephrogenic systemic fibrosis. The use of contrast requires intravenous access and adds extra cost and time to the procedure. Although it may have a role in the staging of OS, its use is not universally accepted and many centers do not currently consider it a standard part of the staging protocol.

5. Computed tomography

CT and MRI are the imaging procedures of choice in locoregional staging as either modality depicts intraosseous and extraosseous spread, skip metastases, growth plate and articular involvement. Thoracic CT is the study of choice in detecting lung metastases [26, 41].

CT is particularly advantageous in clarifying OS is areas with difficult bone structure, such as the maxilla, mandible or pelvis where inconsistent images are seen by conventional radiography. In this setting, CT scans provide a clearer picture of regional anatomy, bone destruction, as well as the extent of soft tissue mass, the nature and extent of parosteal, periosteal, and surface high-grade OS.

CT scanning may render small amounts of mineralized osseous matrix not seen on radiographs and thus alter the differential diagnosis. CT is especially useful, in visualizing flat bones where periosteal changes may be more difficult to recognize.

CT is useful in the evaluation of some OS variants. Telangiectatic osteosarcoma may be confused with an aneurysmal bone cyst especially when associated with fluid/fluid levels. A contrast-enhanced CT scan can be useful in discriminating such a lesion from an aneurysmal bone cyst. Telangiectatic OS is often associated with dense nodular tissue and matrix mineralization at CT in a largely hemorrhagic and/or necrotic osseous lesion with an associated soft-tissue mass, a feature that allows differentiation from aneurysmal bone cyst [42]. The nodular tissue surrounding telangiectatic OS is made up of tumor cells that surround the cystic spaces. This tissue rim shows typically nodular enhancement after the intravenous administration of contrast material.

Periosteal OS and high-grade surface OS may have similar plain film findings. However, histologic and radiological findings are considered together to provide a definitive diagnosis. Prognosis is dictated by tumor size and histologic grade. CT and MRI are more accurate than other imaging for preoperative diagnosis of tumor extent and for assessing tumor relationships to the bone cortex and medullary cavity (Figures 21-26) [43].

A CT guided needle biopsy is a safe and effective technique that is pertinent in the diagnosis and management of musculoskeletal tumours [44, 45].

CT ideally investigates the exclusion of metastatic OS. Lung nodules discovered on CT are biopsied or resected. Solitary nodules represent pseudometastasis in about 25% of cases [46]. Pseudo-metastases should always be confirmed in patients with OS. Some advocate that even if the nodules disappear following chemotherapy, the patient should undergo a thoracotomy. Small foci of residual cancer may occur, and they will most probably reappear in the original CT-positive areas if the patients do not have a thoracotomy and removal of nodules. Calcified/ossified tumors within the lungs have a broad differential diagnosis (see Table 1).

6. Nuclear medicine

OS typically show increased uptake of radioisotope on bone scans obtained by use of technetium-99m (99m Tc) methylene diphosphonate (MDP). The uptake is dependent on the amount of osteoblastic activity within the tumor. The bone uptake is often more than the extent of the tumor due to reactive response surrounding the tumor. The size of the tumor is therefore, difficult to assess on bone scans. Skip lesions and pulmonary metastases may also pick up the radioisotope, but skip lesions are more reliably depicted by MRI. Bone scans are most useful in excluding multifocal disease. The sensitivity of bone scans in the diagnosis of OS is high, but specificity, is low as a multitude of bone lesions show increased isotope uptake including trauma, metabolic bone disease, tumors and infections (Figure 27, 29-30).

Multiple-gated acquisition (MUGA) cardiac scans are often required to monitor the harmful effects of certain chemotherapy, and a baseline line scan is often obtained.

(99m)Tc-MIBI scintigraphy can be used to assess response to chemotherapy in OS. (99m)Tc-MIBI scintigraphy has been compared with (201) Tl scintigraphy, angiography, and conclusions drawn that it could effectively predict the final response to chemotherapy of OS [47].

Increased Tc-99m MDP uptake has been reported in sarcomatous degeneration in a patient with Paget's disease. As expected Tc-99m MDP imaging showed abnormal uptake in both Paget's and the sarcomatous change. However, Tl-201 imaging showed increased uptake in the sarcomatous lesion only. The finding supports the idea that Tl-201 scintigraphy may have a potential role to play in the differentiation of Paget's disease from malignancy [48].

Positron emission tomography (PET) provides physiological understanding of both normal and abnormal body tissues. PET scanning uses a wide range of radiotracers some tissue specific. The most widely used radiotracer is an analogue of glucose specifically F-18 fluoro-2-deoxy-D-glucose (FDG). FDG uptake in body tissues is equivalent to the intensity of glucose metabolism, which increases many folds in malignant tissue. FDG-PET has become the criterion standard in initial staging, monitoring therapeutic response in the management of various cancers. However, the lack of anatomical information has resulted in the complex fusion imaging with CT. Thus, PET-CT not only provides physiological information, but also structural information leading to the diagnosis of sub-centimetre lesions. The detection of smaller lesions has made the procedure useful in the early diagnosis of the disease process and decreasing false-positive lesions [49]. Positron emission tomography imaging is a powerful emerging imaging technique in the management of sarcomas. Its applications include tumor grading, staging, therapy monitoring, and prognostication in both adult and pediatric populations [50]. The degree of tumor necrosis is indicative of progression-free survival, overall survival, and tumor necrosis in OS where (18) F-FDG PET/CT can be used as a prognostic indicator [51]. FDG-PET scanning depicts significant additional information in staging of pediatric sarcoma, which has a relevant impact on treatment planning when compared with other conventional imaging modalities [52]. FDG-PET/CT has a complementary role in the establishment of local recurrence and distant metastases in pediatric sarcomas [53].

The long-term survival with bone sarcomas is closely linked to the response to pre-operative chemotherapy. Response to chemotherapy is assessed in a variety of ways: Clinically, by demonstrating a reduction in pain and swelling of the affected limb. Imaging features of a positive response are a reduction in tumor vascularity and edema on CT or MRI. Conventional radiography is not a reliable indicator of increased vascularity or edema. However, radiologic findings have limitations. The actual size of OS show no change after chemotherapy, and it is difficult to estimate bone response objectively. Therefore, responders can be difficult to distinguish from non-responders by CT or MRI. The histologic response is considered the most reliable prognostic indicator for survival of patients with OS. However, the histologic response can only be obtained after surgery, which might not always be available in inoperable tumors. FDG-PET can be used as a non-invasive surrogate to predict response to chemotherapy in children with bone tumors [54].

7. Ultrasound

Presently there are no advantages of ultrasound over other imaging techniques and ultrasound has not been widely accepted in the diagnosis of OS, but there are certain exceptions where US excels. The US features of bone neoplasia include bone destruction, elevated periosteum and a soft tissue mass. Giant cell tumors, malignant bone tumors, bone cysts, as well as metastatic lesions, have differing sonographic features with one study showing that sonography has equally high accuracy in the diagnosis of these tumors compared with conventional radiography (Figure 28 & 31) [55].

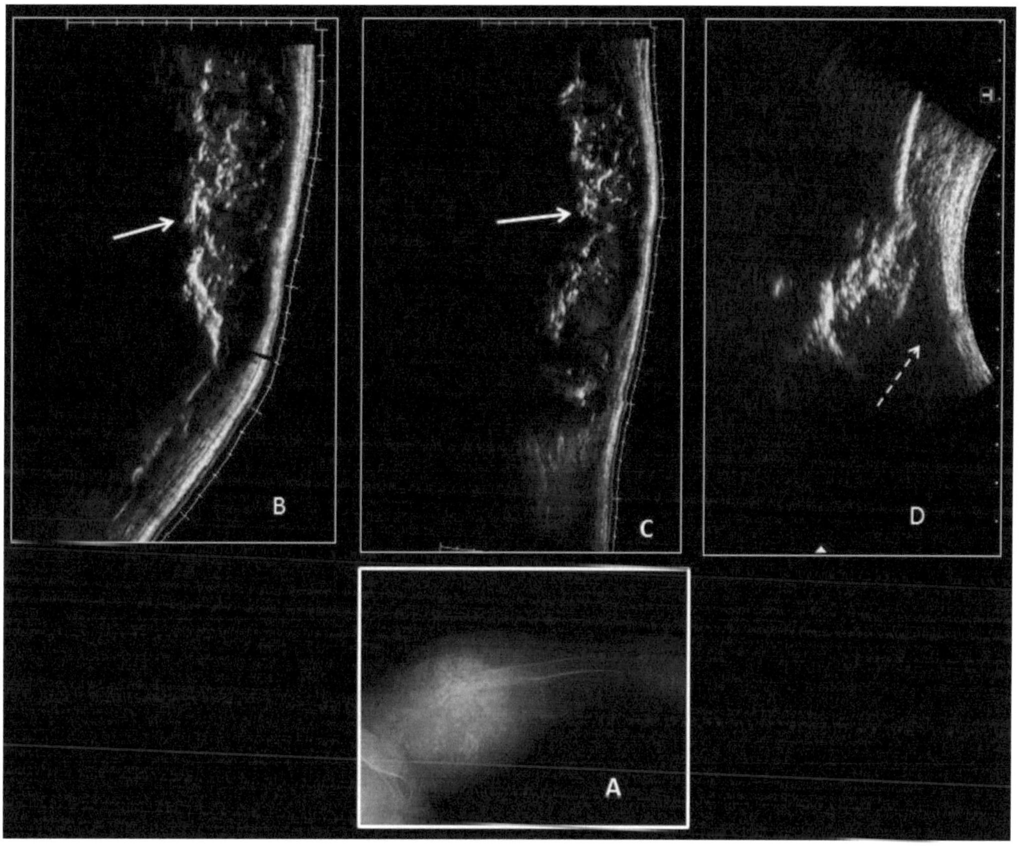

Fig. 31. Ultrasound images of the femur of the same patient as in Figure 33. Note the periosteal reaction (A & B) and a soft tissue window, which can be used for obtaining tissue for biopsy purposes.

Ultrasound features of an OS of the mandible have been described in a young adult. The patient presented with a facial swelling, and an infected lower third molar tooth that was extracted. Subtle signs were missed on dental radiographs. However, an ultrasound examination was crucial in identifying signs of malignancy including a soft tissue mass associated with bone thinning, erosion, expansion, and the "sunray" appearance of the buccal cortex, which were reminiscent of OS. Subsequently other imaging confirmed these findings [56].

Wild et al studied five patients with histologically confirmed OS by US and colour Doppler US. The features included a large soft tissue tumor with echogenic osteosclerotic areas and echo-free caverns within the tumor. Cortical destruction and periosteal elevations were well depicted. Compared to normal tissue there was increased vascularity associated with increased blood flow in colour coded Doppler sonography in the region of the tumor. Sonography and colour coded Doppler sonography are valuable additions of conventional radiology to describe the structure, growth and blood supply of an OS [57].

Lau et al described a parosteal OS that presented 20 years following initial diagnosis, that was treated with wide excision and mega-prosthesis to reconstruct the femur. The tumor recurred in proximity to the femur prosthesis and encased half the femoral stem. Because of a metal prosthesis at the site of recurrence, US was used to detect the lesion. The tumor was eventually treated successfully, with extensive local re-excision. The case emphasise the importance of long-term follow up of parosteal sarcomas and the role of US in the presence of metal prosthesis [58].

Ultrasound is an invaluable skill for guided biopsies. OSs that have broken through the cortex into the soft tissues is receptive to US guided biopsy. Saifuddin and associates have assessed the diagnostic accuracy of US-guided Trucut needle biopsy in patients with suspected primary bone tumors. Of 144 patients, 63 were considered suitable for US-guided biopsy. The results of needle biopsy were compared with those of surgical biopsy. The diagnostic accuracy was 98.4%, with only a single failed biopsy. The authors regard US as a highly reliable method of guidance for percutaneous needle biopsy of bone tumors [59].

US can effectively evaluate the extra-osseous component of malignant and aggressive benign bone tumors arising from bone surfaces. Periosteal reaction, cortical destruction, pathological fractures, matrix mineralization, fluid-fluid levels and involvement of the neurovascular bundle are readily detected. However, ultrasound was found to be of immense help in guiding percutaneous needle biopsy [60].

Ahrar et al took, image guided biopsies on 33 patients with 35 bone lesions suspicious for OS. Of those 35 biopsies, 12 were performed fluoroscopical or with CT guidance. In 23 patients, MRI revealed a soft tissue component; in these cases, biopsies were US guided to target the soft tissue component of the tumor. All 23 US-guided biopsies resulted in positive diagnosis. Two of the 12 fluoroscopy- or CT-guided biopsies (17%) were inconclusive [61].

Soft tissue recurrence of OS may follow limb salvage surgery, and insertion of a metallic endoprosthesis, which is well depicted by US and lends itself to US guided biopsy [62].

Ultrasound has been invaluable in predicting response of OSs to chemotherapy. van der Woude et al have studied the efficacy of sequential color Doppler sonography in predicting histopathologic response to neoadjuant chemotherapy of high-grade bone sarcomas. They concluded that a decreased or unaltered resistive index in the arteries that feed tumors, in addition to continuing, intratumoral flow and high-frequency Doppler shifts after two cycles of chemotherapy suggested a poor histologic response whilst an increased resistive index after two cycles is indicative of significant response [62]. Bramer et al used Color Doppler US in pediatric osteosarcoma and found that it can predict chemotherapy response, but not survival. The method could be useful in planning treatment prior to definitive surgery [63].

High-intensity focused ultrasound has been used in tumor ablation. Chen et al have evaluated US-guided high-intensity focused ultrasound ablation of malignant bone tumors and found it feasible and effective, and have suggested that eventually it may become a part of limb-sparing techniques. Chen et al also concluded that sonographically guided high-intensity focused ultrasound ablation was a safe and practical method of treatment of osteosarcoma which salvages the limb, but large-scale randomized clinical trials are needed for confirmation [64, 65].

8. Radiological intervention to assist tissue diagnosis

Biopsy is always required in a suspected OS as there is a comprehensive clinical and imaging differential more over histology prognosticate the tumor. Orthopedic surgeons choose an open biopsy. However, a large core needle image guided biopsy may suffice. Recently, a fine needle aspirate (FNA) for cytological investigation has been advocated, but there is a margin of error in the interpretation of FNA as under-diagnosis or incorrect diagnosis may occur. The accuracy of FNA in primary malignant bone tumors is 86.9%, and specificity a 100%, and cytological categorization of tumors is possible in the majority of cases. This eliminates the need for bioptic confirmation [66, 67]. Material from FNA may provide additional information from electron microscopy, immunocytochemistry, cytochemistry, DNA-ploidy analysis, chromosomal analysis and molecular genetics [68]. The biopsy tract should be placed where the tract could be excised. Kilpatrick et al reviewed the clinicopathologic features of 145 FNA biopsy specimens from 140 patients without a previous diagnosis of sarcoma. Most FNA specimens are easily recognized as sarcoma, but subtyping is more accurate in bone sarcomas. Histologic subtyping of adult soft tissue sarcomas is often difficult, but this fact by itself has no impact on initial therapy. In contrast, subtyping of pediatric sarcomas by FNA seems most accurate and is essential for proper therapy [69].

Altuntas et al retrospectively studied CT guided core biopsies in a series of 127 patients with musculoskeletal tumors. The accuracy of the CT-guided core needle biopsy was determined by comparing the histology of the biopsy with the final histology of the specimen obtained at open biopsy or surgical resection of the tumor. The effective accuracy was determined, by the accuracy of the biopsy to distinguish between a benign and malignant tumor. The overall accuracy of CT guided core needle biopsy was 80.3%. The effective accuracy as determined by a malignant versus benign lesion was 89%. CT guided core needle biopsy was considered a safe and effective approach to obtain material from musculoskeletal tumors including OS [70].

Histologically differential diagnosis of OS is not immune to erroneous interpretation, as OS may have to be distinguished from a malignant fibrous histiocytoma or a poorly differentiated fibrosarcoma. Rarely an OS may histologically resemble a soft tissue sarcoma or an aneurysmal bone cyst. Therefore, when interpreting histology of bone tumors clinical and radiological correlation is vital [71, 72].

Yang et al retrospectively reviewed data from 508 image-guided needle biopsies of patients with suspected musculoskeletal tumors to determine factors leading to non-diagnostic results. The interpretations of 89% needle biopsies were correct and clinically useful. Nine per cent were non-diagnostic, and 2% were wrong. Bone lesions had a higher non-diagnostic rate than soft tissue lesions (13% vs. 4%). Rare subtypes of OS had higher incorrect rates than other diagnoses. Repeat needle or open biopsies were performed in 14% patients. Bone lesions were more likely than soft tissue lesions to require repeat biopsies. The authors concluded that a high rate of accuracy and clinical usefulness are possible with image-guided needle biopsies of musculoskeletal lesions with an experienced musculoskeletal tumor team with regular communication to correlate clinical, radiographic, and histologic data for each patient [73].

Careful planning of the biopsy site and track must be undertaken to prevent contaminating the soft tissues that the surgeon would not otherwise remove. The biopsy track is usually resected at surgery. If delay is anticipated between biopsy and surgery, the track may be marked with suture, to facilitate eventual safe surgical resection.

9. Angiography

Angiographic findings associated with OSs include neovascularity and hypervascularity, tumor staining, early venous drainage, arterial displacement, and arterial diameter changes. Tumor staining is most familiar with osteolytic OS. These angiographic findings are not specific as similar changes occur in other malignant bone tumors. These angiographic findings are not usually seen with benign tumors with an exception of an occasional arterial displacement. The extra-skeletal part of OS is better depicted by angiography, which is not clearly seen on conventional radiography. Usually, the extra-skeletal part of OS is larger than that in giant cell tumor [74]. During the last three decades, the development of CT and MRI has determined that conventional angiography no longer be routinely performed in the diagnosis of OSs. Conventional angiography, however, is useful as an adjunct to the biopsy of parosteal OS [75]. Occasionaly tumor and vessel relationship may sometimes be better depicted angiography than by CT. Hudson and associates found angiography useful in planning non-ablative resection of bone tumors because they demonstrated the relationships of the tumors to main vessels. Experience with CT indicates that it can accurately describe intra-osseous and soft-tissue extent of bone tumors. If CT does not accurately assess vascular relationships, angiography may still be required. Angiography may sometimes also assist in anticipating operative blood loss, demonstrating variants of vascular anatomy, or organization biopsy [76]. Sellier N and associates studied retrospectively 32 children with malignant bone tumors. All patients underwent conventional arteriography just before surgery. Angiography depicted distal foci of hypervascularity and venous thrombosis, not seen at CT. These findings may vary surgical treatment. Arteriography provides unparalleled characterization of large soft extension of the tumor and remains unchallenged in the assessment of venous involvement [77].

Angiography is an integral part of intra-arterial chemotherapy and embolization before limb salvage surgery in patients with OS of the lower extremity. Zhang HJ et al studied 47 patients that underwent Intra-arterial chemotherapy and embolization 3-7 days preoperatively to evaluate the effectiveness of this procedure on the degree of tumor necrosis and on the amount of blood loss during surgery. Limb salvage was achieved successfully in all cases. The percentage tumor necrosis induced by treatment ranged from 70.2% to 94.2%. The estimated blood loss during surgery, from drains in the postoperative period, and transfusion volumes were significantly lower in the studied patients as compared to the 65 patients who underwent surgery without preoperative intra-arterial chemotherapy and embolization. There is a significant reduction in the mean operative time in the embolized, group when compared to the controls [78]. Angiography has been used to assess response to combined intravenous and intra-arterial neoadjuvant chemotherapy. Cullen JW et al evaluated serial arteriography to evaluate tumor response, predict necrosis, and titrate the duration of combined intravenous and intra-arterial neoadjuvant chemotherapy in patients with histologically proven high-grade OS or malignant fibrohistiocytoma of bone. Serial arteriography was highly sensitive and accurately predicted good responses and individualized and modified, dose-intensified neoadjuvant protocol with an excellent histologic response rate with minimal complications (Figure 32) [79].

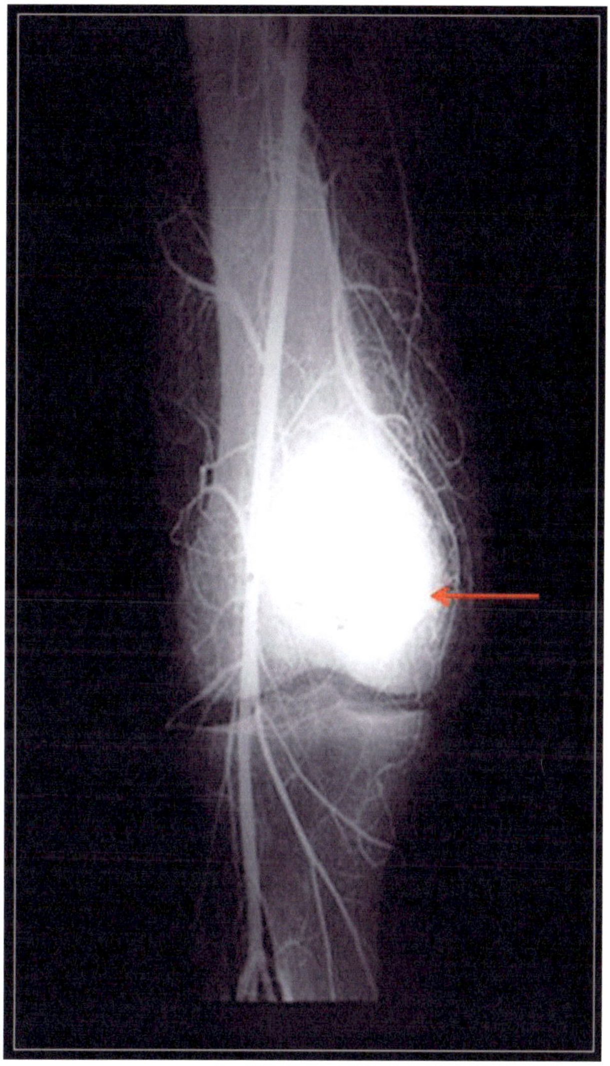

Fig. 32. A peripheral angiogram showing its importance in the management of OS. The angiogram shows intense vascularity in the tumor (arrow). The popliteal artery is displaced medially. These findings are suggestive of OS in the appropriate clinical setting but not specific.

Imaging remains the corner stone of diagnosis, treatment and predicting prognosis in OSs. We have a high diagnostic armamentarium. Each imaging modality has its own indications and limitations. Most OSs are imaged initially by conventional radiographs followed by MRI and a biopsy, which may be image guided. CT, US, radionuclide imaging and angiography have advantages in areas and used if indicated.

Differential Diagnosis Calcified Lung Nodules

Single Large

Pulmonary hamartoma
Calcified granuloma
Primary lung cancer

Carcinoid

Intrathoracic sarcomas

Metastases: Primary sarcomas such as osteogenic, chondrosarcoma, synovial sarcomas, giant cell tumor, malignant mesenchymoma and fibrosarcoma of the breast, papillary and mucinous adenocarcinomas, and occasionally metastases from a medullary carcinoma

Calcifying fibrous pseudotumor

Intralobar pulmonary sequestration

Multiple Large Calcified Nodules

Amyloidosis

Hyalinizing granulomas

Progressive massive fibrosis

Metastatic pulmonary calcifications

Miscellaneous non-neoplastic lung tumors

Many rare non-neoplastic lesions of the lung may mimic lung calcified tumors; these include inflammatory pseudotumor (inflammatory myofibroblastic tumor), placental transmogrification of lung, alveolar microlithiasis and metastatic calcification.

Carney triad

Reference: *Khan AN, Al-Jahdali HH, Allen CM, Irion KL, Al Ghanem S, Koteyar SS. The calcified lung nodule: What does it mean? Ann Thorac Med [serial online] 2010 [cited 2010 Apr 13];5:67-79.*

10. References

[1] Schajowicz F, Sissons HA, Sobin LH. The World Health Organization's histologic classification of bone tumors. A commentary on the second edition. Cancer. 1995;75:1208–1214.

[2] Marcove RC, Mike V, Hajack JV, Levin AG, Hutter RV. Osteogenic sarcoma under the age of twenty-one. A review of one hundred and forty-five operative cases. *J Bone Joint Surg [Am]*. 1970;52:411–23.

[3] McKenna RJ, Schwinn CP, Soonh KY, Higinbotham N. Sarcomata of osteogenic series (osteosarcoma, fibrosarcoma, chondrosarcoma, parosteal osteosarcoma, and sarcomata arising in abnormal bone): an analysis of 552 cases. *J Bone Joint Surg [Am]*. 1966;48–A:1-26.

[4] Murphey MD, Robbin MR, McRae GA, et al. The many faces of osteosarcoma. *Radiographics*. Sep-Oct 1997;17(5):1205-31. [Medline].

[5] Ottaviani G, Jaffe N. The epidemiology of osteosarcoma. Cancer Treat Res. 2009;152:3-13. Review.

[6] Wolden SL, Alektiar KM. Sarcomas across the age spectrum. Semin Radiat Oncol. 2010 Jan;20(1):45-51. Review

[7] Finkel MP, Reilly CA, Jr, Biskis BO. Pathogenesis of radiation and virus-induced bone tumors. Recent Results Cancer Res. 1976:92–103.[PubMed]

[8] Swaney JJ. Familial osteogenic sarcoma. Clin Orthop Relat Res. 1973:64–68. doi: 10.1097/00003086-197311000-00010.[PubMed] [Cross Ref]

[9] McIntyre JF, Smith-Sorensen B, Friend SH, Kassell J, Borresen AL, Yan YX, Russo C, Sato J, Barbier N, Miser J. Germline mutations of the p53 tumor suppressor gene in children with osteosarcoma. J Clin Oncol. 1994;12:925–930.[PubMed]

[10] Wolf RE, Enneking WF. The staging and surgery of musculoskeletal neoplasms. Orthop Clin North Am. 1996;27:473–481.[PubMed]

[11] Mirra JM. Bone Tumors: Clinical, Radiologic and Pathologic Correlations. Philadelphia, Lea & Febiger; 1989. pp. 248–316.

[12] Kim MS, Lee SY, Cho WH, Song WS, Koh JS, Lee JA, Yoo JY, Jung ST, Jeon DG. Relationships between plain-film radiographic patterns and clinicopathologic variables in AJCC stage II osteosarcoma. Skeletal Radiol. 2008 Nov;37(11):997-1001. Epub 2008 Jul 12.

[13] de Santos LA, Edeiken BS.Subtle early osteosarcoma. Skeletal Radiol1985;13(1):44-8.

[14] Rosenberg ZS, Lev S, Schmahmann S, Steiner GC, Beltran J, Present D. Osteosarcoma: subtle, rare, and misleading plain film features. AJR Am J Roentgenol. 1995 Nov;165(5):1209-14.

[15] Campanacci M, Cervellati G.Osteosarcoma: A review of 345 cases. Ital J Orthop Traumatol. 1975 Apr;1(1):5-22.

[16] Bertoni F, Unni KK, McLeod RA, Dahlin DC Osteosarcoma resembling osteoblastoma. Cancer. 1985 Jan 15;55(2):416-26.

[17] Vigorita VJ, Jones JK, Ghelman B, Marcove RC. Intracortical osteosarcoma. Am J Surg Pathol. 1984 Jan;8(1):65-71.

[18] Tsuneyoshi M, Dorfman HD. Epiphyseal osteosarcoma: distinguishing features from clear cell chondrosarcoma, Hum Pathol. 1987 Jun;18(6):644-51

[19] Haworth JM, Watt I, Park WM, Roylance J. Diaphyseal osteosarcoma. Br J Radiol. 1981 Nov;54(647):932-8.

[20] Huvos AG, Sundaresan N, Bretsky SS, Butler A. Osteogenic sarcoma of the skull. A clinicopathologic study of 19 patients.Cancer. 1985 Sep 1;56(5):1214-21.

[21] Giunti A, Laus M. Sarcoma in Paget's disease (11 cases). Ital J Orthop Traumatol. 1979 Dec;5(3):311-20.

[22] Wick MR, Siegal GP, Unni KK, McLeod RA, Greditzer HG 3rd. Sarcomas of bone complicating osteitis deformans (Paget's disease): fifty years' experience. Am J Surg Pathol. 1981 Jan;5(1):47-59.

[23] Greditzer HG 3rd, McLeod RA, Unni KK, Beabout JW. Bone sarcomas in Paget disease. Radiology. 1983 Feb;146(2):327-33.

[24] Torres FX, Kyriakos M.Bone infarct-associated osteosarcoma.Cancer. 1992 Nov 15;70(10):2418-30. Review

[25] Desai P, Perino G, Present D, Steiner GC. Sarcoma in association with bone infarcts. Report of five cases. Arch Pathol Lab Med. 1996 May;120(5):482-9

[26] Spina V, Montanari N, Romagnoli R. Malignant tumors of the osteogenic matrix. Eur J Radiol. 1998 May;27 Suppl 1:S98-109. Review

[27] Panuel M, Gentet JC, Scheiner C, et al. Physeal and epiphyseal extent of primary malignant bone tumors in childhood. Correlation of preoperative MRI and the pathologic examination. *Pediatr Radiol.* 1993;23(6):421-4. [Medline].

[28] Lang P, Honda G, Roberts T. Musculoskeletal neoplasm: perineoplastic edema versus tumor on dynamic postcontrast MR images with spatial mapping of instantaneous enhancement rates. *Radiology.* Dec 1995;197(3):831-9. [Medline].

[29] Iwasawa T, Tanaka Y, Aida N. Microscopic intraosseous extension of osteosarcoma: assessment on dynamic contrast-enhanced MRI. *Skeletal Radiol.* Apr 1997;26(4):214-21. [Medline].

[30] Hoffer FA, Nikanorov AY, Reddick WE. Accuracy of MR imaging for detecting epiphyseal extension of osteosarcoma. *Pediatr Radiol.* May 2000;30(5):289-98. [Medline].

[31] Saifuddin A, Twinn P, Emanuel R. An audit of MRI for bone and soft-tissue tumours performed at referral centres. *Clin Radiol.* Jul 2000;55(7):537-41. [Medline].

[32] Gillespy T 3rd, Manfrini M, Ruggieri P, Spanier SS, Pettersson H, Springfield DS Staging of intraosseous extent of osteosarcoma: correlation of preoperative CT and MR imaging with pathologic macroslides. Radiology. 1988 Jun;167(3):765-7.

[33] Kaufmann GA, Sundaram M, McDonald DJ.Magnetic resonance imaging in symptomatic Paget's disease. Skeletal Radiol. 1991;20(6):413-8.

[34] Sundaram M, Khanna G, El-Khoury GY T1-weighted MR imaging for distinguishing large osteolysis of Paget's disease from sarcomatous degeneration. Skeletal Radiol. 2001 Jul;30(7):378-83. Sundaram

[35] Schima W, Amann G, Stiglbauer R, Windhager R, Kramer J, Nicolakis M, Farres MT, Imhof H. Preoperative staging of osteosarcoma: efficacy of MR imaging in detecting joint involvement. AJR Am J Roentgenol. 1994 Nov;163(5):1171-5.

[36] Dönmez FY, Tüzün U, Başaran C, Tunaci M, Bilgiç B, Acunaş G.MRI findings in parosteal osteosarcoma: correlation with histopathology. Diagn Interv Radiol. 2008 Sep;14(3):142-52.

[37] Geirnaerdt MJ, Bloem JL, van der Woude HJ, Taminiau AH, Nooy MA, Hogendoorn PC. Chondroblastic osteosarcoma: characterisation by gadolinium-enhanced MR imaging correlated with histopathology. Skeletal Radiol. 1998 Mar;27(3):145-53.

[38] Yakushiji T, Oka K, Sato H, Yorimitsu S, Fujimoto T, Yamashita Y, Mizuta H. Characterization of chondroblastic osteosarcoma: gadolinium-enhanced versus diffusion-weighted MR imaging. J Magn Reson Imaging. 2009 Apr;29(4):895-900.

[39] Oka K, Yakushiji T, Sato H, Hirai T, Yamashita Y, Mizuta H. The value of diffusion-weighted imaging for monitoring the chemotherapeutic response of osteosarcoma: a comparison between average apparent diffusion coefficient and minimum apparent diffusion coefficient.Skeletal Radiol. 2010 Feb;39(2):141-6. Epub 2009 Nov 19.

[40] Bajpai J, Gamnagatti S, Kumar R, Sreenivas V, Sharma MC, Khan SA, Rastogi S, Malhotra A, Safaya R, Bakhshi S. Role of MRI in osteosarcoma for evaluation and prediction of chemotherapy response: correlation with histological necrosis. Pediatr Radiol. 2011 Apr;41(4):441-50. Epub 2010 Oct 27.

[41] Picci P. Osteosarcoma (osteogenic sarcoma). Orphanet J Rare Dis. 2007 Jan 23;2:6. Review

[42] Murphey MD, wan Jaovisidha S, Temple HT, Gannon FH, Jelinek JS, Malawer MM.Telangiectatic osteosarcoma: radiologic-pathologic comparison. Radiology. 2003 Nov;229(2):545-53. Epub 2003 Sep 25.

[43] Levine E, De Smet AA, Huntrakoon M. Juxtacortical osteosarcoma: a radiologic and histologic spectrum. Skeletal Radiol. 1985;14(1):38-46.

[44] Altuntas AO, Slavin J, Smith PJ, Schlict SM, Powell GJ, Ngan S, Toner G, Choong PF Accuracy of computed tomography guided core needle biopsy of musculoskeletal tumours. ANZ J Surg. 2005 Apr;75(4):187-91.

[45] Schaller RT Jr, Schaller JF, Buschmann C, Kiviat N. The usefulness of percutaneous fine-needle aspiration biopsy in infants and children. J Pediatr Surg. 1983 Aug;18(4):398-405.

[46] Picci P, Vanel D, Briccoli A, Talle K, Haakenaasen U, Malaguti C, Monti C, Ferrari C, Bacci G, Saeter G, Alvegard TA. Computed tomography of pulmonary metastases from osteosarcoma: the less poor technique. A study of 51 patients with histological correlation. Ann Oncol. 2001;12:1601–1604. doi: 10.1023/A:1013103511633.[PubMed]

[47] Miwa S, Shirai T, Taki J, Sumiya H, Nishida H, Hayashi K, Takeuchi A, Ooi A, Tsuchiya H. Use of (99m)Tc-MIBI scintigraphy in the evaluation of the response to chemotherapy for osteosarcoma: comparison with (201)Tl scintigraphy and angiography. Int J Clin Oncol. 2011 Feb 18. [Epub ahead of print]

[48] Colarinha P, Fonseca AT, Salgado L, Vieira MR. Diagnosis of malignant change in Paget's disease by Tl-201. Clin Nucl Med. 1996 Apr;21(4):299-301.

[49] Kumar R, Chauhan A, Vellimana AK, Chawla M. Role of PET/PET-CT in the management of sarcomas. Expert Rev Anticancer Ther. 2006 Aug;6(8):1241-50.

[50] Benz MR, Tchekmedyian N, Eilber FC, Federman N, Czernin J, Tap WD. Utilization of positron emission tomography in the management of patients with sarcoma. Curr Opin Oncol. 2009 Jul;21(4):345-51.

[51] Costelloe CM, Macapinlac HA, Madewell JE, Fitzgerald NE, Mawlawi OR, Rohren EM, Raymond AK, Lewis VO, Anderson PM, Bassett RL Jr, Harrell RK, Marom EM. 18F-FDG PET/CT as an indicator of progression- free and overall survival in osteosarcoma. J Nucl Med. 2009Mar;50(3):340-7.

[52] Völker T, Denecke T, Steffen I, Misch D, Schönberger S, Plotkin M, Ruf J, Furth C, Stöver B, Hautzel H, Henze G, Amthauer H. Positron emission tomography for staging of pediatric sarcoma patients: results of a prospective multicenter trial. J Clin Oncol. 2007 Dec 1;25(34):5435-41.

[53] Arush MW, Israel O, Postovsky S, Militianu D, Meller I, Zaidman I, Sapir AE, Bar-Shalom R. Positron emission tomography/computed tomography with 18fluoro-deoxyglucose in the detection of local recurrence and distant metastases of pediatric sarcoma. Pediatr Blood Cancer. 2007 Dec;49(7):901-5.

[54] Kim DH, Kim SY, Lee HJ, Song BS, Kim DH, Cho JB, Lim JS, Lee JA. Assessment of Chemotherapy Response Using FDG-PET in Pediatric Bone Tumors: A Single Institution Experience. Cancer Res Treat. 2011 Sep;43(3):170-5. Epub 2011 Sep 30.

[55] Kang B, Du J, Huang J. Sonographic diagnosis of bone tumors. J Tongji Med Univ. 1997;17(2):106-9.

[56] Ng SY, Songra A, Ali N, Carter JL. Ultrasound features of osteosarcoma of the mandible--a first report. Oral Surg Oral Med Oral Pathol Oral Radiol Endod. 2001 Nov; 92(5):582-6.

[57] Wild F, Erhardt J, Beck JD, Deeg KH, Stehr K. Sonographic and Doppler color sonographic findings in osteosarcoma. Klin Padiatr. 1991 May-Jun;203(3):155-7. [Article in German]

[58] Lau TW, Wong JW, Yip DK, Chien EP, Shek TW, Wong LL. Local recurrence of parosteal osteosarcoma adjacent to prosthesis after 20 years: a case report. J Orthop Surg (Hong Kong). 2004 Dec;12(2):263-6.

[59] Saifuddin A, Mitchell R, Burnett SJ, Sandison A, Pringle JA .Ultrasound-guided needle biopsy of primary bone tumours. J Bone Joint Surg Br. 2000 Jan; 82(1):50-4.

[60] Saifuddin A, Burnett SJ, Mitchell R. Pictorial review: ultrasonography of primary bone tumours. Clin Radiol. 1998 Apr; 53(4):239-46.

[61] Ahrar K, Himmerich JU, Herzog CE, Raymond AK, Wallace MJ, Gupta S, Madoff DC, Morello FA Jr, Murthy R, McRae SE, Hicks ME. Percutaneous ultrasound-guided biopsy in the definitive diagnosis of osteosarcoma. J Vasc Interv Radiol. 2004 Nov; 15(11):1329-33.

[62] Garant M, Sarazin L, Cho KH, Chhem RK. Soft-tissue recurrence of osteosarcoma: ultrasound findings. Can Assoc Radiol J. 1995 Aug;46(4):305-7.

[63] van der Woude HJ, Bloem JL, van Oostayen JA, Nooy MA, Taminiau AH, Hermans J, Reynierse M, Hogendoorn PC. Treatment of high-grade bone sarcomas with neoadjuvant chemotherapy: the utility of sequential color Doppler sonography

in predicting histopathologic response. AJR Am J Roentgenol. 1995 Jul;165(1):125-33.

[64] Bramer JA, Gubler FM, Maas M, Bras H, de Kraker J, van der Eijken JW, Schaap GR. Colour Doppler ultrasound predicts chemotherapy response, but not survival in paediatric osteosarcoma. Pediatr Radiol. 2004 Aug;34(8):614-9. Epub 2004 May 18.

[65] Chen W, Zhu H, Zhang L, Li K, Su H, Jin C, Zhou K, Bai J, Wu F, Wang Z.Primary bone malignancy: effective treatment with high-intensity focused ultrasound ablation. Radiology. 2010 Jun;255(3):967-78.

[66] Li C, Wu P, Zhang L, Fan W, Huang J, Zhang F. Osteosarcoma: limb salvaging treatment by ultrasonographically guided high-intensity focused ultrasound. Cancer Biol Ther. 2009 Jun;8(12):1102-8. Epub 2009 Jun 27.

[67] Jayaram G, Gupta M. Fine needle aspiration cytology in the diagnosis of bone tumours. Malays J Pathol. 1994 Dec;16(2):137-44.

[68] Fleshman R, Mayerson J, Wakely PE Jr. Fine-needle aspiration biopsy of high-grade sarcoma: a report of 107 cases. Cancer. 2007 Dec 25;111(6):491-8.

[69] Willén H. Acta Orthop Scand Suppl. 1997 Feb;273:47-53. Fine needle aspiration in the diagnosis of bone tumors.

[70] Kilpatrick SE, Cappellari JO, Bos GD, Gold SH, Ward WG. Is fine-needle aspiration biopsy a practical alternative to open biopsy for the primary diagnosis of sarcoma? Experience with 140 patients. Am J Clin Pathol. 2001 Jan;115(1):59-68

[71] Altuntas AO, Slavin J, Smith PJ, Schlict SM, Powell GJ, Ngan S, Toner G, Choong PF. Accuracy of computed tomography guided core needle biopsy of musculoskeletal tumours. ANZ J Surg. 2005 Apr;75(4):187-91.

[72] Campanacci M. Bone and Soft Tissue Tumors: Clinical Features, Imaging, Pathology and Treatment. 2. Wien, Austria: Springer-Verlag; 1999. pp. 464–491.

[73] Mirra JM. Bone Tumors: Clinical, Radiologic and Pathologic Correlations. Philadelphia, Lea & Febiger; 1989. pp. 248–316.

[74] Yang J, Frassica FJ, Fayad L, Clark DP, Weber KL. Analysis of nondiagnostic results after image-guided needle biopsies of musculoskeletal lesions. Clin Orthop Relat Res. 2010 Nov;468(11):3103-11. Epub 2010 Apr 10.

[75] Hu YG. [Arteriographic findings in bone tumors: experience with 170 cases]. Zhonghua Wai Ke Za Zhi. 1990 Apr;28(4):195-7, 251.[Article in Chinese]

[76] Carrasco CH. Angiography of osteosarcoma. Hematol Oncol Clin North Am. 1995 Jun;9(3):627-32.

[77] Hudson TM, Enneking WF, Hawkins IF Jr.The value of angiography in planning surgical treatment of bone tumors. Radiology. 1981 Feb;138(2):283-92.

[78] Sellier N, Vecchierini A, Kalifa G.[Malignant bone tumors in children. Is there still a role for arteriography?].[Article in French] J Radiol. 1988 Jan;69(1):7-11.

[79] Zhang HJ, Yang JJ, Lu JP, Lai CJ, Sheng J, Li YX, Hao Q, Zhang SM, Gupta S. Use of intra-arterial chemotherapy and embolization before limb salvage surgery for osteosarcoma of the lower extremity. Cardiovasc Intervent Radiol. 2009 Jul;32(4):672-8. Epub 2009 Mar 19.

[80] Cullen JW, Jamroz BA, Stevens SL, Madsen W, Hinshaw I, Wilkins RM, Cullen P, Camozzi AB, Fink K, Peck SD, Kelly CM. The value of serial arteriography in osteosarcoma: delivery of chemotherapy, determination of therapy duration, and prediction of necrosis. J Vasc Interv Radiol. 2005 Aug;16(8):1107-19.

Part 2

Osteosarcoma Treatment

3

Misdiagnosis and Mistreatment for Osteosarcoma: Analysis of Cause and Its Strategy

Yao Yang and Lin Feng
Department of Medical Oncology,
Sixth People's Hospital of Shanghai Jiaotong University, Shanghai
China

1. Introduction

Objective To investigate various kinds of causes and consequences for misdiagnosis and mistreatment of osteosarcoma (OS). **Methods** The data from 94 patients with osteosarcoma undergoing misdiagnosis and mistreatment were collected and their clinical causes and consequences were analyzed retrospectively. **Results** The causes contributing to the misdiagnosis among 94 patients, including that patients delayed to consult physician (36 cases, 38.3%), patients underwent medical misdiagnosis (34 cases, 36.17%) and both of components occurred simultaneously (24 cases, 25.53%). The average duration of misdiagnosis was 72.15 d, 7.34 d and 100.68 d, respectively. 28 cases (29.79%) accepted traditional Chinese medicine therapy, 22 (23.40%) cases were treated by incorrect operation. Perhaps there were 56 patients (59.57%) losting limb-salvage procedure opportunity, 16 patients (17.02%) had recurrence after limb-salvage operation, 40 patients (42.55%) underwent metastasis induced by misdiagnosis and mistreatment. **Conclusion** the main cause of misdiagnosis and mistreatment of OS is that doctors, patients and their parents have deficient professional knowledge of OS. CT and MRI examinations are the effective to prevent the misdiagnosis of early OS. The probability of all kinds of diagnoses should be estimated sufficient, the therapeutic protocol should be made consummately and any other treatment procedures should not be taken blindly for atypical cases before question or biopsy.

Osteosarcoma is the most common bone cancer occurred by teenage, and its onset is more occult, higher malignant, and rapid progress, and even early stage lung metastases may occur. In recent years, the integrated treatment including chemotherapy, limb-salvage and technology-based reconstruction is developed rapidly, which is not only improving the survival of patients, but also the quality of life. However its efficacy, quality of life and survival mainly depend on the treatment of clinical stage. But it is found practically that various kinds of causes and consequences for misdiagnosis and mistreatment of osteosarcoma, which lead some patients to amputate and even metastasis of lung and other organ. Therefore, here are the analysis and treatment strategies for the 94 patients with osteosarcoma undergoing misdiagnosis and mistreatment.

2. Materials and methods

2.1 Case choice

The data from 94 patients with pathological diagnosis, osteosarcoma undergoing misdiagnosis and mistreatment from department of Medical Oncology, Sixth People's Hospital of Shanghai Jiaotong University from Janrary, 2002 to December, 2004 were collected and their clinical causes and consequences were analyzed retrospectively. Among these 94 patients, the youngest is 5 years old, the eldest is 54 years old and the average is 21.48 years old; male is 62 cases and female is 32 cases; primary lesions in the distal femur is 40 cases (42.6%), proximal tibia is 28 cases (29.8%), proximal humerus is 10 cases (10.6%), proximal femur is 6 cases (6.4%) and distal humerus, distal ulna, calcaneus, iliac crest and maxilla is 2 cases respectively, 10 cases totally; according to Enneking & Wolf (1996), stage IIB below is 20 cases (21.3%), stage IIB is 36 cases (38.3%), stage IIB above is 18 cases (19.1) and unknown stage is 20 cases (21.3%).

2.2 Measure of remedial treatment

Most patients had received confirmation of Pathology again in our hospital and meantime accepted MRI for localized lesions, CT for chest, bone scan for whole body, B-mode ultrasound for abdominal and pelvic and serum LDH and AKP check. Chemotherapy before operation was 56 cases, who accepted HD-MTX-CFR,IFO,E-ADM,DDP intravenous chemotherapy 3 times and limb-salvage patients should add E-ADM+DDP intravenous chemotherapy. Chemotherapy after operation was 92 cases (2 case has given up chemotherapy). Among these 90 cases, there were 88 patients operated in our hospital, including 34 cases limb-salvage (40.5%) with 20 cases allograft (23.8%), 4 cases autologous bone graft (4.8%) and 10 cases artificial joint replacement(11.9%), 54 cases amputation (61.1.%) in our hospital and 2 case amputation outside.

3. Result

3.1 Causes of misdiagnosis

Table 1 shows the causes of misdiagnosis for these 94 cases. The factor contribute to misdiagnosis of patients was mainly due to the mild and not typical character of the early clinical symptoms of osteosarcoma. Patients delayed to consult physician because of the

Reasons of misdiagnosis	Cases	Male	Female
Patients	36(28.30)	26(27.66)	10(10.64)
Motion injury	16(17.02)	12(12.77)	4(4.25)
Individual delay	20(21.28)	14(14.89)	6(6.39)
Doctors	34(36.17)	24(25.53)	10(10.64)
Individual delay	18(19.15)	12(12.77)	6(6.38)
Misdiagnosis by X-ray	12(12.77)	10(10.64)	10(2.13)
Misdiagnosis by pathology	4(4.25)	2(2.13)	2(2.13)
Both	24(25.53)	12(12.77)	12(12.77)

Table 1. The analysis of the reasons of misdiagnosis in 47 cases of osteosarcoma [n(%)]

intense of study and work which is 21.28%, and the other reason is about 12.77% because of the misunderstanding of the motion injuries particularly men's. The factor contribute to patients underwent medical misdiagnosis is 36.17% including the misdiagnosis of motion injuries or arthritis particularly men's. The factor contribute to the physicians' delay is 19.15% including the delay of the X-ray examination for patients in time. The misdiagnosis of the X-ray examination is 12.77% for the X-ray examination is lack of the typical X-ray for osteosarcoma at the same time CT and MRI examination haven't been taken. Among these 47 patients, the misdiagnosis contribute to both patients and physicians is 24 cases (25.53%) and the average misdiagnosis time reached to 100.68 d, and significantly higher than the patients or physician individually.

3.2 Consequent analysis and mistreatment

Table 2 analyzed amputation, local recurrence and distant metastasis contribute to misdiagnosis and mistreatment. Among these 94 patients, the ratio of amputation was 56 cases (59.57%) including 44 local amputated cases at a late stage of disease; the ratio of distant metastasis was 40 cases (42.55%) including 30 distant metastasis cases before treatment and 10 cases after operation, and 8 cases reached CR after chemotherapy; the ration of recurrence after operation is 16 cases(17.02%) including 6 re-amputated cases after bone graft and 4 amputated cases because of local recurrence. 28 cases (29.79%) of misdiagnosis treated as massage, TCM herbs cupping and other traditional Chinese medicine treatment. 22 cases (23.40%) took incorrect surgical procedure, and 4 cases (14.25%) took intra-articular infection with antibiotic up to 3 weeks.

Consequences of misdiagnosis or mistreatment	case	misdiagnosis			Mistreatment with misdiagnosis		
		Factor of patient	Factor of doctor	Bilateral factors	Traditional medicine therapy	Incorrect surgery	Others
Amputation	56(59.57)	24(25.53)	20(21.28)	12(12.76)	18(19.15)	12(12.77)	2(2.13)
Distant metastasis	40(42.55)	16(17.02)	14(14.89)	10(10.64)	10(10.64)	4(4.25)	2(2.13)
Recurrence after operation	16(17.02)	8(8.51)	6(6.38)	6(6.38)	0	6(6.38)	0

Table 2. The analysis of consequences of misdiagnosis or mistreatment in 94 cases of osteosarcoma [n (%)]

4. Discussion

Osteosarcoma at the early stage has no typical clinical symptom and the most common symptom is the local pain, redness and/or mild dysfunction similar to injury. As osteosarcoma occurs in younger's metaphysis with joint particularly in lower limb joints. Those male adolescents who like sports and their parents are likely to mistake the osteosarcoma as motion injuries. In addition, most of young patients had heavy burdern of learning and lack of the medical knowledge of this disease was the main cause of misdiagnosis. Our study showed that the misdiagnosis due to the patients is 38.30% especially the misdiagnosis of the male adolescents is 27.06%, and the average misdiagnosis time is 72.15 days. Author thought that it was important to enhance the osteosarcoma knowledge disseminate, and if the pain and red around joints has occurred for one week particular at night whatever with or withour motion and injured history, X-ray should be taken timely in the hospital that has the diagnosis conditions for osteosarcoma. If there is any doubt, CT or MRI examinations should be taken in time.

The misdiagnosis due to the doctors is 36.17%, and the average misdiagnosis day is 57.34 d. Most of the doctors especially the doctors from primary hospitals should pay more attention to the clinical symptom of osteosarcoma. When some patients had the typical clinical symptom as treatment, doctors should not be still subjective to misdiagnose as injury or other benign tumors without any imaging. Reviewing 12 osteosarcoma patients with X-ray as treatment, author found that almost cases were lack of the typical osteosarcoma's features for the most X-ray with only small range of bone destruction or Codman triangle. Daylight occurred rarely and another misdiagnosis of x-ray contributed to poor X-ray rates, poor light conditions, incorrect camera position and perspective and other technical factors in the primary hospital. Analyzing 4 cases of pathological misdiagnosis, the main factor was less needle biopsy material or the material from tumor necrosis zone without tumor cells. In addition to educate the knowledge of osteosarcoma to all level of physicians, the combination among clinic, imaging and pathology should be emphasized. Although X-ray clearly shows the size of the tumor lesions and bone destruction and periosteal reaction, it is short of sensitivity and only up to 30% of bone destruction can be detected. So X-ray examination cannot check osteosarcoma at the early stage. CT and MRI examinations have more resolution than X-ray, and they are the prior methods to exam osteosarcoma. They can show the tumor size, location and the relationship to normal tissue more clearly. Furthermore they provide the most important evidence to osteosarcoma clinical stage, surgical approach[2,3]. Author thought those osteosarcoma suspected in clinic should be checked routine lateral X-ray compared with the healthy side. If necessary, an experienced physician should be asked to observe the focus repeatedly under the lesion site. The suspicious cases should be taken CT or MRI examination and that is the most effective method to prevent misdiagnosis. It is worth mentioned that the biopsy-negative patients who are diagnosed as osteosarcoma probable by clinic and imaging should not be biopsied repeatedly, to avoid artificial compartment open, clinical stage from stage IIA to IIB and cutting tumor cells metastasis. Those cases that are difficult to diagnose should be frozen biopsy before surgery by experienced physicians. Mistreatment is in the premise of misdiagnosis.

The misdiagnosis and mistreatment of osteosarcoma at the early stage commonly occur in China. Misdiagnisis is relative to patients,relatives and doctors and mistreatment is the responsibility of the doctors'. Among 94 cases, 28 patients had massage, TCM herbs cupping and other traditional Chinese medicine treatments before diagnosing osteosarcoma; 18 patients should be operated as local tumor has violated the outdoor and soft tissue; 10 patients had distant metastasis; 22 patients (23.40%) has taken surgery in local as benign tumors or injury; 2 patient has the indications for limb salvage of the proximal humerus osteosarcoma as stage IIB, who has freed the line shoulder surgery; 4 patients has been treated with antibiotics for arthritic.

Overtreatment is another question. Neoadjuvant chemptherapy increased survival in patients without metastasis, however, the patient who benefit from neoadjvant chemotherapy are those had good histopathological response to chemotherapy [1-5]. Therefore, it's important to develop an effective method to evaluate tumor response to chemotherapy, so that we can choose right patient to surgery and avoid overtreatment. Fluorine-18-fluorodeoxyglucose positron emission tomography with computed tomography (PET-CT) is now widely used with promising results in the initial diagnosis, staging, and detection of recurrence in many kinds of cancer [6]. Furthermore, some studies revealed that the change of 18F-FDG uptake after chemotherapy is associated with pathological response, providing a good option to noninvasively monitor effectiveness of treatment[7-18]. We meta-analyzed eleven studies comprising 233 patients. By analyzing two parameters of PET: SUV (standardized uptake value) or TBR (tumor to background ratios), we found that the ratio of TBR after treatment (TBR2) to TBR before treatment (TBR1) (TBR2/1), the SUV after therapy (SUV2) and the ratio of SUV after treatment (SUV2) to SUV before treatment (SUV1)(SUV2/1) have relatively good predicting performance(Table 3, Figure 1a,b,c, unpublished data). Therefore, if we want to make decision that when the patient should undergo surgical treatment after chemotherapy to avoid overtreatment, the PET-CT scan might be the choice.

Studies	N	Positive LR(95% CI)	Q	Negative LR(95% CI)	Q
TBR2:1	57	4.26(2.01-9.04)	0.2	0.11 (0.03-0.36)	0.63
SUV2	138	3.56(1.80-7.0)	1.37	0.56(0.39-0.80	5.72
SUV2:1	233	1.90(1.27-2.85)	15.13	0.47(0.34-0.66)	7.54

Table 3. Likelihood ratios for the association between PET and histological response to chemotherapy (unpublished).

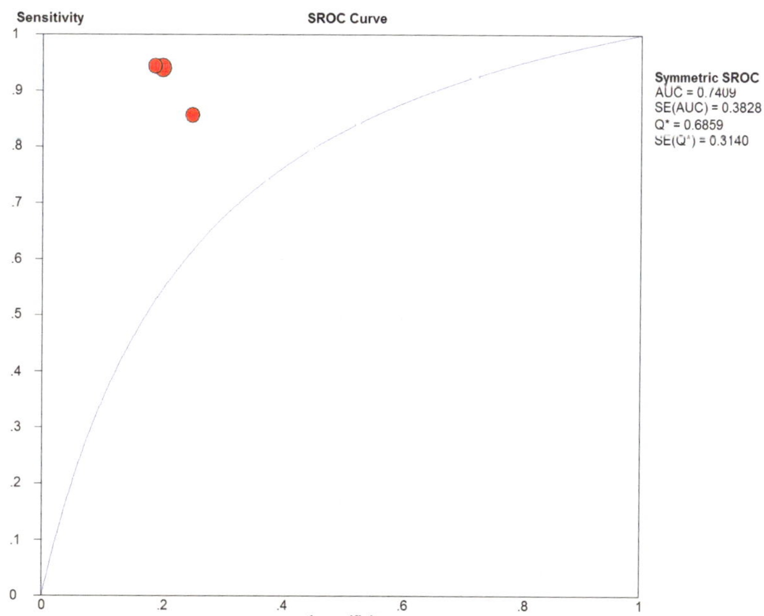

a)

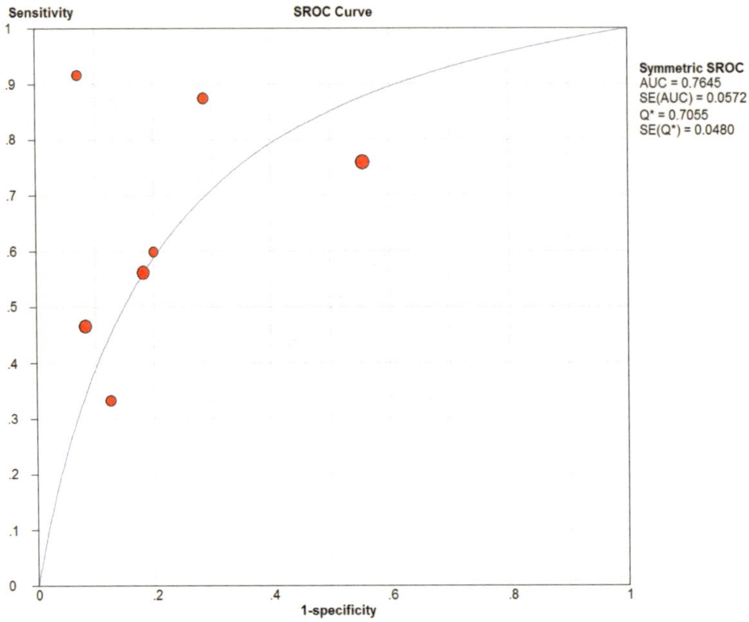

b)

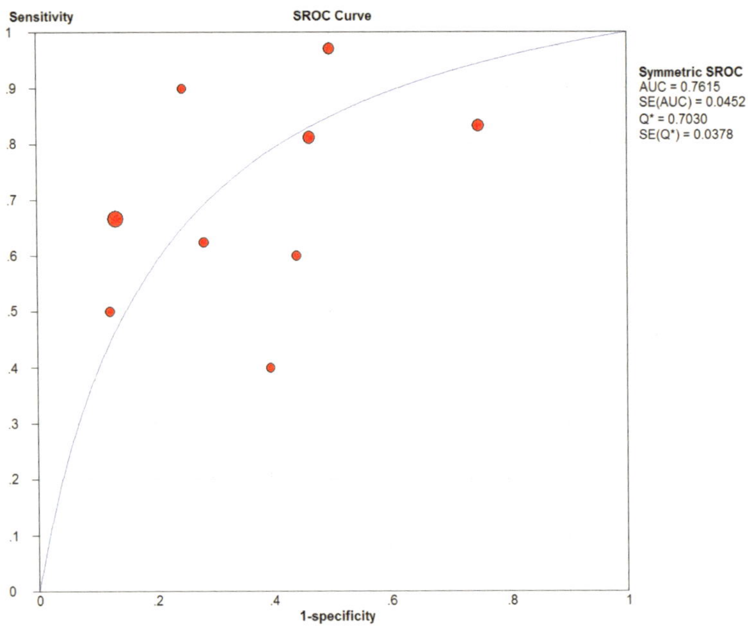

c)

Fig. 1. The summary receiver operating characteristic (SROC) curves for TBR2:1(a), SUV2 (b) and SUV2:1(c) on a per-patient basis. Each solid circle represents each study in the meta-analysis. The size of the circle indicates the study size. The *Q indexes estimate for TBR2:1, SUV2 and SUV2:1 were 0.6859, 0.7055 and 0.7030 respectively. AUC: area under the curve; SE, standard error. (unpublished).

It is analyzed retrospectively that all misdiagnosed patients have the limb-salvage instructions by X-ray film before treatment. Lung was the distant metastasis location for 40 case and almost cases hadn't taken Chest CT as treatment. Data of our study shows mistreatment not only delay the best time of treatment, but also stimulate the growth of tumor cell directly and leading to osteosarcoma cells partial or/and distant metastasis. Reviewing previous data, it is commonly misdiagnosed malignancy as carcinoid or inflammatory disease with Chinese medical treatment or surgical debridement and bone graft, and the main reason of misdiagnosis is the lack of clinical knowledge by physicians. Our study indicates the diagnosis of osteosarcoma should combine clinic, imaging and pathology as practice. For those atypical clinical manifestations or bone destruction of X-ray not clearly for early diagnosis, clinical physicians should read X-ray film carefully and even enhance the relationship with radiated and pathological doctor. Before treatment or surgery, clinical physicians should estimate all kinds of diagnosis and develop comprehensive treatment program , and Chinese medicine treatment can be considered after completely getting rid of bone cancer. If the diagnosis of ostemsarcoma has been clearly, chest CT should be taken to avoid distant metastasis and develop treatment program before surgery. In addition, those patients of extremity osteosarcoma that has the indication for limb salvage as stage IIA, in the premise of preoperative chemotherapy, direct surgery may affect life quality of patients and the long-term survival may not be improved further.

5. References

[1] Picci, P., et al. Relationship of chemotherapy-induced necrosis and surgical margins to local recurrence in osteosarcoma. *Journal of clinical oncology : official journal of the American Society of Clinical Oncology*. 1994; 12:12: 2699-705.

[2] Bielack, S.S., et al. Prognostic factors in high-grade osteosarcoma of the extremities or trunk: an analysis of 1,702 patients treated on neoadjuvant cooperative osteosarcoma study group protocols. *Journal of clinical oncology : official journal of the American Society of Clinical Oncology*. 2002; 20:3: 776-90.

[3] Rosen, G., et al. Primary osteogenic sarcoma of the femur: a model for the use of preoperative chemotherapy in high risk malignant tumors. *Cancer Invest*. 1984; 2:3: 181-92.

[4] Picci, P., et al. Prognostic significance of histopathologic response to chemotherapy in nonmetastatic Ewing's sarcoma of the extremities. *Journal of clinical oncology : official journal of the American Society of Clinical Oncology*. 1993; 11:9: 1763-9.

[5] Rosen, G., et al. Proceedings: Disease-free survival in children with Ewing's sarcoma treated with radiation therapy and adjuvant four-drug sequential chemotherapy. *Cancer*. 1974; 33:2: 384-93.

[6] Quarles van Ufford, H.M., et al. Added value of baseline 18F-FDG uptake in serial 18F-FDG PET for evaluation of response of solid extracerebral tumors to systemic cytotoxic neoadjuvant treatment: a meta-analysis. *Journal of nuclear medicine : official publication, Society of Nuclear Medicine*. 2010; 51:10: 1507-16.

[7] Gaston, L.L., et al. (18)F-FDG PET response to neoadjuvant chemotherapy for Ewing sarcoma and osteosarcoma are different. *Skeletal radiology*. 2011.

[8] Hawkins, D.S., et al. Evaluation of chemotherapy response in pediatric bone sarcomas by [F-18]-fluorodeoxy-D-glucose positron emission tomography. *Cancer*. 2002; 94:12: 3277-84.

[9] Hawkins, D.S., et al. [18F]Fluorodeoxyglucose positron emission tomography predicts outcome for Ewing sarcoma family of tumors. *Journal of clinical oncology : official journal of the American Society of Clinical Oncology*. 2005; 23:34: 8828-34.

[10] Denecke, T., et al. Assessment of histological response of paediatric bone sarcomas using FDG PET in comparison to morphological volume measurement and standardized MRI parameters. *European journal of nuclear medicine and molecular imaging*. 2010; 37:10: 1842-53.

[11] Costelloe, C.M., et al. 18F-FDG PET/CT as an indicator of progression-free and overall survival in osteosarcoma. *Journal of nuclear medicine : official publication, Society of Nuclear Medicine*. 2009; 50:3: 340-7.

[12] Nair, N., et al. Response of Osteosarcoma to Chemotherapy. Evaluation with F-18 FDG-PET Scans. *Clinical positron imaging : official journal of the Institute for Clinical P.E.T.* 2000; 3:2: 79-83.

[13] Franzius, C., et al. Prognostic significance of (18)F-FDG and (99m)Tc-methylene diphosphonate uptake in primary osteosarcoma. *Journal of nuclear medicine : official publication, Society of Nuclear Medicine*. 2002; 43:8: 1012-7.

[14] Schulte, M., et al. Evaluation of neoadjuvant therapy response of osteogenic sarcoma using FDG PET. *Journal of nuclear medicine : official publication, Society of Nuclear Medicine*. 1999; 40:10: 1637-43.

[15] Franzius, C., et al. Evaluation of chemotherapy response in primary bone tumors with F-18 FDG positron emission tomography compared with histologically assessed tumor necrosis. *Clinical nuclear medicine*. 2000; 25:11: 874-81.

[16] Ye, Z., et al. Response of osteogenic sarcoma to neoadjuvant therapy: evaluated by 18F-FDG-PET. *Annals of nuclear medicine*. 2008; 22:6: 475-80.

[17] Iagaru, A., et al. F-18 FDG PET and PET/CT evaluation of response to chemotherapy in bone and soft tissue sarcomas. *Clinical nuclear medicine*. 2008; 33:1: 8-13.

[18] Huang, T.L., et al. Comparison between F-18-FDG positron emission tomography and histology for the assessment of tumor necrosis rates in primary osteosarcoma. *Journal of the Chinese Medical Association : JCMA*. 2006; 69:8: 372-6.

4

Chemotherapy in Osteosarcoma

Kapadia Asha, Almel Sachin and Shaikh Muzammil
P.D. Hinduja National Hospital & Medical Research CentreV.S. Marg, Mahim, Mumbai India

1. Introduction

Osteosarcoma is the most frequent primary solid malignancy of bone. It is defined by the presence of malignant mesenchymal cells which produce osteoid or immature bone[1,2]. The incidence of osteosarcoma in the general population is only 2-3 per million per year. It is much higher in adolescents, where the annual incidence peaks at 8-11 per million at age 15-19 years and the tumor accounts for more than 10% of all solid malignancies. Males are affected approximately 1.4 times more often than females[3,4]. High-grade osteosarcomas have a great propensity to metastasize. Primary as well as metachronous metastases usually involve the lungs or, less frequently, distant bones, while other sites are only rarely affected[1,2,5,6]. At diagnosis, even the most accurate staging procedures detect metastases in only 10-20% of patients, but without adequate treatment, most patients with seemingly localized disease will develop secondary metastases and die within one to two years[1,2,5,6]. With present day multimodality treatment, approximately 50- 70% of patients can hope to achieve long-term survival with an interdisciplinary treatment including surgery and multidrug chemotherapy[7].

Amputation had been the standard method of treatment for most bone sarcomas, but the 1980s witnessed the development of limb-sparing surgery for most malignant bone tumors. Kenneth C. Francis at New York University and Ralph C. Marcove performed the original limb-sparing procedures in the United States[8,9]. Today, limb-sparing surgery is considered safe and routine, but demanding, for approximately 90% to 95% of patients with extremity osteosarcomas. Before routine use of systemic chemotherapy for the therapy of osteosarcoma, fewer than 20% of patients survived more than 5 years. Further, recurrent disease developed in 50% of patients, almost exclusively in the lungs, within 6 months of surgical resection. The findings of two randomized clinical studies completed in the 1980s comparing surgery alone to surgery followed by chemotherapy demonstrated conclusively that the addition of systemic chemotherapy improved survival in patients presenting with localized high-grade osteosarcoma.

Prior to the use of neoadjuvant or adjuvant chemotherapy, 80 to 90 percent of patients with bone sarcomas developed metastases despite achieving local tumor control and died of their disease. It was demonstrated[10] that subclinical metastatic disease was present at the time of diagnosis in the majority of patients and the use of chemotherapy can successfully eradicate these deposits if initiated at a time when disease burden is low. The benefit of adjuvant chemotherapy was demonstrated in two prospective randomized trials conducted in the

1980s in which the addition of postoperative chemotherapy improved survival in patients presenting with localized high-grade osteosarcoma when compared to surgery alone[11,12,13]. Chemotherapy is now considered a standard component of osteosarcoma treatment, both in children and in adults. In addition, up to 35 to 40 percent of those with limited pulmonary metastases may be cured with multimodality therapy. In contrast, long-term survival can be expected in less than 20 percent of all other patients who present with or develop overt metastatic disease.

2. Historical aspect of chemotherapy in osteogenic sarcoma

Neoadjuvant chemotherapy evolved in concert with the use of limb-salvage surgical approaches. At Memorial Sloan-Kettering Cancer Center, customized endoprosthetic devices in limb-salvage procedures often required several months to manufacture. Rather than delaying treatment, investigators began to administer chemotherapy while waiting for the endoprosthesis to be made. This approach led to suggestions that preoperative chemotherapy improved survival of the patients. In addition, orthopedic oncologists developed their own opinions regarding the advantages and disadvantages of presurgical chemotherapy

3. Neoadjuvant versus adjuvant chemotherapy

Chemotherapy is now considered a standard component of osteosarcoma treatment, both in children and in adults. The choice of regimen and optimal timing (i.e., preoperative versus postoperative) are controversial; however, many centers preferentially utilize preoperative chemotherapy, particularly if a limb-sparing procedure is being contemplated for an extremity osteosarcoma.

These observations ultimately led to a randomized clinical study conducted between 1986 and 1993 by the Pediatric Oncology Group (POG trial 8651) that compared immediate surgery and postoperative chemotherapy versus 10 weeks of the same chemotherapy regimen followed by surgery in 100 patients under the age of 30 with nonmetastatic high-grade osteosarcoma[14]. Chemotherapy consisted of alternating courses of HDMTX with leucovorin rescue, cisplatin plus doxorubicin, and bleomycin, cyclophosphamide, and dactinomycin (BCD). The five-year relapse-free survival rates were similar between the two groups (65 versus 61 percent for adjuvant and neoadjuvant therapy, respectively) as was the limb salvage rate (55 and 50 percent for immediate and delayed surgery, respectively).

The study was criticized for the relatively low rate of limb-sparing surgery in both groups (by modern standards) and the inclusion of BCD as a component of the regimen. The contribution of BCD to the therapeutic efficacy of this regimen is unclear, while it can clearly contribute to long-term bleomycin-related pulmonary toxicity

Limb-sparing surgery – Due to its success in killing cancer cells (although actual tumor shrinkage during treatment is not common, particularly with chondroblastic osteosarcomas), neoadjuvant chemotherapy has evolved to a method of increasing the proportion of patients who are suitable candidates for limb-salvage surgery. The majority of limb-sparing surgical procedures for extremity osteosarcomas are now performed at institutions using presurgical chemotherapy. Neoadjuvant chemotherapy is never a substitute for sound surgical principles.

4. Response to neoadjuvant chemotherapy and its implications

Initial chemotherapy response and individualizing postoperative therapy – One of the most compelling rationales for neoadjuvant chemotherapy is its ability to function as an in vivo drug trial to determine the drug sensitivity of an individual tumor and to customize postoperative therapy. Many grading system for assessing the effect of preoperative chemotherapy on the tumor has been developed. (Table 1)[15]

Picci et al	Huvos et al
Total response-No viable tumour	IV-No histological viable tumour
Good response- 90%-99% necrosis	III- Scattered foci of viable tumour
Fair response- 60%-89% necrosis	II-Areas of necrosis with viable tumour
Poor response-<60% necrosis	I-Little or no chemotherapy effect

Table 1.

A consensus has emerged that uses greater than 90% necrosis and less than 90% necrosis as separating good and poor responses, respectively. Furthermore, most current studies use 10 to 12 weeks of preoperative chemotherapy (Fig 1).

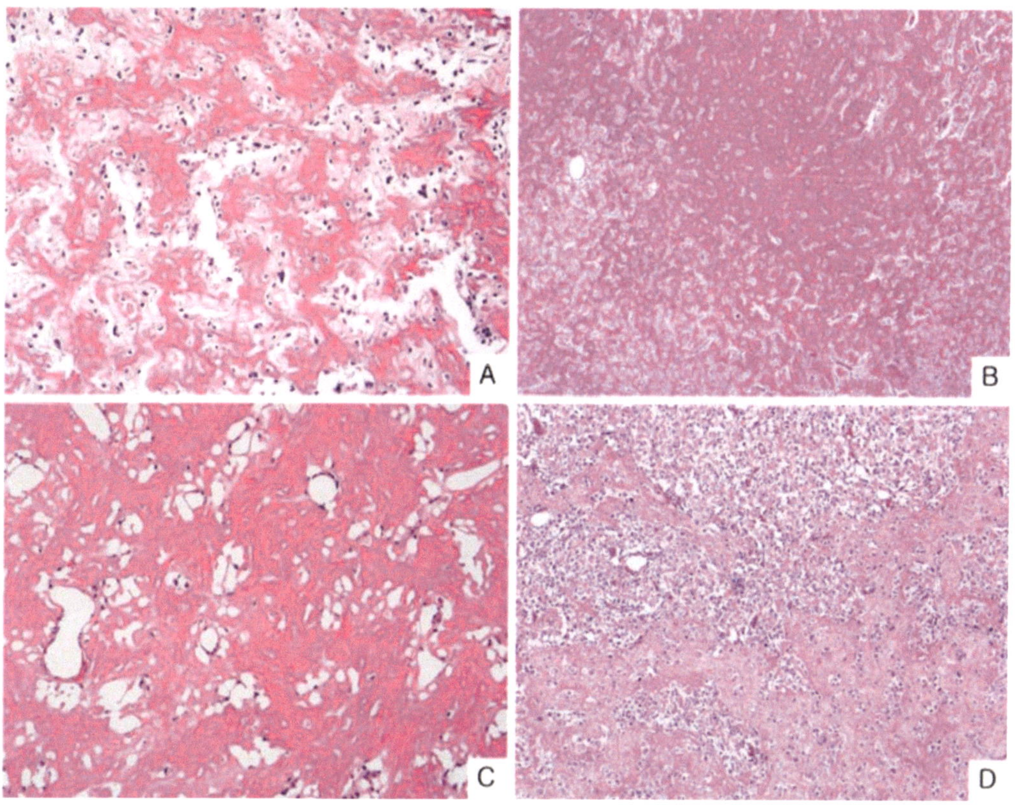

Fig. 1. The preoperative biopsy demonstrates osteoblastic osteosarcoma that contains malignant spindle cells with abundant well-formed osteoid matrix (**A**). The sclerotic sheet-like osteoid matrix with vascular channels is observed after chemotherapy (**B**, **C**), and viable tumor cells are remained among abundant eosinophilic matrix (**D**).

The IOR reviewed data on localized-extremity osteosarcoma in patients less than 40 years of age over the 19-year period from 1983 to 2002[16]. More than 1,000 patient records were analyzed. Fifty-nine percent of all patients had a good response to chemotherapy, and 41% had a poor response. Patients with a good histologic response to chemotherapy had a 5-year survival of 76%, whereas those with a poor response had a 5-year survival rate of 56%.

The COSS database was similarly reviewed and included 1,700 patients entered on study between 1980 and 1998. This analysis included all sites, ages, and presence or absence of metastases[17]. The data look remarkably similar to those of the Italian study, with 55.6% of patients classified as having a good response to therapy and 44.4% having a poor response. The 5-year survival rate was 77.8% for good responders and 55.5% for poor responders. Of further note, all the patients in both of these analyses received HD-MTX, and the majority also received ADM, CDDP, with or without IFOS.

The European Osteosarcoma Intergroup (EOI) analyzed data for two consecutive studies between 1983 and 1986 and 1986 and 1991[18]. A total of 570 patients were analyzed in the report. This analysis is notable for several differences compared to the COSS and IOR analyses. Only 28% of patients had a good histologic response, whereas 72% of patients had a poor histologic response. Patients with a good histologic response had a 5-year survival of 75%, whereas those with a poor response had a 5-year survival of 45%. Of note, many of the patients included in the analysis did not receive HD-MTX because many were treated on a randomized study comparing two drugs, ADM and CDDP, to more intensive therapy including HD-MTX, similar to the COSS and IOR studies [Table 2]. The large randomized study failed to show an advantage of multiagent therapy compared to ADM and CDDP alone[19].

Trials	No of PTS	Good responders	Poor responders	HD-MTX used
COSS	1700	56.6%	44.4%	YES
IOR	1000	59%	41%	YES
EOI	570	28%	72%	NO

Table 2.

A factor that could possibly influence histologic response to therapy and its predictive value on survival is the histologic subtype of the tumor. In both studies, fibroblastic tumors had a higher rate of good histologic response (approximately 80% in the IOR study), whereas chondroblastic tumors had a lower rate of good responders (43% in the IOR study). Perhaps even more important, unlike other histologies, 5-year survival rates were identical for good and for poor responders in chondroblastic histology, at 68%.

5. Modification of chemotherapy based on necrosis

By knowing the histologic response to neoadjuvant therapy an exciting avenue of modifying post operative chemotherapy and hence attempting to improve survival in poor responders has opened. This has been earlier proven in hematolymphoid malignancy. In the early 1980s at Memorial Sloan-Kettering Cancer Center, poor responders had CDDP substituted for HD-MTX in addition to continuing BCD (bleomycin, cyclophosphamide, and dactinomycin) and ADM[20]. Patients who had adjustments in their postoperative chemotherapy based on poor initial response did not have improvement in survival compared to those who had no modifications[21]. Several other reports have also failed to demonstrate an ability to rescue poor responders[22,23]. Although tumor necrosis correlates with outcomes, detection of this feature at such a late stage may not offer the chance to target therapy, and therefore, better methods to identify chemoresistant tumors at diagnosis are needed. Thus, to date, it has not been possible to improve the outcome of poor responders by altering postoperative chemotherapy.

6. Development of chemotherapy regimens

The choice of chemotherapeutic agents has largely been empirical with most groups using ADM, CPL or High dose methotrexate(HD-MTX).

Role of methotrexate – The role of HDMTX has been questioned (particularly in adults). There are no randomized studies that have shown an advantage for higher as compared to intermediate doses of methotrexate[24] or for HDMTX plus doxorubicin and cisplatin versus doxorubicin/cisplatin alone[25]. Furthermore, investigators at St. Jude's Hospital have demonstrated good outcomes (five-year event free and overall survival rates 66 and 75 percent) with a non-methotrexate-containing chemotherapy regimen consisting of carboplatin plus ifosfamide and doxorubicin[26].

On the other hand, a benefit for HDMTX is supported by at least one series that demonstrates a superior outcome with high-dose as compared to intermediate-dose methotrexate in the context of a multiagent chemotherapy regimen. Furthermore, many studies have shown a correlation between peak serum levels of methotrexate, tumor response, and outcome[27-30]. Thus, it is possible that determining a benefit for HDMTX has been compromised by the use of insufficient doses[31] or administration schedules. The role of HDMTX in chemotherapy for osteosarcoma requires further study[32].

Benefit of ifosfamide-based therapy and mifamurtide – The upfront addition of ifosfamide with or without etoposide to HDMTX, doxorubicin, and cisplatin improves initial tumor response rates, but the influence on overall and event-free survival is unclear[33-37]. The benefit of ifosfamide and the liposomal formulation of immune stimulant muramyl tripeptide phosphatidylethanolamine (MTP-PE, mifamurtide, Junovan) were evaluated in a large phase III study involving 677 patients with nonmetastatic osteosarcoma[33]. All patients received doxorubicin, cisplatin, and methotrexate, and were randomized in a 2 x 2 scheme to receive or not receive ifosfamide, and then to receive or not receive liposome encapsulated mifamurtide.

The addition of ifosfamide-based therapy improved the relapse-free survival rate, but only when used in conjunction with the mifamurtide. Thus, the routine addition of ifosfamide to adjuvant chemotherapy for osteosarcoma is not recommended outside of a clinical trial However, the use of mifamurtide improved survival, which led to European regulatory approval of this agent for patients with osteosarcoma[38].

Chemotherapy for adults - In many (but not all series, adults, especially older adults, have a worse prognosis than children with osteosarcoma. This was shown in a population-based series from the Surveillance, Epidemiology, and End Results (SEER) database of the National Cancer Institute[39]. Adults are most often offered doxorubicin plus cisplatin, although the role of HDMTX remains a major unanswered question. For patients under the age of 35, we often employ all three agents, while for older patients, in whom the biology of the tumor may be somewhat different, we generally employ doxorubicin and cisplatin only, given the lack of difference between cisplatin/doxorubicin and the more complex T10-type regimen in the adjuvant setting in one study.

7. Chemotherapy in metastatic disease

Optimal management for patients who present with metastatic osteosarcoma has not been defined by randomized clinical trials, and thus, there is no single standard approach. The most active drugs in patients with measurable disease (HDMTX, doxorubicin, cisplatin, ifosfamide) have single-agent response rates between 20 and 40 percent[40-45]. Response rates are higher with multiagent regimens but a lower proportion of patients treated for metastatic disease show a good histological response to neoadjuvant chemotherapy as compared to those with apparently localized disease This suggests an underlying difference in the biological behavior.

In an effort to improve outcomes, the Pediatric Oncology Group and others have utilized a strategy of applying novel agents to patients with newly diagnosed metastatic disease prior to standard therapy (termed the "therapeutic window" approach)[40,42,46,47]. Using this approach, POG identified the combination of ifosfamide/etoposide as effective induction therapy, particularly for those with metastatic bone disease. Thus, although there is no accepted standard approach for the treatment of newly diagnosed metastatic patients, available data would suggest that such patients should be treated with currently available aggressive multiagent chemotherapy with complete surgical resection of all sites of disease if at all possible.

Nevertheless, few patients with metastatic osteosarcoma are cured, and new therapeutic approaches are needed. For patients who present with overt metastatic disease, participation in experimental trials should be encouraged.

A study evaluating the feasibility of adding trastuzumab to standard chemotherapy for patients whose tumors are HER2 positive was just completed by the Children's Oncology Group (COG)[48]. The results of this study are not yet available.Numerous in vitro and xenograft studies support the concept that bisphosphonates have activity against osteosarcoma alone or in combination with chemotherapy[49].

8. Treatment of recurrent disease

Patients with a disease recurrence after resection alone can often be salvaged with additional surgery and chemotherapy, although their long-term survival is inferior to that of patients who received conventional multiagent chemotherapy in conjunction with surgery upfront[50,51].

Treatment of relapse in patients who have already received adjuvant and/or neoadjuvant chemotherapy is a more difficult situation. Such patients usually have received most of the effective drugs, and presumably their tumors are more chemotherapy-resistant than those that have never been exposed to antineoplastic agents[52].

Salvage is still possible and is more likely in patients with a longer relapse-free interval. In a large database of 565 osteosarcoma patients who relapsed after being treated on one of three different neoadjuvant chemotherapy protocols within the European Osteosarcoma Intergroup, five year survival postrelapse in those whose disease recurred after two years versus within two years of randomization was 35 versus 14 percent, respectively[53]. Other favorable prognostic factors in recurrent osteosarcoma include no more than one or two pulmonary nodules, the presence of unilateral pulmonary involvement, lack of pleural disruption, and achieving a second surgical remission,[50,54-56]. In general, patients should be treated with any of the four most active agents noted earlier if initial therapy did not include one or more of these agents. Patients who have recurrences more than 1 year after completing prior systemic therapy may benefit from reintroduction of at least some of the same drugs in a salvage regimen. The use of high-dose chemotherapy with autologous hematopoietic stem cell rescue has been applied to salvage therapy. However, at least two small pilot studies failed to demonstrate an advantage to standard salvage therapy approaches[57,58].

9. Newer and investigational approaches

A study of the mTOR inhibitor ridaforolimus in patients with metastatic sarcoma suggests potential activity for this class of compounds in patients with osteosarcoma[59], raising the possibility of using these and other kinase-targeted agents in patients with metastatic disease. If activity is confirmed, it is expected that these agents will be studied in the adjuvant setting as well.

Among other interesting agents that may have clinical utility are inhibitors of insulin-like growth factor I receptor (IGF IR), since IGF signaling is critical for bone formation during development. Early studies with a variety of monoclonal antibodies and small molecule inhibitors of the IGF IR are underway.

Immunotherapy – Immune responses may influence the survival of patients with osteosarcoma. Cytotoxic lymphocytes are present in such patients[60,61], and in at least one study, the degree of lymphocytic infiltration correlated with survival[61]. These findings have prompted investigators to explore a variety of immunotherapeutic approaches for patients with advanced osteosarcoma.

The addition of Bacille Calmette-Guerin (BCG) and interferon did not improve survival when added to multiagent chemotherapy[62,63]. However, encouraging preliminary results were obtained using liposomal muramyl tripeptide-phosphatidyl-ethanolamine (mifamurtide), an agent derived from BCG that activates macrophages and increases circulating cytokine levels[64,65]. These data led to a randomized study, described above, in which patients were assigned, using a 2 x 2 factorial design, to standard chemotherapy with or without ifosfamide and then to receive or not receive mifamurtide. The addition of mifamurtide to standard chemotherapy resulted in a statistically significant improvement in overall survival (78 versus 70 percent at six years) and a trend toward improved event-free survival (67 versus 61 percent)

However, when the analysis was restricted to the 91 patients with metastatic disease at diagnosis, there was only a nonstatistically significant trend toward improved five-year event free survival (42 versus 26 percent) and overall survival (53 versus 40 percent) that favored mifamurtide[66]. The drug is not available in the United States. Thus, the role of mifamurtide in patients with metastatic osteosarcoma remains uncertain and a further randomized trial seems warranted.

Another immunotherapeutic approach that is being pursued for pulmonary metastatic disease is inhalation of aerosolized granulocyte macrophage colony-stimulating factor (GM-CSF). GM-CSF stimulates the proliferation and differentiation of hematopoietic progenitor cells and augments the functional activity of neutrophils, monocytes, macrophages, and dendritic cells. Recombinant GM-CSF has been used primarily to enhance neutrophil recovery after chemotherapy.

Preclinical as well as early clinical studies suggest that locally applied GM-CSF may provide antitumor effects[67,68]. These data form the basis for novel therapeutic vaccine approaches using irradiated tumor cells or dendritic cells that are genetically engineered to produce GM-CSF locally and provide the rationale to explore local application of GM-CSF in other diseases.

Local application to the lungs (the most common site of metastatic disease) through inhalation of GM-CSF has been studied. Early data using aerosolized GM-CSF (250 micrograms per dose, twice daily) in a variety of cancers with pulmonary metastases suggest that this approach is safe and possibly effective; in one study, a patient with metastatic Ewing sarcoma had a complete response to therapy[69,70]. In at least one case, upregulation of tumor-specific cytotoxic T lymphocytes has been shown.

Inhaled GM-CSF was evaluated in 43 patients with pulmonary relapse from osteosarcoma in the American Osteosarcoma Study Group [AOST] protocol 0221[71]. Inhaled G-CSF was administered at doses from 250 to 1750 microg twice daily every other week; after four weeks, resection was performed, and G-CSF was resumed for an additional 24 weeks or until progression. Although doses as high as 1750 microg twice daily were feasible with no dose-limiting toxicity, there was no detectable immunostimulatory effect on the pulmonary metastases or suggestion of improved outcomes post relapse (three-year event-free and overall survival rates were 8 and 35 percent, respectively).

10. Intra-arterial chemotherapy

The introduction of neoadjuvant chemotherapy into the multi-modality of treatment of osteosarcoma is the most important advancement in treatment of the disease. However, for the last 10 years, there has been less significant improvement in survival with the use of multiagent neoadjuvant chemotherapy. In these patients, the extent of chemotherapy-induced tumor necrosis is strictly correlated with prognosis. To increase the rate of chemotherapy-induced tumor necrosis, delivery of larger doses of drugs to the primary tumor has been attempted using intraarterial chemotherapy. Of the drugs which are effective in osteosarcoma, cisplatin is considered the most suitable for intraarterial infusion because intraarterial cisplatin is not associated with a significant local reaction and systemic drug levels are not compromised by intraarterial infusion[72,73].

The COSS-86 study was the only prospective controlled study designed to verify whether intraarterial infusion of cisplatin was more effective than intravenous infusion in a multiagent pre-operative chemotherapy setting. In this study, intraarterial or intravenous cisplatin were given with HD-MTX, adriamycin and ifosfamide and the response rate and 10-year event free survival were also identical. The authors themselves suggested that a selection bias may have influenced outcome.

In Bacci et al's study, the doses and the time infusion of cisplatin were the same for patients treated intraarterially and intravenously. When used within a three-drug regimen (HD-MTX, cisplatin, adriamycin), intraarterial cisplatin was significantly more effective on the primary tumor than the intravenous infusion. When cisplatin was delivered within a four-drug regimen (HD-MTX, cisplatin, adriamycin and ifosfamide), which significantly increased the good responses, the advantage of intraarterial cisplatin disappeared[74]. Therefore, it seems that the addition of another active drug to cisplatin and adriamycin concealed the difference. The Instituto Ortopedico Rizzoli (IOR-OS) 2 and 3 studies demonstrated that the rate of histological response was significantly higher in the intraarterial cisplatin regimen than the IV regimen[75]. Apart from histologic necrosis, response evaluation can also be done with pre and post chemotherapy angiograms [Fig. 2].

However there is lack of randomized trials of intraarterial chemotherapy in osteogenic sarcomas to draw any definitive conclusions on this promising modality of treatment. Future endeavors should involve a multi-institutional randomized study comparing this approach with another multiagent intravenous neoadjuvant protocol.

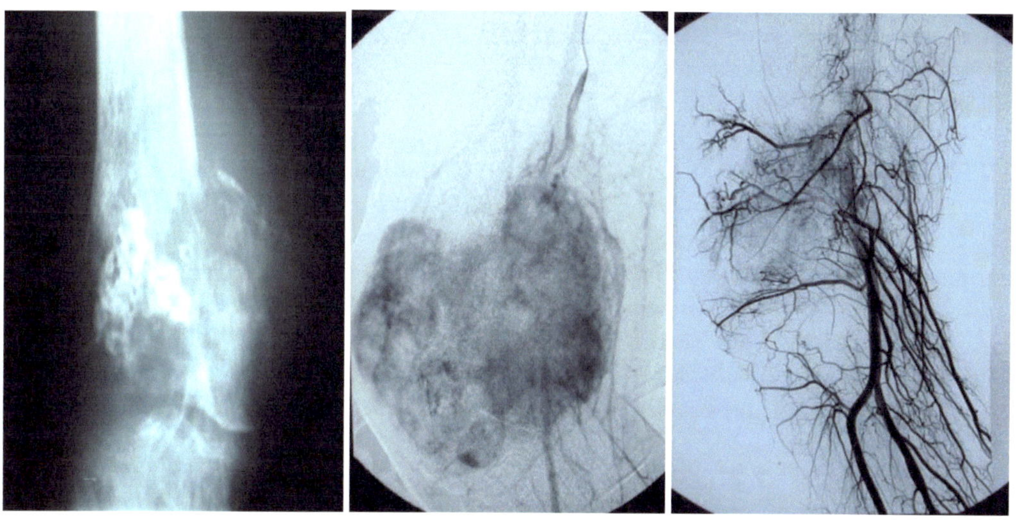

Fig. 2. (A) A radiogram of a man with osteosarcoma of the distal femur.
(B) An arteriogram after the first course of chemotherapy shows viable tumor area with tortuous vessels and intense contrast uptake.
(C) An arteriogram after the fourth course shows a decrease in contrast uptake with little evidence of residual tumor staining. It was estimated that there was > 90% decrease in neovascularity.

11. Conclusion

Chemotherapy in osteogenic sarcoma has remarkable impact evident by the fact that survival has increased from dismal 20% in pre-chemotherapy era to respectable 60% in present era.The impact of chemotherapy in Limb salvage approach is tremendous with limb salvage rates around 90-95% at most referral centres. The optimal regimen and timing (Neoadjuvant vs Adjuvant) of chemotherapy needs to be defined. The strategy of chemotherapy modification based on percentage necrosis after pre-op chemotherapy needs further clarification.

Despite impressive 60% survival in most western centers, the survival data of osteogenic sarcoma is not so encouraging in developing countries. The overall 5- and 10-year survival rates in the Brazilian osteosarcoma study group were lower than the rates reported in North American and European trials. A pattern of advanced disease at diagnosis was often present, with a high proportion of patients having metastases (20.8%) and large tumor size (42.9%)[76].The developing countries have low limb salvage rates secondary to non availability of costly hardware along with few referral centers with expertise to administer high dose Methotrexate. Development of indigenous, low cost and durable implants[77] and less costly effective chemotherapy[78] is needed to optimally treat this disease in developing countries. More patients need to be enrolled in randomized clinical trials testing optimal regimen, timing and low cost implants. Newer molecules in research pipeline provide ray of hope for metastatic and relapsed osteogenic sarcoma.

12. References

[1] Huvos A. *Bone tumors. Diagnosis, treatment, and prognosis.* Philadelphia: W.B.Saunders Company, 1991.

[2] Arndt CA, Crist WM. Common musculoskeletal tumors of childhood and adolescence. *N.Engl.J.Med.* (1999) 341(5): 342-352.

[3] Stiller CA, Craft AW, Corazziari I. Survival of children with bone sarcoma in Europe since 1978: results from the EUROCARE study. *Eur.J.Cancer* (2001) 37(6): 760-766.

[4] Kaatsch P, Spix C Michaelis M. Jahresbericht 1999. Deutsches Kinderkrebsregister. Mainz, Johannes-Gutenberg-Universität Institut für Medizinische Statistik and Information. 2000. Report.

[5] Link MP, Goorin AM, Miser AW et al. The effect of adjuvant chemotherapy on relapse-free survival in patients with osteosarcoma of the extremity. *N.Engl.J.Med.* (1986) 314(25): 1600-1606.

[6] Eilber F, Giuliano A, Eckardt J, Patterson K, Moseley S, Goodnight J. Adjuvant chemotherapy for osteosarcoma: a randomized prospective trial. *J.Clin.Oncol.* (1987) 5(1): 21-26.

[7] Bielack SS, Kempf-Bielack B, Delling G et al. Prognostic factors in high-grade osteosarcoma of the extremities or trunk: an analysis of 1,702 patients treated on neoadjuvant cooperative osteosarcoma study group protocols *J.Clin.Oncol.* (2002) 20(3): 776-790.

[8] Francis K, Worcester JJ. Radical resection for tumors of the shoulder with preservation of a functional extremity. *J Bone Joint Surg Am* 1962;44:1423.

[9] Marcove RC, Miké V, Hajek JV, Levin AG, Hutter RV. Osteogenic sarcoma under the age of twenty-one. A review of one hundred and forty-five operative cases. *J Bone Joint Surg Am* 1970;52(3):411.

[10] Bruland OS, Høifødt H, Saeter G, et al. Hematogenous micrometastases in osteosarcoma patients. Clin Cancer Res 2005; 11:4666.

[11] Eilber F, Giuliano A, Eckardt J, et al. Adjuvant chemotherapy for osteosarcoma: a randomized prospective trial. J Clin Oncol 1987; 5:21.

[12] Link MP, Goorin AM, Miser AW, et al. The effect of adjuvant chemotherapy on relapse-free survival in patients with osteosarcoma of the extremity. N Engl J Med 1986; 314:1600.

[13] Link MP, Goorin AM, Horowitz M, et al. Adjuvant chemotherapy of high-grade osteosarcoma of the extremity. Updated results of the Multi-Institutional Osteosarcoma Study. Clin Orthop Relat Res 1991; :8.

[14] Goorin AM, Schwartzentruber DJ, Devidas M, et al. Presurgical chemotherapy compared with immediate surgery and adjuvant chemotherapy for nonmetastatic osteosarcoma: Pediatric Oncology Group Study POG-8651. J Clin Oncol 2003; 21:1574.

[15] Rosen G, Marcove RC, Huvos AG, et al. Primary osteogenic sarcoma: eight-year experience with adjuvant chemotherapy. J Cancer Res Clin Oncol 1983; 106 Suppl:55.

[16] Bacci G, Bertoni F, Longhi A, et al. Neoadjuvant chemotherapy for high-grade central osteosarcoma of the extremity. Histologic response to preoperative chemotherapy correlates with histologic subtype of the tumor. *Cancer* 2003;97(12):3068.

[17] Bielack SS, Nishida Y, Nakashima H, Shimoyama Y, Nakamura S, Ishiguro N. Prognostic factors in high-grade osteosarcoma of the extremities or trunk: an analysis of 1,702 patients treated on neoadjuvant cooperative osteosarcoma study group protocols. *J Clin Oncol* 2002;20(3):776.

[18] Hauben EI, Weeden S, Pringle J, Van Marck EA, Hogendoorn PC. Does the histological subtype of high-grade central osteosarcoma influence the response to treatment with chemotherapy and does it affect overall survival? A study on 570 patients of two consecutive trials of the European Osteosarcoma Intergroup. *Eur J Cancer* 2002;38(9):1218.

[19] Souhami RL, Craft AW, Van der Eijken JW, et al. Randomised trial of two regimens of chemotherapy in operable osteosarcoma: a study of the European Osteosarcoma Intergroup. *Lancet* 1997;350(9082):911.

[20] Rosen G, Caparros B, Huvos AG, et al. Preoperative chemotherapy for osteogenic sarcoma: selection of postoperative adjuvant chemotherapy based on the response of the primary tumor to preoperative chemotherapy. *Cancer* 1982;49(6):1221.

[21] Meyers PA, Heller G, Healey J, et al. Chemotherapy for nonmetastatic osteogenic sarcoma: the Memorial Sloan-Kettering experience. *J Clin Oncol* 1992;10(1):5.

[22] Winkler K, Beron G, Delling G, et al. Neoadjuvant chemotherapy of osteosarcoma: results of a randomized cooperative trial (COSS-82) with salvage chemotherapy based on histological tumor response. *J Clin Oncol* 1988;6(2):329.

[23] Provisor AJ, Ettinger LJ, Nachman JB, et al. Treatment of nonmetastatic osteosarcoma of the extremity with preoperative and postoperative chemotherapy: a report from the Children's Cancer Group. *J Clin Oncol* 1997;15(1):76.

[24] Krailo M, Ertel I, Makley J, et al. A randomized study comparing high-dose methotrexate with moderate-dose methotrexate as components of adjuvant chemotherapy in childhood nonmetastatic osteosarcoma: a report from the Childrens Cancer Study Group. Med Pediatr Oncol 1987; 15:69.

[25] Bramwell VH, Burgers M, Sneath R, et al. A comparison of two short intensive adjuvant chemotherapy regimens in operable osteosarcoma of limbs in children and young adults: the first study of the European Osteosarcoma Intergroup. J Clin Oncol 1992; 10:1579.

[26] Daw NC, Neel MD, Rao BN, et al. Frontline treatment of localized osteosarcoma without methotrexate: results of the St. Jude Children's Research Hospital OS99 trial. Cancer 2011; 117:2770.

[27] Saeter G, Alvegård TA, Elomaa I, et al. Treatment of osteosarcoma of the extremities with the T-10 protocol, with emphasis on the effects of preoperative chemotherapy with single-agent high-dose methotrexate: a Scandinavian Sarcoma Group study. J Clin Oncol 1991; 9:1766.

[28] Bacci G, Ferrari S, Delepine N, et al. Predictive factors of histologic response to primary chemotherapy in osteosarcoma of the extremity: study of 272 patients preoperatively treated with high-dose methotrexate, doxorubicin, and cisplatin. J Clin Oncol 1998; 16:658.

[29] Delepine N, Delepine G, Jasmin C, et al. Importance of age and methotrexate dosage: prognosis in children and young adults with high-grade osteosarcomas. Biomed Pharmacother 1988; 42:257.

[30] Graf N, Winkler K, Betlemovic M, et al. Methotrexate pharmacokinetics and prognosis in osteosarcoma. J Clin Oncol 1994; 12:1443.

[31] Zelcer S, Kellick M, Wexler LH, et al. Methotrexate levels and outcome in osteosarcoma. Pediatr Blood Cancer 2005; 44:638.

[32] van Dalen EC, de Camargo B. Methotrexate for high-grade osteosarcoma in children and young adults. Cochrane Database Syst Rev 2009; :CD006325.

[33] Meyers PA, Schwartz CL, Krailo MD, et al. Osteosarcoma: the addition of muramyl tripeptide to chemotherapy improves overall survival--a report from the Children's Oncology Group. J Clin Oncol 2008; 26:633.

[34] Patel SJ, Lynch JW Jr, Johnson T, et al. Dose-intense ifosfamide/doxorubicin/ cisplatin based chemotherapy for osteosarcoma in adults. Am J Clin Oncol 2002; 25:489.

[35] Bacci G, Briccoli A, Ferrari S, et al. Neoadjuvant chemotherapy for osteosarcoma of the extremity: long-term results of the Rizzoli's 4th protocol. Eur J Cancer 2001; 37:2030.

[36] Zalupski MM, Rankin C, Ryan JR, et al. Adjuvant therapy of osteosarcoma--A Phase II trial: Southwest Oncology Group study 9139. Cancer 2004; 100:818.
[37] Ferrari S, Smeland S, Mercuri M, et al. Neoadjuvant chemotherapy with high-dose Ifosfamide, high-dose methotrexate, cisplatin, and doxorubicin for patients with localized osteosarcoma of the extremity: a joint study by the Italian and Scandinavian Sarcoma Groups. J Clin Oncol 2005; 23:8845.
[38] Bielack, S, Carrle, D, Casali, PG. Osteosarcoma: ESMO Clinical Recommendations for diagnosis, treatment and follow-up. Ann Oncol 2009; 20:iv137.
[39] Mirabello L, Troisi RJ, Savage SA. Osteosarcoma incidence and survival rates from 1973 to 2004: data from the Surveillance, Epidemiology, and End Results Program. Cancer 2009; 115:1531.
[40] Ferguson WS, Harris MB, Goorin AM, et al. Presurgical window of carboplatin and surgery and multidrug chemotherapy for the treatment of newly diagnosed metastatic or unresectable osteosarcoma: Pediatric Oncology Group Trial. J Pediatr Hematol Oncol 2001; 23:340.
[41] Meyers PA, Heller G, Healey JH, et al. Osteogenic sarcoma with clinically detectable metastasis at initial presentation. J Clin Oncol 1993; 11:449.
[42] Harris MB, Gieser P, Goorin AM, et al. Treatment of metastatic osteosarcoma at diagnosis: a Pediatric Oncology Group Study. J Clin Oncol 1998; 16:3641
[43] Benjamin RS, Baker LH, O'Bryan RM, et al. Chemotherapy for metastic osteosarcoma--studies by the M.D. Anderson Hospital and the Southwest Oncology Group. Cancer Treat Rep 1978; 62:237.
[44] Edmonson JH, Creagan ET, Gilchrist GS. Phase II study of high-dose methotrexate in patients with unresectable metastatic osteosarcoma. Cancer Treat Rep 1981; 65:538.
[45] Baum ES, Gaynon P, Greenberg L, et al. Phase II study of cis-dichlorodiammineplatinum(II) in childhood osteosarcoma: Children's Cancer Study Group Report. Cancer Treat Rep 1979; 63:1621
[46] Goorin AM, Harris MB, Bernstein M, et al. Phase II/III trial of etoposide and high-dose ifosfamide in newly diagnosed metastatic osteosarcoma: a pediatric oncology group trial. J Clin Oncol 2002; 20:426.
[47] Harris MB, Cantor AB, Goorin AM, et al. Treatment of osteosarcoma with ifosfamide: comparison of response in pediatric patients with recurrent disease versus patients previously untreated: a Pediatric Oncology Group study. Med Pediatr Oncol 1995; 24:87.
[48] Website for children's cancer trials www.curesearch.org/our_research/clinical_trials.
[49] Meyers PA, Healey JH, Chou AJ, et al. Addition of pamidronate to chemotherapy for the treatment of osteosarcoma. Cancer 2011; 117:1736.
[50] Hawkins DS, Arndt CA. Pattern of disease recurrence and prognostic factors in patients with osteosarcoma treated with contemporary chemotherapy. Cancer 2003; 98:2447.
[51] Bacci G, Forni C, Longhi A, et al. Local recurrence and local control of non-metastatic osteosarcoma of the extremities: a 27-year experience in a single institution. J Surg Oncol 2007; 96:118.

[52] Goorin AM, Shuster JJ, Baker A, et al. Changing pattern of pulmonary metastases with adjuvant chemotherapy in patients with osteosarcoma: results from the multiinstitutional osteosarcoma study. J Clin Oncol 1991; 9:600.

[53] Gelderblom H, Jinks RC, Sydes M, et al. Survival after recurrent osteosarcoma: data from 3 European Osteosarcoma Intergroup (EOI) randomized controlled trials. Eur J Cancer 2011; 47:895.

[54] Kempf-Bielack B, Bielack SS, Jürgens H, et al. Osteosarcoma relapse after combined modality therapy: an analysis of unselected patients in the Cooperative Osteosarcoma Study Group (COSS). J Clin Oncol 2005; 23:559.

[55] Ferrari S, Briccoli A, Mercuri M, et al. Postrelapse survival in osteosarcoma of the extremities: prognostic factors for long-term survival. J Clin Oncol 2003; 21:710.

[56] Chou AJ, Merola PR, Wexler LH, et al. Treatment of osteosarcoma at first recurrence after contemporary therapy: the Memorial Sloan-Kettering Cancer Center experience. Cancer 2005; 104:2214.

[57] Sauerbrey A, Bielack S, Kempf-Bielack B, Zoubek A, Paulussen M, Zintl F. High-dose chemotherapy (HDC) and autologous hematopoietic stem cell transplantation (ASCT) as salvage therapy for relapsed osteosarcoma. *Bone Marrow Transplant* 2001;27(9):933.

[58] Fagioli F, Aglietta M, Tienghi A, et al. High-dose chemotherapy in the treatment of relapsed osteosarcoma: an Italian sarcoma group study. *J Clin Oncol* 2002;20(8):2150.

[59] Chawla SP, Sankhala KK, Chua V, et al. A phase II study of AP23573 (an mTOR inhibitor) in patients (pts) with advanced sarcomas (abstract). J Clin Oncol 2005; 24: 833.

[60] Trieb K, Lechleitner T, Lang S, et al. Evaluation of HLA-DR expression and T-lymphocyte infiltration in osteosarcoma. Pathol Res Pract 1998; 194:679.

[61] Goorin AM, Perez-Atayde A, Gebhardt M, et al. Weekly high-dose methotrexate and doxorubicin for osteosarcoma: the Dana-Farber Cancer Institute/the Children's Hospital--study III. J Clin Oncol 1987; 5:1178.

[62] Winkler K, Beron G, Kotz R, et al. Adjuvant chemotherapy in osteosarcoma - effects of cisplatinum, BCD, and fibroblast interferon in sequential combination with HD-MTX and adriamycin. Preliminary results of the COSS 80 study. J Cancer Res Clin Oncol 1983; 106 Suppl:1

[63] Rosenburg SA, Chabner BA, Young RC, et al. Treatment of osteogenic sarcoma. I. Effect of adjuvant high-dose methotrexate after amputation. Cancer Treat Rep 1979; 63:739.

[64] Kleinerman ES, Jia SF, Griffin J, et al. Phase II study of liposomal muramyl tripeptide in osteosarcoma: the cytokine cascade and monocyte activation following administration. J Clin Oncol 1992; 10:1310.

[65] Kleinerman ES, Gano JB, Johnston DA, et al. Efficacy of liposomal muramyl tripeptide (CGP 19835A) in the treatment of relapsed osteosarcoma. Am J Clin Oncol 1995; 18:93.

[66] Chou AJ, Kleinerman ES, Krailo MD, et al. Addition of muramyl tripeptide to chemotherapy for patients with newly diagnosed metastatic osteosarcoma: a report from the Children's Oncology Group. Cancer 2009; 115:5339.

[67] Dranoff G, Jaffee E, Lazenby A, et al. Vaccination with irradiated tumor cells engineered to secrete murine granulocyte-macrophage colony-stimulating factor stimulates potent, specific, and long-lasting anti-tumor immunity. Proc Natl Acad Sci U S A 1993; 90:3539.

[68] Kumar R, Yoneda J, Fidler IJ, Dong Z. GM-CSF-transduced B16 melanoma cells are highly susceptible to lysis by normal murine macrophages and poorly tumorigenic in immune-compromised mice. J Leukoc Biol 1999; 65:102.

[69] Rao RD, Anderson PM, Arndt CA, et al. Aerosolized granulocyte macrophage colony-stimulating factor (GM-CSF) therapy in metastatic cancer. Am J Clin Oncol 2003; 26:493.

[70] Anderson PM, Markovic SN, Sloan JA, et al. Aerosol granulocyte macrophage-colony stimulating factor: a low toxicity, lung-specific biological therapy in patients with lung metastases. Clin Cancer Res 1999; 5:2316.

[71] Arndt CA, Koshkina NV, Inwards CY, et al. Inhaled granulocyte-macrophage colony stimulating factor for first pulmonary recurrence of osteosarcoma: effects on disease-free survival and immunomodulation. a report from the Children's Oncology Group. Clin Cancer Res 2010; 16:4024.

[72] Steward DJ, Benjamin RS, Zimerman S, Caprioli RM, Wallace S, Chuang V, Calvo D 3rd, Samuels M, Bonura J, Loo TL. Clinical pharmacology of intraarterial cisdiammine dichloroplatinum (II). Cancer Res 1983;43:917-20.

[73] Bielack S, Ertman R, Looft G, Purfürst C, Delling G, Winkler K, Landbeck G. Platinum disposition afterintraarterial and intravenous infusion of cisplatinum for osteosarcoma. Cancer Chemother Pharmacol 1988;24:376-80.

[74] Bacci G, Ferrari S, Tienghi A, Bertoni F, Mercuri M, Longhi A, Fiorentini G, Forni C, Bacchini P, Rimondini S, De Giorgi U, Picci P. A comparison of methods of loco-regional chemotherapy combined with systemic chemotherapy as neoadjuvant treatment of osteosarcoma of the extremity. Eur J Surg Oncol 2001;27:98-104.

[75] Ferrari S, Mercuri M, Picci P, Bertoni F, Brach del Prever A, Tienghi A, Mancini A, Longhi A, Rimondini S, Donati D, Manfrini M, Ruggieri P, Biagini R, Bacci G. Nonmetastatic osteosarcoma of the extremity: results of a neoadjuvant chemotherapy protocol (IOR/OS-3) with high-dose methotrexate, intraarterial or intravenous cisplatin, doxorubicin and salvage chemotherapy based on histologic tumor response. Tumori 1999;85:458-64.

[76] Results of the Brazilian Osteosarcoma Treatment Group Studies III and IV: Prognostic Factors and Impact on Survival. *Sérgio Petrilli, Beatriz de Camargo, Vicente Odone Filho,JCO* VOLUME 24 _ NUMBER 7 _ MARCH 1 2006,pg 1161-1168.

[77] Limb salvage surgery for osteosarcoma: effective low-cost treatment. Agarwal M, Anchan C, Shah M, Puri A, Pai S. Source Department of Surgery, Tata Memorial Hospital, Mumbai, India.PMID:17417098 [PubMed - indexed for MEDLINE].

[78] Non-methotrexate based triple drug combination chemotherapy for untreated osteosarcoma. S. S. Hingmire, S. K. Pai, A. V. Bakshi, R. Bharath, M. Agarwal, A. Puri, U. Dangi, S. Mandhaniya, T. Maksud and P. M. Parikh. Journal of Clinical Oncology, 2007 ASCO Annual Meeting Proceedings (Post-Meeting Edition). Vol 25, No 18S (June 20 Supplement), 2007: 20512.

5

Limb Salvage for Osteosarcoma: Current Status with a Review of Literature

Manish G. Agarwal* and Prakash Nayak
Department of Orthopaedics
P.D Hinduja National Hospital & Medical Research Centre
India

1. Introduction

Osteosarcoma is the most common primary bone tumor. These tumors have long been known to be very aggressive in their natural history and therefore for a very long time amputation was considered to be the only way to achieve local control of the tumor in the limb. Even after an amputation, only 10-20%survived[1,2], the rest succumbing to systemic disease[3,4].

In the last 30 years a sea of change has occurred in the outlook for these cancers. Chemotherapy has allowed better local and systemic control[5, 6]. Better imaging with CT and MRI has allowed the surgeon to accurately define the extent and therefore plan tumor resection. Advances in bioengineering have provided exciting options for reconstruction and the world has moved from amputation to limb salvage. In osteosarcoma, survival improved from dismal 10-20% to 50-70%[7, 8]. Long term studies showed that limb salvage operations, performed with wide margins and chemotherapy did not compromise the survival or local control compared to an amputation[9-14].

Cheaper and yet effective chemotherapy protocols and low cost indigenously manufactured megaprosthesis have allowed limb salvage surgery to develop even in the poorer countries. Good surgical technique has improved functional results and made limb salvage today, the standard of care for osteosarcoma.

2. Evaluation

The patient is first assessed clinically and a mental impression formed whether the limb is salvageable, borderline or non salvageable. All patients undergo an imaging workup for local extent and distant spread. This is done prior to a biopsy. An MRI of the local area helps further define the extent and relationships to vital structures like the neurovascular bundle. The MRI helps us plan the margins of resection. The commonest site of distant metastases is the chest. An xray of the chest and where limb salvage is considered a CT scan of the chest (if the x-ray is clear) helps to screen for pulmonary metastases. A bone scan is used to screen for skip lesions and osseous metastases. A PET-CT scan is now being increasingly used for staging instead of

* Corresponding Author

CT chest and bone scan. Presence of distant metastases decreases cure rates but with effective treatment when the metastases are resectable, cure rates of 20-40% have been reported.

3. Biopsy

Irrespective of how typical the imaging appearance, a histopathological diagnosis is a vital step in the diagnostic work up of bone tumors. Fine needle aspiration provides only cytologic material and is not the preferred method for diagnosis of primary bone tumors like osteosarcoma[15]. For bone tumors, the cellular architecture as well as the quality of matrix has to be studied for a proper diagnosis which FNAC cannot provide. A tissue sample may be obtained either by an open incisional biopsy or a closed core biopsy. Traditionally an open biopsy has been used. Various complications related to open biopsy like incorrect placement of incision, large scale contamination of tissues, infection and pathological fracture have often forced an amputation when otherwise a limb salvage was feasible. This happens more frequently when the open biopsy procedure is performed by individuals not experienced in managing tumors. A badly done biopsy can negatively impact overall survival[16-21]. We therefore recommend that open biopsy should only be performed in specialized units by surgeons experienced in managing tumors.

Percutaneous core biopsy of bone lesions provides early and definitive diagnosis. The biopsy site chosen should be such that the tract can be excised en bloc with the tumour. The periphery of the tumour is the best site and the pre biopsy MRI may help in localizing the most representative area. Necrotic or heavily calcified or ossified areas are avoided. A soft tissue mass is adequately representative for a biopsy. Where necessary an imaging C-arm or CT guidance is used.

4. Patient education

The patient and the patient's family participate in the decision making process. They are counseled in detail especially when limb salvage is considered regarding the costs, change in lifestyle and mobility and risks involved. The possibility of an amputation and other complications is explained. Amputation as an alternative is also offered in an unbiased way and the patient is encouraged to make his own decision. An attempt is made to facilitate a meeting between the prospective limb salvage candidate and a patient who has already undergone the procedure. Photographs and videos are also shown to the patients and their families.

When the patient and the family are fully informed and participate in the choice of treatment, they are much more likely to be satisfied with the ultimate outcome, even if complications and problems arise at a later stage. It is important to stress to patient and their family that limb salvage may require additional procedures either in near or distant future to manage some of the complications.

5. Indications for limb salvage surgery

Long term clinical case studies have shown that a limb salvage procedure has the same survival as an amputation[9-14]. Therefore every patient with a malignant tumor of the extremity is considered for limb salvage if the tumor can be removed with an adequate margin and the resulting limb has satisfactory function. An adequate margin is one that results in an acceptably low rate of local recurrence of the tumor. An adequate margin is generally wide in most areas. It may be close in some areas for example in the case of a distal femur resection, the popliteal vessels may be on the pseudocapsule but can be easily separated and experience has shown an acceptable low rate of local recurrence. After salvage the limb should have an acceptable degree of function and cosmetic appearance with a minimal amount of pain, and should be capable of withstanding the demands of normal daily activities. It must look and function comparable or better than an artificial limb after amputation. Balancing these sometimes conflicting requirements is what makes limb salvage surgery a complex and difficult, but rewarding process.

In selected cases, limb salvage can be combined with metastatectomy. For patients with uncontrollable disease, limb salvage should be considered if the surgery can be accomplished with minimum morbidity and rapid return to function. These patients can enjoy relief from pain, improved quality of life, and intact body image that limb salvage can offer, even if they may not survive long term.

6. Barriers to limb salvage

Barriers to limb salvage include poorly placed biopsy incisions, major vascular involvement, encasement of a major motor nerve, pathological fracture of the involved bone, infection and inadequate motors after resection. These adverse factors are barriers but not absolute contraindications. For example in pathological fractures, the fracture often heals with chemotherapy and the specimen can be removed with adequate margins. Ability to transfer motors, graft nerves and vessels and provide skin cover with microsurgical methods have allowed successful limb salvage despite many barriers. If the patient has limited financial resources, it is better to spend the money on chemotherapy and do an amputation rather than doing limb salvage and not giving chemotherapy.

7. Surgical resections and reconstructions

For successful local tumor control it is essential to achieve a complete resection of the tumor with an adequate margin (Fig 1). As stated earlier, an adequate margin in any particular case remains controversial[25]. For high grade sarcomas, a wide margin is considered adequate and will achieve successful control of the primary tumor approximately 95% of the time, whereas marginal or intralesional margins are associated with higher rate of local recurrence and poor outcomes[26]. For bone 3cm away from the extent on T1-MRI image is adequate[27-32]. The marrow is always sent from the cut end for frozen section evaluation for tumour. If positive the resection is revised. For the soft tissue 1-2cm margin is preferred wherever possible. In practice, the line between a wide and a marginal margin is sometimes difficult to define as the surgeon strives to control the tumor while still leaving the patient with a useful limb. However, when in doubt, the surgeon errs on the side of excess tissue removal. The adequacy of the margin can be judged by bivalving the specimen. If there is any doubt about margins, a frozen section can be done and a decision for an amputation can be made on table. This is the reason that any patient undergoing a limb salvage procedure is forewarned about this possibility and a consent for amputation always obtained.

After completion of the tumor resection, the surgeon must reconstruct the resulting surgical defect. The surgeon must eliminate potential dead space and transfer tissues if necessary to allow an effective closure. Occasionally, the reconstruction or substitution of a segment of artery or nerve may be required.

Most osteosarcomas occur in the metaphyseal portion of the bone, so that the typical resection involves the whole proximal or distal part of the bone. If the joint is not contaminated by the tumor, an intraarticular resection is performed through the joint. If the joint is contaminated, then an extraarticular resection is required, taking the entire joint and joint capsule, and cutting through the uninvolved bone on the other side of the joint to achieve a wide margin. The gap remaining needs reconstruction either with metal or with bone or a composite of the two. For tumors that involve the diaphyseal portion of a bone, an intercalary resection and reconstruction can be performed that saves the joints at either end. It is now possible to save the joint even if only 1.5-2cms of condyle thickness remain[27]. For low grade osteosarcoma, a hemicortical excision which removes only a part of the bone circumference is effective in disease control. The reconstruction done often depends on the kind of defect (fig 2).

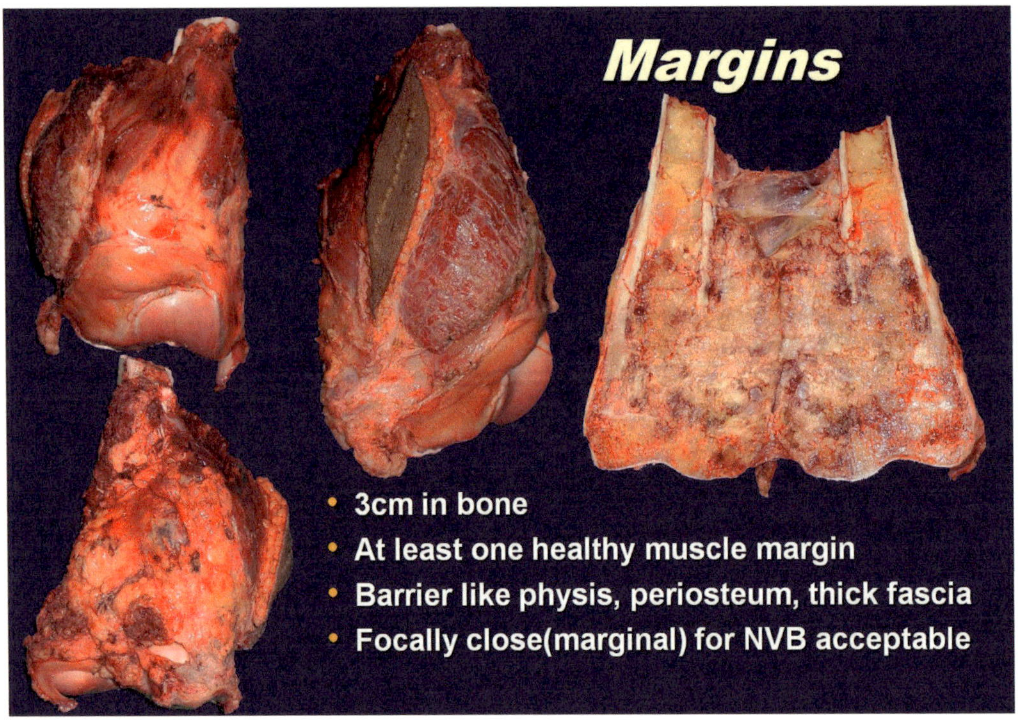

Fig. 1. Margins considered adequate for high grade osteosarcoma excision.The figure shows a resection specimen of the distal femur osteosarcoma. It is covered by an uninvolved muscle layer. The biopsy track has been completely excised enbloc with skin. There is 3cm margin from marrow extent of tumor at proximal end and the joint cartilage as margin for the distal end.

7.1 Hemicortical defects

These result generally from partial circumferential excision of benign or low grade tumors like a parosteal osteosarcoma. Reconstruction of these defects can be done by a shaped allograft or by fibula or iliac crest strut autograft.[28] Because of the large contact area and vascularity of the bed, usual complications associated with allografts like infection, non-union and fracture are rare. We reported our results in ten cases with complete incorporation of the graft in all the cases and no local recurrence.[28]

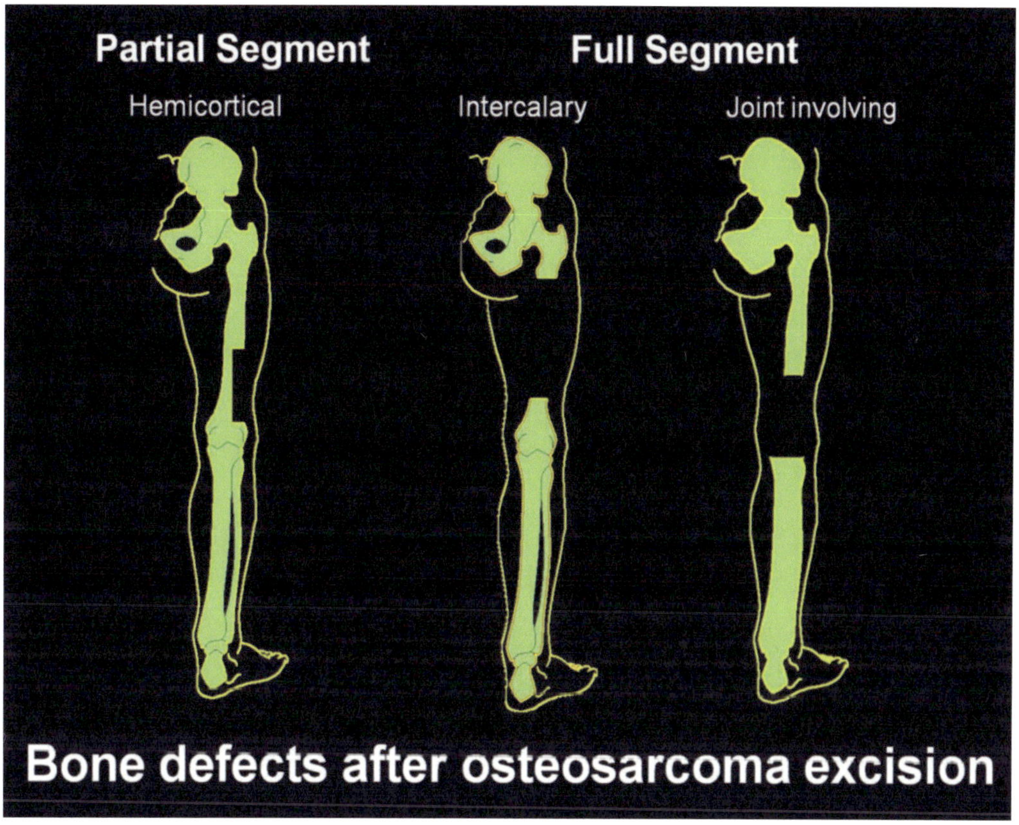

Fig. 2. The various kinds of bone defects resulting from an excision of an osteosarcoma. Hemicortical excision can be done for a low grade osteosarcoma like parosteal osteosarcoma. For all others, a full segment resection is advised.

7.2 Full segment defects

These are a result of complete circumferential excision of bone segments. These can be intercalary or joint involving (Fig 2). Since most tumors occur around the metaphysis, joint involving defects are more common.

7.2.1 Joint involving defects

7.2.1.1 Megaprosthesis

Megaprosthesis is a large metallic joint designed to replace the excised length of bone and the adjacent joint. These are fully constrained hinge joints. They provide an immediate return to function and are not affected by ongoing adjuvant treatment like chemotherapy and radiotherapy. They thus form the mainstay in limb salvage surgery for reconstruction after tumor resection.

Advances in metallurgy and fabrication have tremendously improved these joints. Joint breakage is now rare and aseptic loosening rates are also very low with the use of rotating hinges and with extracortical bridging between the bone and implant collar.[29] Infection and local recurrence are the commonest cause of prosthesis failure and happen in around 15% of cases.

A customised joint has to be ordered as per individual patient's dimensions. It takes 4-6 weeks for fabrication. In contrast modular systems (Fig 3) allow for immediate availability. They also allow intraoperative flexibility. The drawback is that they are expensive and a large inventory of the components has to be kept. A customized prosthesis can be improved with every joint but this is not possible for a modular system. Currently modular systems are used for most adults and children near skeletal maturity as adequate modularity ensures a good fit into the defect for almost all patients. In children or in places where anatomy is distorted, customized implants are used to adjust for smaller or abnormal bone size and to allow expansion.

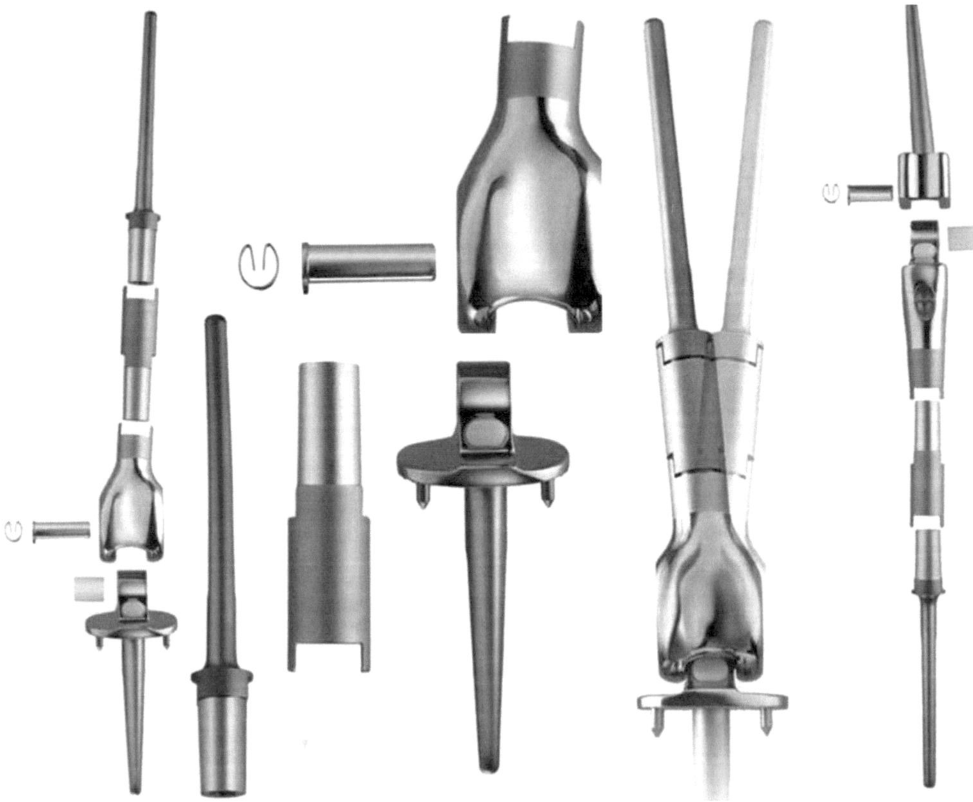

Fig. 3. Figure showing a modular megaprosthetic system for distal femur or proximal tibia resection (RESTOR, Adler Mediquip Pvt Ltd, India). Note that numerous components linked to assemble the complete prosthesis. The modularity allows the implant to be matched to the defect as well as to the bone in which it is to be implanted.

Special attention is paid during closure to ensure that the prosthesis is fully covered by a healthy soft tissue envelope. Wherever possible, as in proximal tibia, tendons are reattached to the construct. In the proximal femur, wherever possible, reattachment of the abductors reduces the limp. In the shoulder, the rotator cuff is lost and the proximal humerus implant works as a mere spacer to allow function of the elbow and hand. Wherever the deltoid and axillary nerve can be preserved, a reverse shoulder implant can be used.[30] This allows active flexion and abduction which was not possible with the conventional implant. Scapular endoprosthesis after a scapulectomy may provide better function than simple humeral suspension of the latissimus dorsi, trapezius, deltoid and rhomboids can be preserved with better abduction and flexion.[31]

It is now possible to reconstruct the entire humerus or femur (fig 4)with prosthesis. Though the surgery involves a massive exposure and long duration, the functional results have been superior to that after an amputation and external prosthesis.

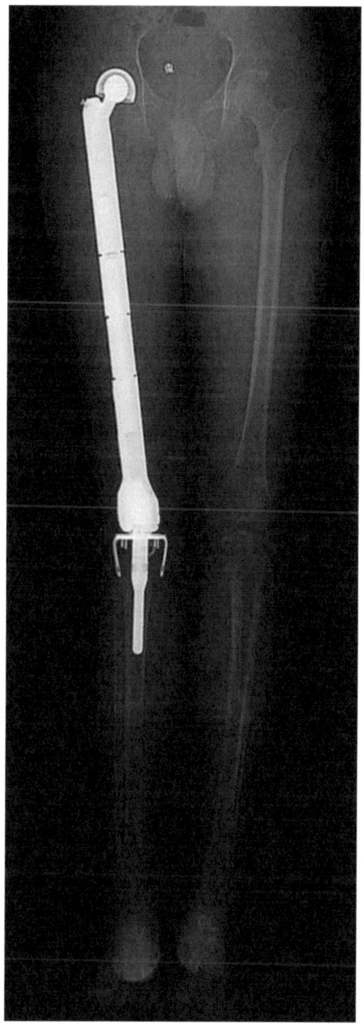

Fig. 4. A total Femoral endoprosthetic replacement

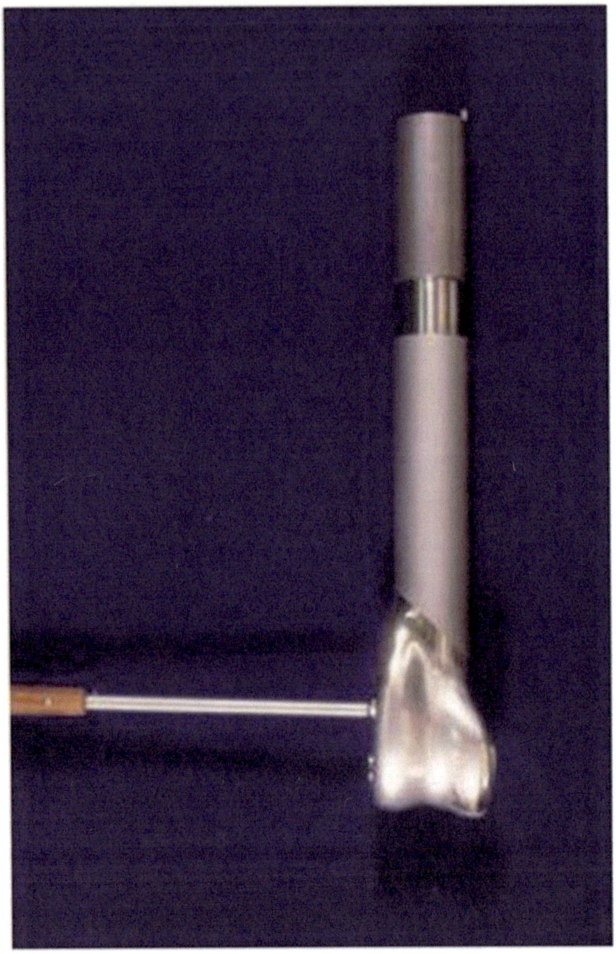

Fig. 5. An expandable distal femur megaprosthesis. This is a minimally invasive expandable system. The screwdriver drives a wormgear mechanism to drive out a telescoping cylinder resulting in lengthening.

Regardless of the method of fixation to the host bone, the prosthesis may loosen over time. Mechanical wear of the polyethylene bearing surfaces can lead to failure of the reconstruction. Rebushing is required more commonly in the fixed hinge implant and generally after five years.[29, 32] Using an hydroxyapatite coated or porous coated collar to allow extracortical bone bridging between host bone and implant has reduced the rates of aseptic loosening to almost zero.[29] Breakages are now rare with the use of stronger metals and superalloys like titanium and Chrome-cobalt. When these implants fail, revision procedures though complex have generally been successful after implantation of a new prosthesis.[33]

7.2.1.2 Expandable prosthesis

Managing limb lengths is a challenge in young children treated with limb saving surgery. While they are cured of cancer, the operated leg becomes shorter as the normal leg continues to grow while the operated leg does not. This required the child to use shoes with a thick heel to compensate for limb length discrepancy but also resulted in limp and poor function. To overcome these problems, a special prosthesis was designed which could be lengthened periodically (expandable prosthesis). The prosthesis had a worm-gear mechanism which allowed a telescoping cylinder to increase the length when a screw was turned (Fig 5). This was done surgically by a small operation in which a small cut was made and a screw driver used on the prosthesis to turn a screw which allowed a tube to telescope out. This had to be done repeatedly as the child grew to keep pace with the growth of the normal side. Though surgery was involved, the fact was that now length could be maintained in these children.

Even with all these advances, it means that the child has to undergo multiple surgical procedures for lengthening. It means admission to hospital, anaesthesia and surgery, all of this adding to the costs of treatment. Also, since we want to minimize the number of operations required, we lengthen more at each operation. We try to lengthen 1cm or more depending on the child and the need. Every surgery results in some stiffness, pain and time to rehabilitate to come to normal as this much growth is not easily adjusted to by the body. Each surgery also increases the risk of infection which is estimated to be about 8% in the current era.[34]

In order to solve some of the problems above, prostheses have been developed which can be expanded remotely without the need of any surgery. We have used the implant made by stanmore implants worldwide, U.K. The prosthesis has a very sophisticated mechanism sealed inside it which allows lengthening to happen with the help of an electromagnetic field.[35] A rare earth magnet is placed along with a motor and a gear system inside the prosthesis. A coil from outside around the implant can now generate an electromagnetic field to turn the motor. Through a system of miniature gears, the movement of the motor can allow the expansion of the implant by moving the telescoping tube out just like it was done with a screw driver. The biggest advantage is that now surgery is not required for lengthening. Small amounts of lengthening are done more like normal growth. There is no pain or stiffness, no hospitalization and no risk of infection. In the long run this turns out to be cheaper than the minimally invasive implant.

7.2.1.3 Osteoarticular allografts

Allografts offer the surgeon additional reconstructive options in bridging large bone defects after tumor excision. Osteoarticular allografts have shown a success rate of 70% at long term follow-up.[42]. Allografts have the advantage of providing biological bed for soft tissue anchorage. The attachment of muscle insertions is more successful in allografts than in prostheses, yielding better function in some sites. Initial enthusiasm for allografts has been tempered by a variety of problems as experience has accumulated. While it was initially hoped that massive allografts would become fully incorporated into the host, retrieval data show that only a small percentage of the allograft actually becomes revascularized, while the rest remains necrotic [43, 44]. Rather than a biologic replacement for the excised bone segment, the allograft functions as a biologic spacer. Massive allografts are susceptible to infection (5-15%), fracture (15-20%), Non-union (15-20%) and osteoarthritis from collapse of the articular surface (with osteoarticular graft) [45-49]. Chemotherapy and radiotherapy can adversely affect the union rates[48-52]. An additional concern is the potential for the transmission of bacterial or viral disease.

7.2.1.4 Alloprosthetic composite and others

Sometimes a composite of an allograft and an endoprosthesis is used for certain limb-salvage reconstructions. An appropriate allograft is selected and implanted to replace the segment of bone resected. The articular surfaces of the graft are excised and replaced using conventional techniques of total joint arthroplasty. The allograft provides a source of bone stock and a site for tendon insertions, while the prosthesis provides a reliable and stable articulation and some support for the allograft. The surgeon can customize the implant for any particular need. An allo-prosthesis construct has a lower fracture rate than allograft alone[49] and is not susceptible to osteoarthritis.

7.2.1.5 Resection arthrodesis

Arthrodesis for the knee, though disabling can provide a practical low cost option for reconstruction after bone tumor resection especially if patient is likely to engage in heavy manual labour. Even in a developing country it causes difficulty with squatting, traveling in bus, etc. It is therefore not easily accepted and done only occasionally by us. The principles of surgery involve bone grafts coupled with internal fixation, very similar to those of intercalary resections. Allografts alone, unlike in intercalary resections have shown a high failure rate due to infection, fracture and non-union.[53-54] Autografts vascularised or non-vascularised are used along with fixation which is either a locked long nail, or a long plate or sometimes an external fixator.[55] Distraction osteogenesis has been another option used particularly in benign tumors. An intramedullary nail, double osteotomy, fewer rings and early fixator removal have reduced the complication rates.[55] We have preferred to use a double barrel live fibula or an allograft combined with a live fibula and neutralized with a long plate.(fig 6)

The defect can be bridged by using autograft or an allograft or a combination. A vascularised live fibula with allograft supplementation is a good alternative and our method of choice. A non vascularised graft always has the risk of fracture. Fixation is either with a plate spanning the defect or with a long customized nail. These patient have to be immobilized for a long time till union. Besides, radiotherapy and chemotherapy can interfere with union. An intercalary long segment allograft can be used with implant fixation but has a high rate of complications[45]. Even with an autograft, non union and fracture rates are high and it is almost a year before arthrodesis is sound. Till this time the patient has to be protected and load bearing restricted.

Functionally, the gait of these patients with knee arthrodesis is a little awkward due to the stiff knee and sitting is difficult. However these patients are not afraid of loading their limb and can engage in strenuous activities[56].

Very few of our patients opted for an arthrodesis. The ones that did, did it for reasons of cost. The low cost of the megaprosthesis made it easier for patients to opt for a mobile reconstruction. Occasionally a nail and cement arthrodesis is used in cases where long term survival is unlikely (palliative limb salvage). A long K nail is used with cement to bridge the defect. The cement provides rotational stability. In these cases patient can be ambulant immediately.

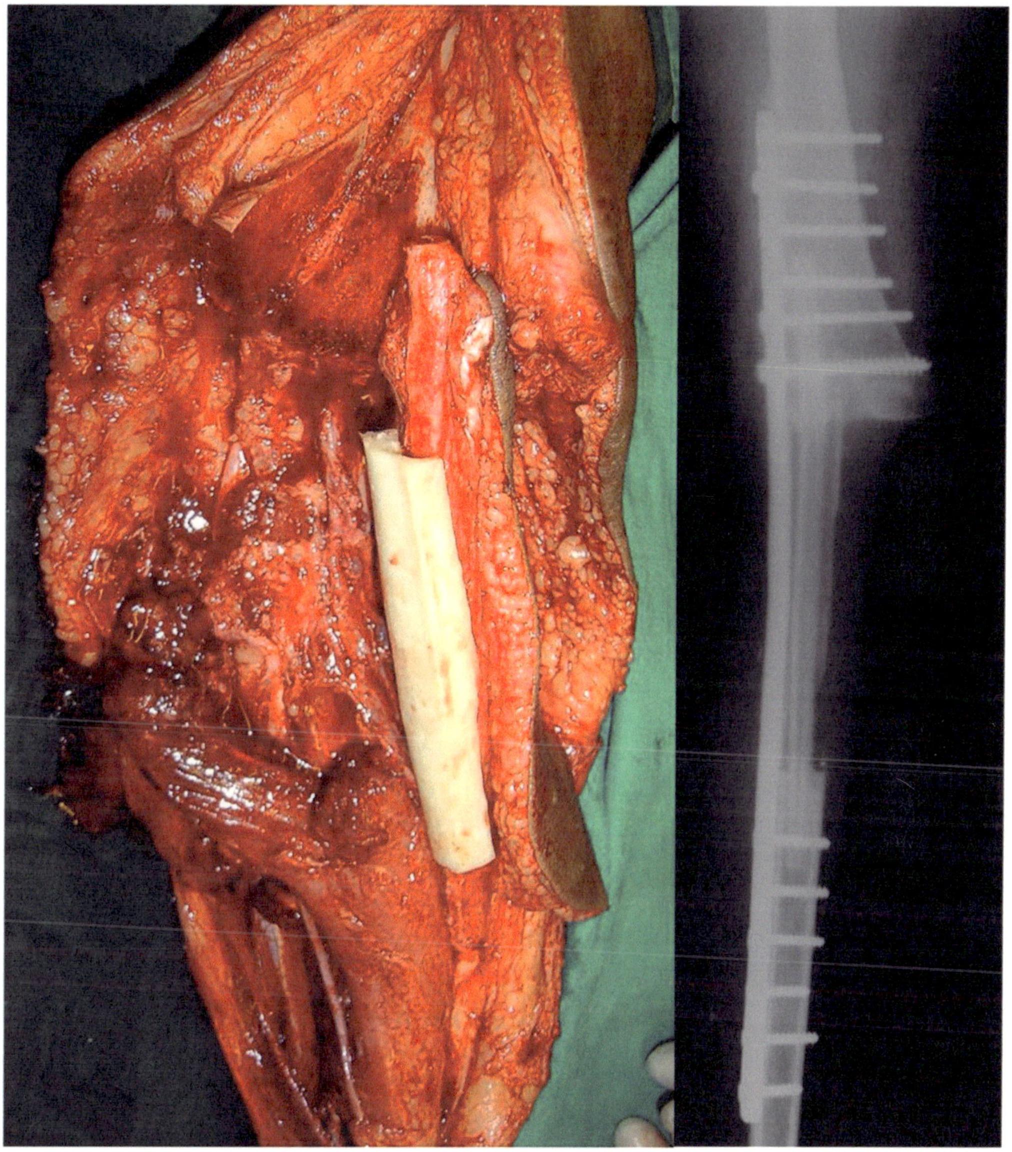

Fig. 6. An allograft with a pedicled (vascularised) fibula for a resection arthrodesis of the knee. The allograft is hemicylindrical to avoid any compression of the pedicle or skin attached to the fibula. The xray shows the union at junctions which happened uneventfully in less than 6 months.

7.2.1.6 Rotationplasty

Rotationplasty is a procedure which allows the ankle to substitute as the knee after 180^0 rotation of the limb. The original idea was conceived by Borggreve in 1927 to treat a shortened lower limb with stiff knee after tuberculosis and popularized by Van Ness for management of proximal focal femoral deficiency[57]. Salzer in 1974 first used it for malignant tumors around the knee[58]. It is essentially an intercalary limb resection preserving the continuity of the neurovascular bundle. The limb continuity is established by fusing the Tibia with the proximal femoral remnant after 180^0 external limb rotation. This allows the ankle joint to come to the level of the knee and its axis of motion corresponding with the original knee. A special external prosthesis then is fitted allowing the patient to ambulate. Ankle movements now simulate knee movements (Fig 7). This reconstruction therefore functions like a below-knee amputation. A big advantage is that the sole being the normal weight bearing area, there is no phantom pain. The stump can be left longer in children to account for subsequent shortening with growth. These patients are able to walk normally, run, participate in leisure outdoor sporting activities, ride a bicycle and drive a car etc.

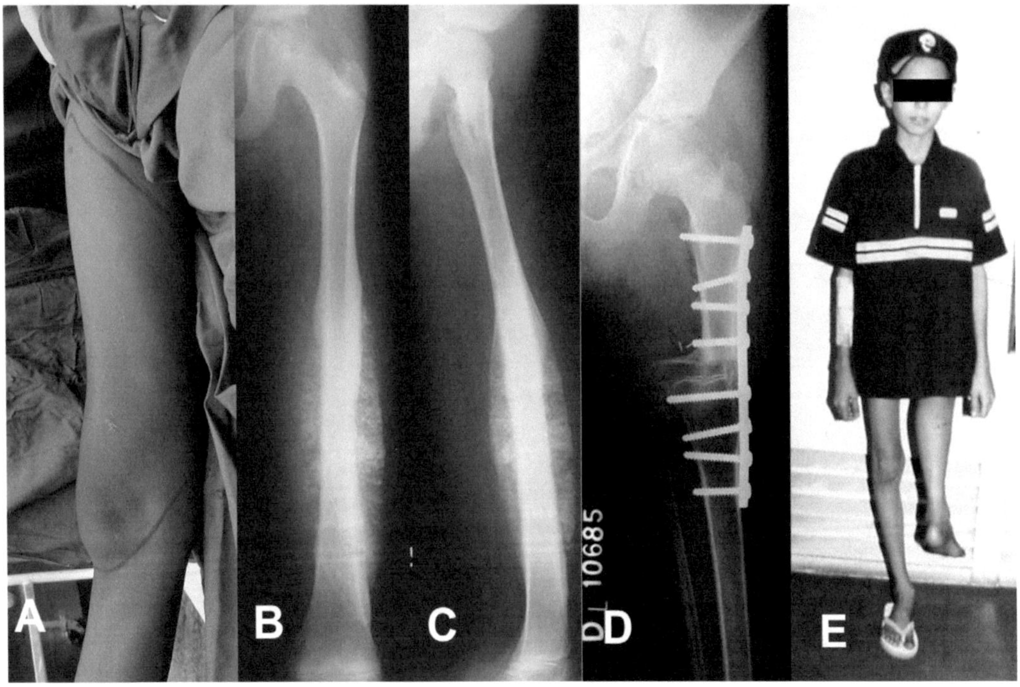

Fig. 7. Rotationplasty. A: the rhomboid incision taken. B &C : The Anteroposterior and lateral xrays of a femoral osteosarcoma after induction chemotherapy. D: postoperative xray showing the osteosynthesis between the proximal femur and proximal tibia using a plate. E: The clinical appearance of rotationplasty

Though very well described in literature with functional results comparable to an endoprosthetic reconstruction[59-62], the limb disfigurement produced has been a psychological barrier to widespread acceptance especially in the developed world. Most series for functional evaluation have shown superior functional results compared to megaprostheses, but small numbers in rotationplasty group have made statistical evaluation difficult.[62-63] Patients with rotationplasty are reported to have less pain and are more likely to participate in sports as compared to megaprostheses.[61] Akahane et al[64] in a small group of 17 patients reported better function and quality of life results with a rotationplasty than with an endoprosthesis. Rotationplasty is a low cost alternative to prosthesis in a developing country like India.[65] The surgical procedure is straightforward, the external orthoses cheap and easily available and with no revisions necessary coupled with the ability to squat and load the limb make it an easily accepted alternative over amputation for the economically backward. In children one can adjust the stump length for growth and avoid all the problems and costs associated with expandable prosthesis and expansions. It also works as an excellent salvage option for a failed megaprosthesis, especially after infection.[66] Another advantage is that with large tumors and extensive quadriceps involvement (common in a developing country like India), it can still provide functionally good outcome. An osteotomy of the femur early in the procedure allows limb rotation and makes dissection of the neuro-vascular bundle easier.[66] A specially designed jig helps to cut the bone perfectly perpendicular to the long axis and makes osteosynthesis between tibia and femur easier.[65-66]. Rotationplasty can be performed in even in smaller hospital setups without need for complex instrumentation. Long term results have not shown any arthroses in the ankle joint proving excellent adaptation.[67]

We have found excellent functional scores and patient satisfaction with this method. This has to be compared with an high above knee amputation or hip disarticulation where even with an artificial limb the function is inferior. Walking speeds, gait, oxygen consumption and general efficiency were better or comparable with other procedures like arthrodesis, endoprosthesis & amputation[68-70]. Though cosmetically unappealing, functional benefits overshadow the appearance. Prior to surgery the patient is shown photographs and videos and wherever possible meets another similar patient. The mental preparation goes a long way in ultimate acceptance by the patient.

7.3 Intercalary defects

Intercalary defects are broadly classified as diaphyseal, metaphyseo-diaphyseal, or epiphyseodiaphyseal (fig 8).[68]

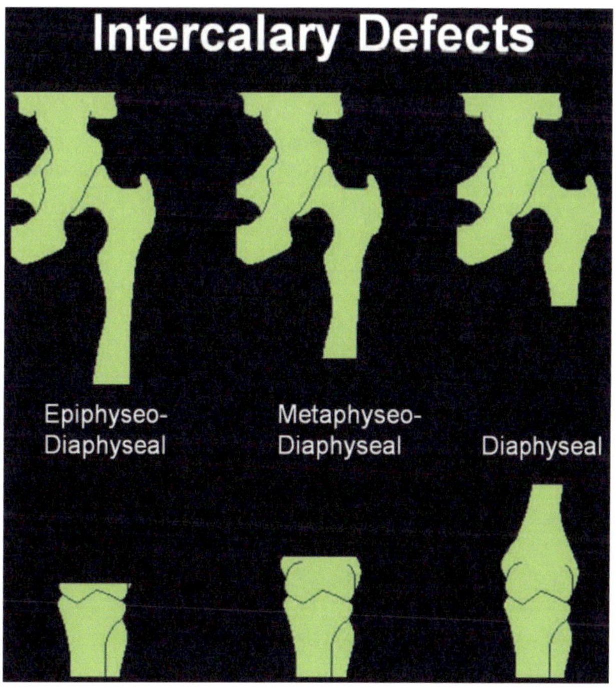

Fig. 8. Various types of intercalary defects depending on the level of distal and proximal cut

7.3.1 Autografts and allografts

Although numerous problems continue to limit the success of allograft reconstructions, they remain a viable choice for selected uses, especially in the upper extremity, for intercalary resections, and for patients who will not need chemotherapy. Intercalary allografts have shown higher success than the osteoarticular ones[46]. Reconstruction of epiphyseo-diaphyseal defects with allografts is challenging. Despite the large cancellous bony contact surface, lack of rigid fixation at the epiphyseal end delayed the average time to union to 18 months compared to 13 months at metaphyseal end.[68] Vascularised fibula (VF) is a good alternative for intercalary defects especially for longer gaps.[69-70] VF showed 93% union rate with only 15% delayed union as compared to allografts which have had 68-90% union rates with 51-57% delayed union rates.[69] Most of VF patients could return to athletic activity. Donor site morbidity was not a serious problem with most complications resolving with conservative treatment.

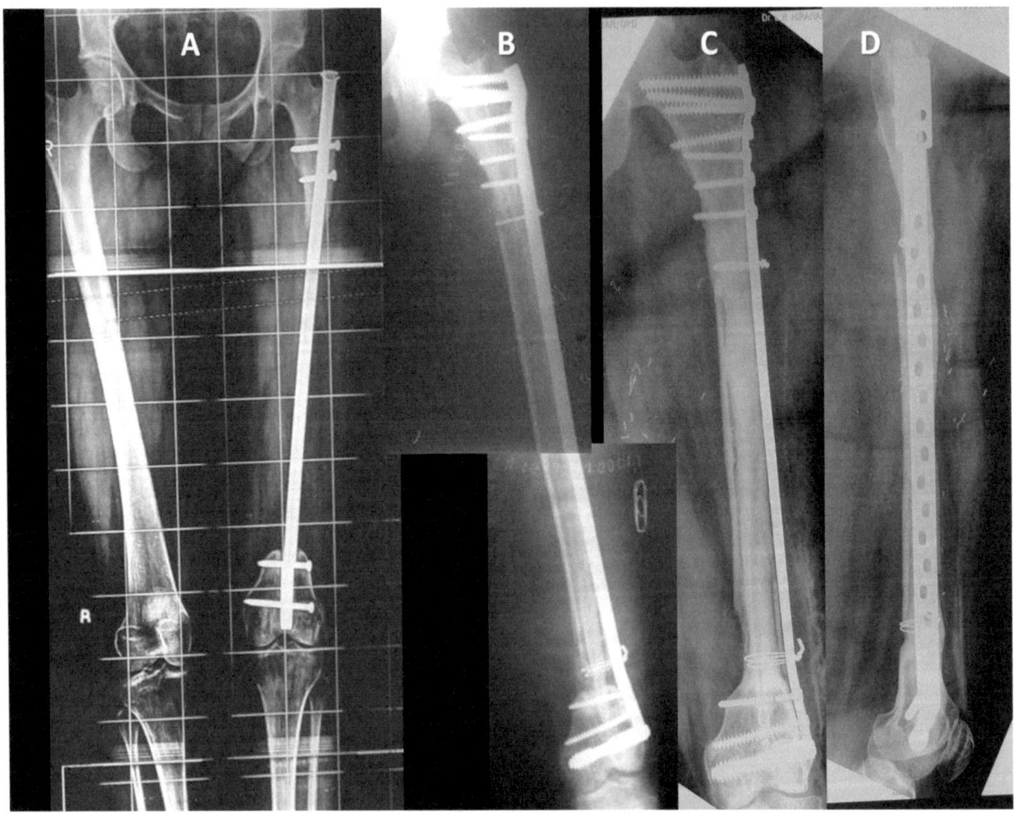

Fig. 9. A: Osteosarcoma of the femur treated by an intercalary resection. The surgeon reconstructed the defect with an interlocking nail only which broke in 2 years. This was replaced by an Allograft with a vascularised fibula placed in the intramedullary canal (B). C & D show the follow up xray at one year showingthe excellent incorporation of graft and fibular hypertrophy

Non vascularised fibular autograft can be a simple low cost and yet effective alternative to Allograft or VF. Krieg et al[71] reported from their experience of 31 cases using a non vascularised fibula a primary union rate of 89% in a median time of 24 weeks. 15% had a fatigue fracture with no fractures where a double or triple strut was used. Hypertrophy of the graft was similar to that in VF.

The results of allograft can be improved by combining them with a vascularised fibula either placed in the medullary canal of the allograft or as an onlay by providing vascularity in the centre of the allograft.[72-73] The healing of the junctions is quick and reliable and the fibula hypertrophies over a period of time. The allograft provides the initial strength and the vascularised autograft provides speed of union. Our experience with radiated allograft alone has been rather disappointing with only about 40% grafts incorporating. Radiation and chemotherapy have probably resulted in poorer incorporation. A single fibula especially in defects over 20cm was prone to fracture. We therefore recommend an allograft combined with a live fibula rather than an allograft alone for long full segment defects. The faster incorporation results in fewer failures and earlier return to full function. For smaller defects with strong and rigid fixation, a VF alone may be adequate.

7.3.2 Reimplantation of tumor bearing bone

Reimplanting the tumor bearing bone after some form of treatment (autoclaving, pasteurization, freezing with liquid nitrogen, or extracorporeal radiation) to kill the tumor cells is another exciting low cost option. Though dead like an allograft, it is perfectly matched to the defect. Autoclaved bone has provided fairly good results as reported from 12 cases from Pakistan with only one non-union and no fractures with an average MSTS score of 70% at a mean follow-up of 49 months.[74] Yamamoto et al[75] histologically examined a specimen of autoclaved and reimplanted bone in femur retrieved after 24 months and found most of the graft not incorporated. New bone formation was thin and superficial over the graft and bone scan exaggerated the bone formation. This does not seem to match the clinical experience cited above. In future it may be possible to improve the osteoinductivity of autoclaved bone by coating with rhBMP-2.[76] A combination of dehydration and thermal denaturing can prevent loss of strength and improve clinical performance.[77]

High temperatures associated with autoclaving are known to damage the collagen matrix leading to loss of strength as well as BMP and osteoinductivity. Pasteurisation involves heating the bone to 60 deg C for 30 min in a water bath and is an effective way of killing all tumor without affecting strength and osteoinductivity. Clinical results with pasteurized graft have shown results at least comparable to allografts.[78-79] Freezing in liquid nitrogen is another way of killing the tumor and yet being able to reimplant the bone. Tsuchiya et al[80] reported bony union at a mean of 6.7 months after the operation in 26/28 patients. There were three deep infections, two fractures, and two local recurrences.

Extracorporeal irradiation (FIG 10) with doses of 5000rad (equivalent to 25kgy of conventional radiation) is also effective in killing all tumor.[81] The rate of non union (7%) is significantly lower with ECRT as compared to allografts (43%).[82] The fracture rates were similar and there were no infections. Histological evaluation of specimens from failed ECRT cases show changes of repair and viable osteoblasts after 2-3 years.[83]

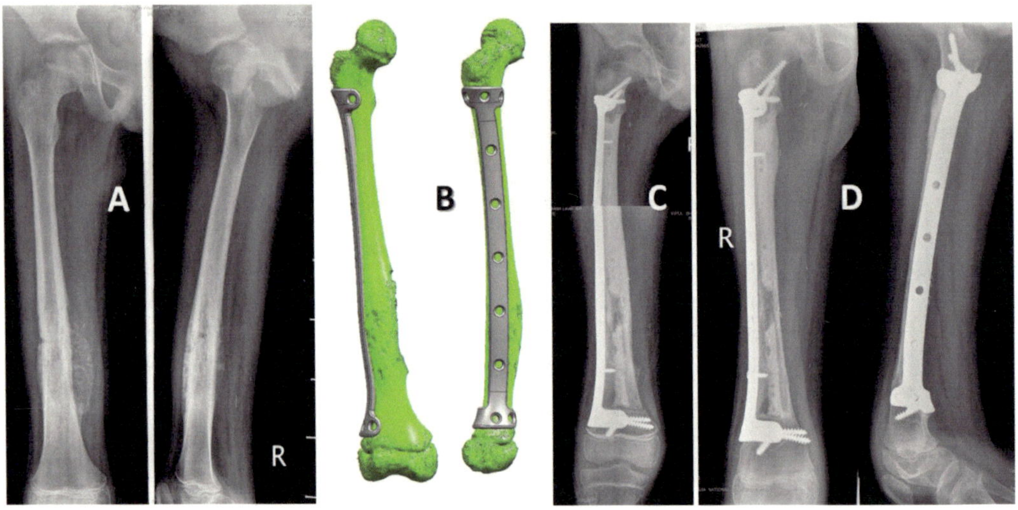

Fig. 10. A: Preoperative xrays of an osteosarcoma of the femur treated with extracorporeal irradiation and reimplantation(ECRT). B: schematic view showing the custom plates made to fix the construct. C: The postoperative xray showing the radiated autograft construct. Note the screws close to the distal physis. D: followup xray showing incorporation of the graft and growth from the distal femoral physis.

As in an allograft, a live fibula improves the results with pasteurized as well as radiation treated bone.[71, 73, 84]

7.3.3 Prosthesis

Prosthesis can be used to reconstruct non-joint defects. These can be used as physis sparing or joint saving implants.[27] Endoprosthetic reconstruction of a diaphyseal defect avoids the donor site morbidity of autograft and the fracture and non-union risk of allograft especially for patients on chemotherapy. It also shortens surgical time significantly as compared to a VF. Clinical results have been at least as good as allografts.[85, 86] The higher rate of loosening in the upper limb may be due to rotational stresses. The aseptic loosening may be reduced with hydroxyapatite (HA) or porous titanium bead coating.[29] Customised HA coated implants have been used for epiphyseo-diaphyseal defects. (fig 5) Early stability is obtained by extracortical plate fixation. No loosening or fractures were reported from 8 cases studied with a short follow up of 3 years.[87] This implant can be expandable where the physis is resected to maintain limb length with growth.(fig 11) The early results are promising and this could become the method of choice for intercalary reconstruction.

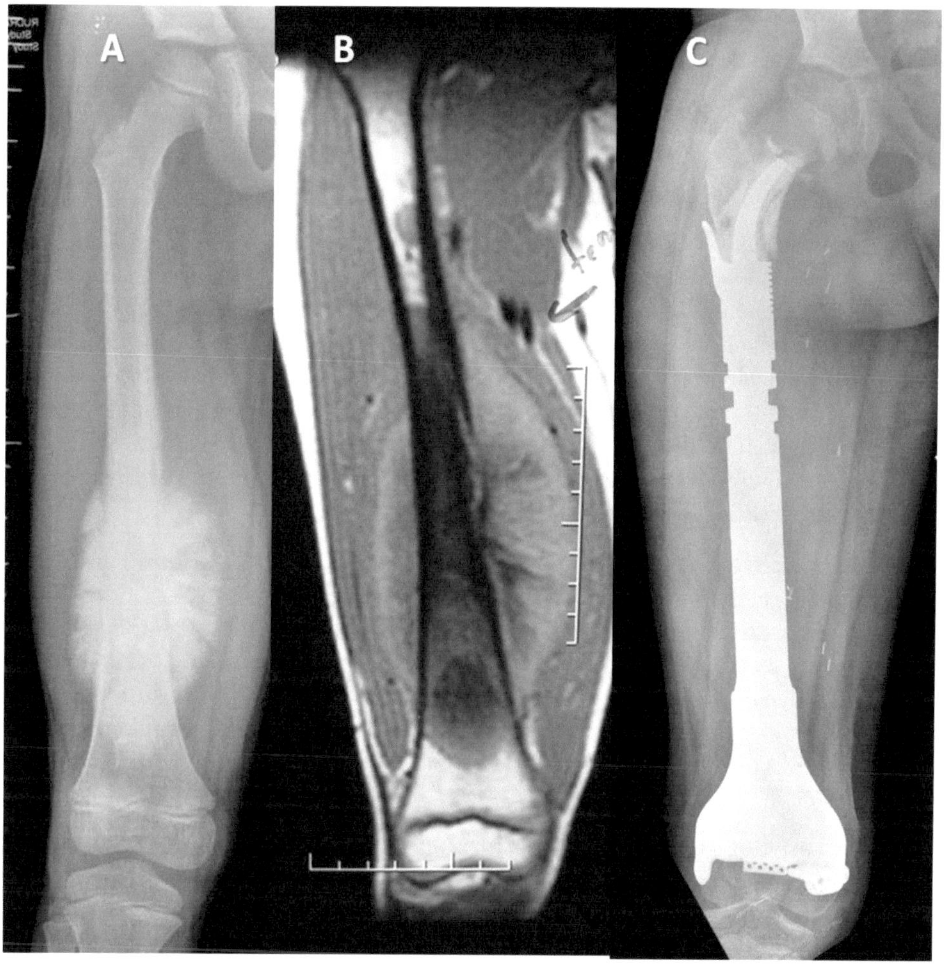

Fig. 11. A: Preoperative xray of a distal femur osteosarcoma. B: The MRI shows the extent just proximal to the distal femoral physis. Note the skip lesion proximally. C: The defect was constructed with a custom prosthesis designed to fit into the small distal and proximal fragment. The distal fixation is with an hydroxyapatite coated surface and small extracortical plates. The proximal fixation is with a curved short intramedullary stem. This prosthesis could be lengthened with a noninvasive expansion mechanism (STANMORE implants, UK)

8. Pelvis

Any tumor in the pelvis is a challenge to an orthopaedic oncologist for resection and osteosarcoma being a high grade malignant tumor is even more challenging. Tumors are often large at presentation and do not always respond well to the preoperative chemotherapy. Osteosarcomas of the pelvis are rare accounting for 7-9% of all osteosarcomas.[88] Prognosis has been reported to be dismal with 18% 5 year survival[88,89,90] . Recent report indicates a 50% 5 year survival.[91] Since osteosarcoma does not respond well to radiation, surgical resection with a tumor free margin is the only reliable method for cure.

The surgery is extensive and has the potential for many complications. An external hemipelvectomy has therefore been the standard of care in the past. Though it causes major disfigurement and extensive functional handicap, it was the safest way of getting a chance of cure in a pelvic osteosarcoma. With improvement in imaging as well as surgical technique and technology, limb saving resections have now become feasible and are the standard of care.

Pelvic resections for tumors are amongst the most challenging of operations for any surgeon. A detailed knowledge of anatomy and preparedness and ability to deal with large blood losses is a prerequisite. Pelvic resections are any one or the combination of the following four types. Type I (Iliac), Type II (periacetabular), Type3 (anterior arch) and type IV (sacrum). Classically, internal hemipelvectomy means resection of the entire hemipelvis from the SI joint to the pubic symphysis. Today, the term has come to include resections of the pelvis which include the acetabulum with varying portions of the Ilium & the anterior arch. Resections involving the acetabulum leave behind significantly more instability than the other types of partial pelvic resections.

Pelvic resections are extensive operations associated with the risks of major blood loss as well as wound problems from the extensive exposure and long surgical time. Resection without any reconstruction was done in the past to minimize these complications. With improvement in technique and results, reconstruction using arthodesis (iliofemoral and ischiofemoral fusion)(fig 12), surgical pseudarthrosis (mesh reconstruction), pelvic allografts, custom-made endoprostheses, the saddle prosthesis and reimplantation of the excised hemipelvis after sterilisation by radiation have been used with better cosmetic and functional results.[92]

It is logical to use these extensive surgical procedures only in those with a chance of cure. To minimize the incidence of local recurrence, only those patients should be selected where the extent of the tumor (judged by a preoperative workup) is such that it is possible to provide adequate margins for local control by surgery.; ie, tumors involving the innominate bone without extension into soft tissue or with minimal or moderate extension into soft tissue such that would permit an en bloc resection through clean planes and allow preservation of the major nerves and vessels for the ipsilateral extremity. Also, the general physical condition and life expectancy of the patient should justify the procedure because of the prolonged rehabilitation period (9-15mo). Involvement by the tumor of one of the major nerves, ie, sciatic or femoral, requiring its sacrifice, should revise the operative plan to that of a standard hemipelvectomy. Of course, such an eventuality should be explained beforehand to the patient, and the appropriate consent obtained.

Tumors located near the sacroiliac joints or pubic symphysis present a special problem in that positive margins of resection may occur unless the procedure is extended to the sacral ala or the contralateral side of the symphysis, respectively. Also, lesions medial to the pelvic bones may be adjacent to the neurovascular bundle and result in positive margins of excision. Induction chemotherapy may be useful to shrink these tumors prior to their surgical removal and thereby facilitate removal with more adequate resection margins.

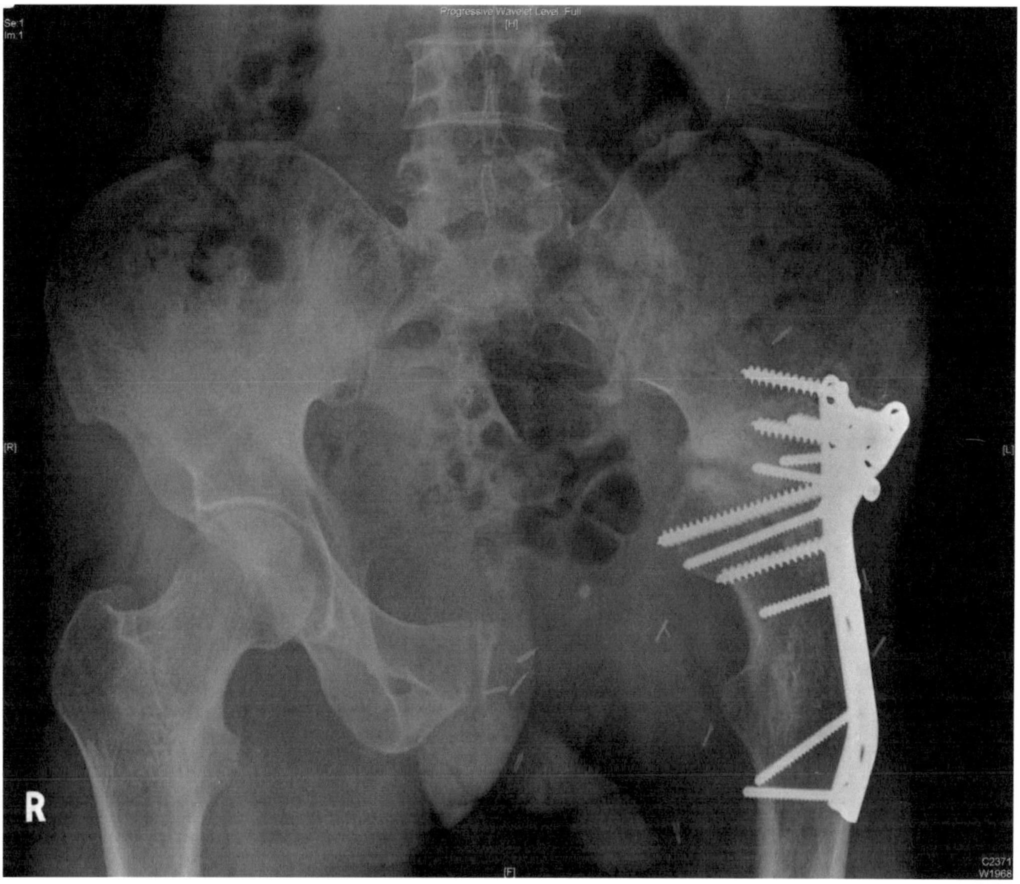

Fig. 12. An Iliofemoral fusion held with a distal femur condyle buttress plate. This is contoured to match the bone contour.

The incisions needed for each case may be different depending on the resection and reconstruction planned. A wrongly done biopsy is very likely to compromise the chance of limb salvage. It is therefore recommended that biopsy be best done by the surgeon who will be performing the final procedure.

In acetabulum involving resection without reconstruction, a 2-3" shortening of the ipsilateral extremity occurs. The patient has normal function at the ankle and knee joints, but no function at the hip area. As fibrosis occurs, these patients can walk in 6-9 months with help of some support like a crutch or walking stick. The functional results could be improved by stabilising the pelvis by reconstructing. Hip transposition (mesh pseudoarthrosis) has given acceptable results with lower complication rates than other methods like prosthesis and allografts.[93] Type II resections(periacetabular) have a better outcome with allograft and prosthesis composite as compared to more massive complete hemipelvic resections.[94] Saddle prosthesis provides better function than a hemipelvectomy but has a considerable complication rate.[95, 96] Infection (37%), dislocation (22%), fractures (22%), and heterotopic ossification (37%) were the commonest reported complications.[97] Vertical migration has been noted in some cases. Pelvic allografts have been reported to give

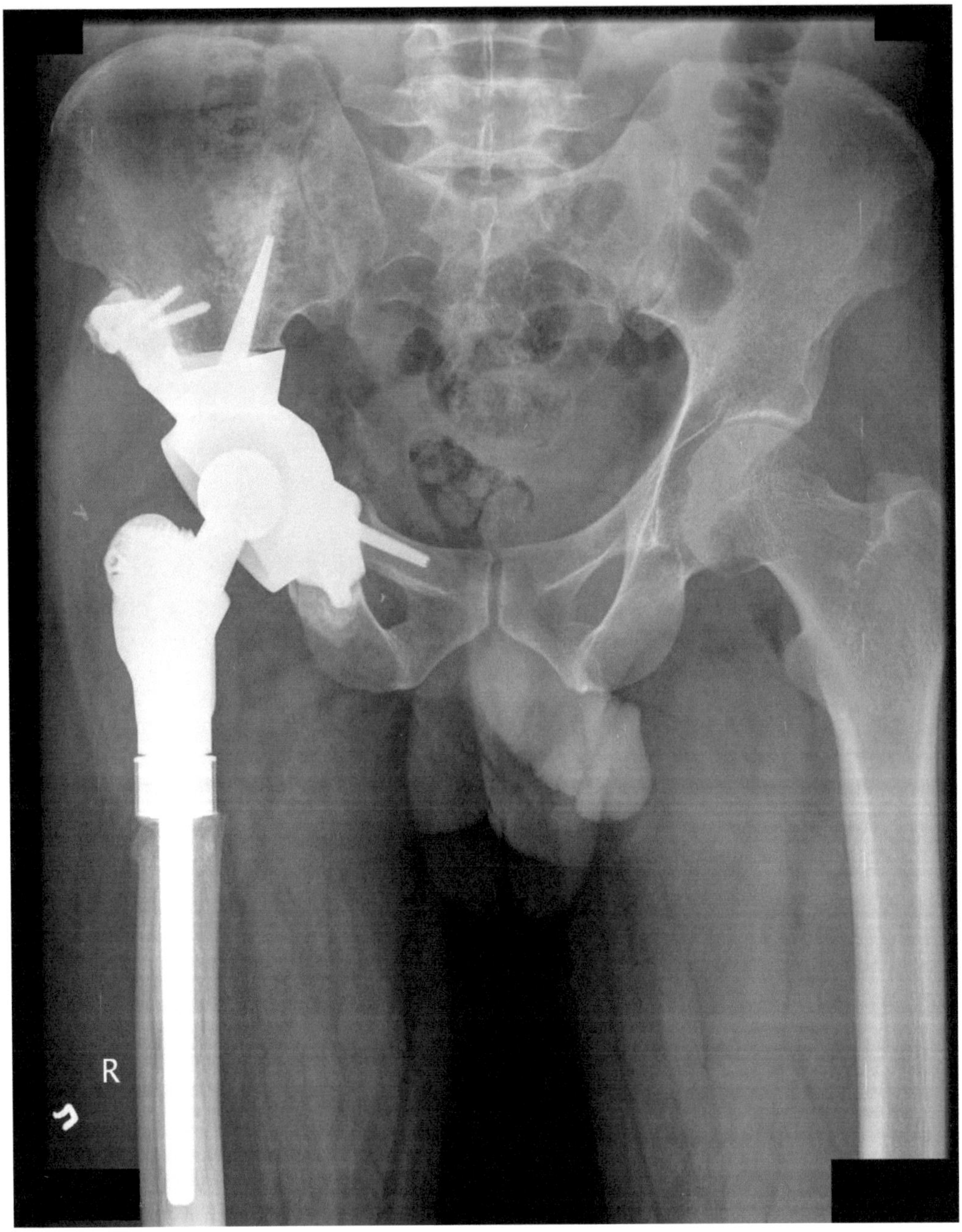

Fig. 13. Reconstruction after an extraarticular resection of the proximal femur. The acetabulum is reconstructed with a custom acetabular prosthesis and femur with a modular proximal femoral megaprosthesis (ISIQU Orthopaedics, Capetown, South Africa). The acetabular prosthesis anchors into the posterior ilium, pubis and ischium with small stems which are cemented.

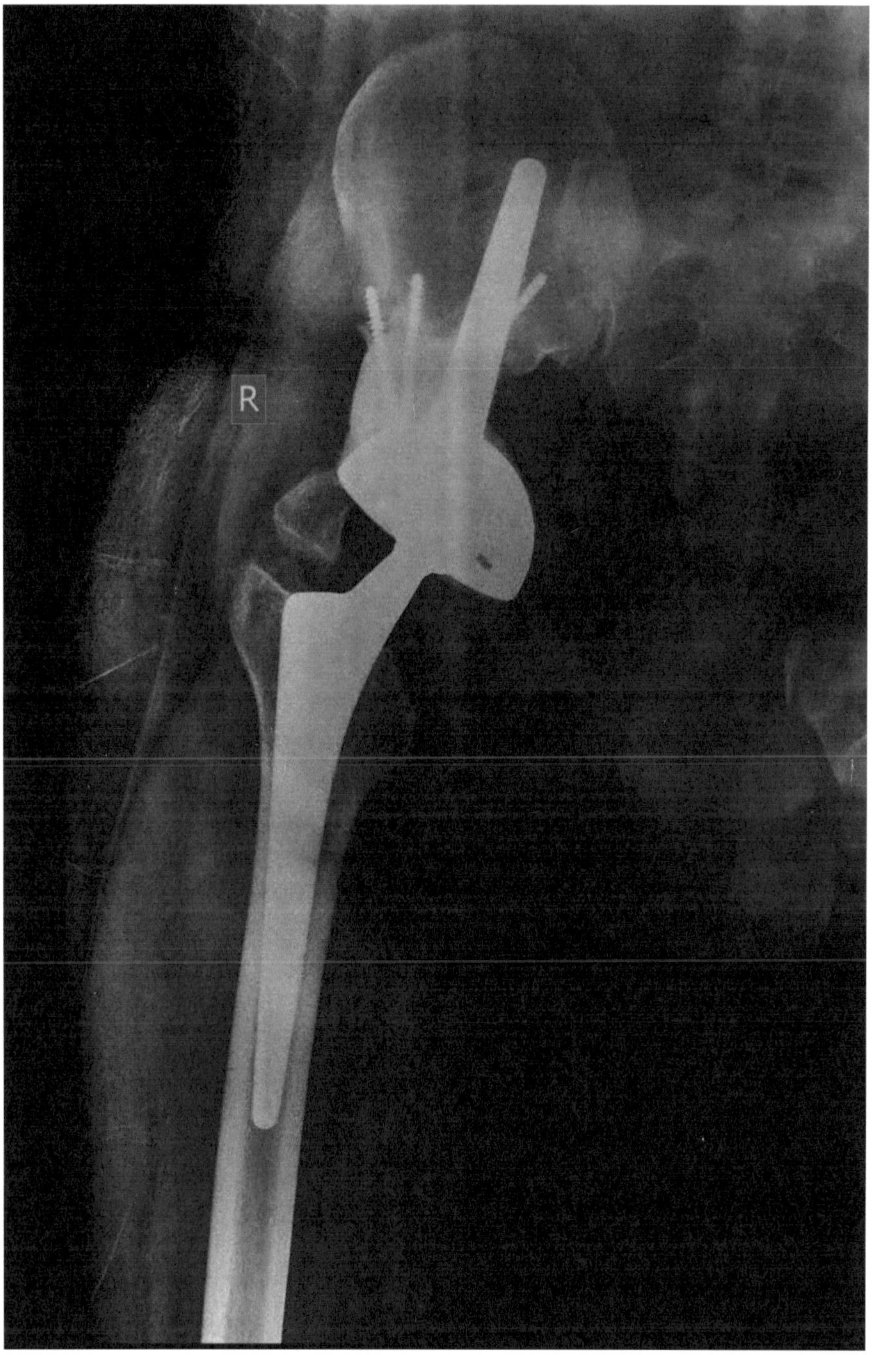

Fig. 14. Acetabulum reconstructed with a modular coned hemipelvic implant (Stanmore implants worldwide, UK). The stem is uncemented and fits into the thick posterior ilium remnant. Additional screws pass into the ilium and the defect is bridged with cement. An uncemented standard femoral component used in hip replacement surgery is placed in the proximal femur and mated to the cup with a constrained liner.

good functional results though the complication rate has been high.[97] Nonunion, infection and local recurrence were the commonest complications.[97] Custom or modular acetabular prosthesis have also been used with satisfactory functional results in some reports[98,99,100] and poor results in others.[101] Similarly custom or modular hemipelvic prosthesis have been reported with poor[101] or satisfactory results.[102]

Complication rates in various series varies from 42-65%. Infection and local recurrence are the biggest complications. Injury to NV bundle, ureter, bladder & rectum are the other complications described. Injury to the sciatic nerve would severely compromise the functional result. Sciatic and femoral nerve palsies have been reported frequently after pelvic resections and reconstructions.[93, 95, 97]

We have preferred to use either modular coned hemipelvis (fig 14) from Stanmore implants or extracorporeal irradiation and reimplantation with or without a hip prosthesis. Wherever enough bone stock is present, an arthrodesis like iliofemoral or ischiofemoral fusion is used.(fig 12)

9. Conclusions

The first decade of the new millennium has been globally recognized by the orthopaedic fraternity as the decade of improvements in the treatment of bone and joint disorders. An ideal situation in the management of bone tumors is when the disease can be successfully removed without an amputation and the resulting loss of bone and muscle compensated by a method which retains near normal limb function. Patient survivals have dramatically improved following the availability of newer chemotherapy drugs and this has accentuated the need for durable methods of reconstruction of large musculoskeletal defects. Orthopaedic surgeons have risen to the challenge and it is now possible to offer limb salvage to a large majority of patients with bone tumors. Ever increasing advances in technology and biomaterials combined with a better understanding of biomechanics will further help in increasing the durability of and refining limb salvage procedures.

10. References

[1] Dahlin DC, Coventry MB : Osteosarcoma – a study of 600 cases. J Bone Joint Surg 49A:101-110.1967.
[2] Marcove RC, Mike V, Hajeh JV, et al : Osteosarcoma under the age of twenty one: A review of one hundred and forty five operative cases. J Bone Joint Surg 52: 411-423, 1970
[3] Huth JF, Eilber FR : Patterns of recurrence after resection of osteosarcoma of the extremity: strategies for treatment of metastases. Arch Surg 124: 122-126, 1989.
[4] Bacci G, Avella M, Picci P et al: Metastatic patterns in osteosarcoma. Tumori 74:421-427,1988.
[5] Link MP, Goorin AM, Miser AW et al : The effect of adjuvant chemotherapy on relapse free survival in patients with osteosarcoma of the extremity. New Eng J Med 314(25): 1600-1606.1986.
[6] Eilber F, Giuliano A, EckhardtJ et al: Adjuvant chemotherapy for osteosarcoma: a randomized prospective trial. J. Clin. Oncol.5(1): 21-26,1987.

[7] Meyers PA, Heller G, Healy J et al :Chemotherapy for non-metastatic osteogenic sarcoma: the Memorial Sloan-Kettering experience : J. Clin. Oncol. 10(11): 5-15,1992.

[8] Baci G, Ferrari S, Bertoni F, Ruggieri P et al : Long term outcome for patients with non-metastatic osteosarcoma of the extremity treatment at the istituto ortopedico Rizzoli according to the istituto ortopedico Rizzoli / osteosarcoma-2 protocol: an updated report. J. Clin. Oncol. 2000 Dec 15;18(24):4016-27.

[9] Sim, F. H.; Ivins, J. C.; Taylor, W. F.; and Chao, E. Y. S.: Limb-Sparing Surgery for Osteosarcoma: Mayo Clinic Experience. Cancer Treat. Sympos., 3: 139-154, 1985.

[10] Lane, J. M.; Glasser, D. B.; Duane, Karen; Healey, J. H.; McCormack, R. R., Jr.; Rosen, Gerald; Sison, Brenda; Huvos, A. G.; Marcove, R. C.; and Cammisa, F. P., Jr.: Osteogenic Sarcoma: Two Hundred Thirty-three Consecutive Patients Treated with Neoadjuvant Chemotherapy. Orthop. Trans., 11: 495, 1987.

[11] Goorin, A. M.; Perez-Atayde, Antonio; Gebhardt, Mark; Andersen, J. W.; Wilkinson, R. H.; Delorey, M. J.; Watts, Hugh;Link, Michael; Jaffe, Norman; Frei, Emil, III; and Abelson, H. T.: Weekly High-Dose Methotrexate and Doxorubicin for Osteosarcoma: The Dana-Farber Cancer Institute/The Children's Hospital -- Study III.J. Clin. Oncol., 5: 1178-1184, 1987.

[12] Simon, M. A.; Aschliman, M. A.; Thomas, Neal; and Mankin, H. J.: Limb-Salvage Treatment versus Amputation for Osteosarcoma of the Distal End of the Femur. J. Bone and Joint Surg., 68-A: 1331-1337, Dec. 1986.

[13] Winkler, K.; Beron, G.; Kotz, R.; Salzer-Kuntschik, M.; Beck, J.; Beck, W.; Brandeis, W.; Ebell, W.; Erttmann, R.; Gobel, U.; Havers, W.; Henze, G.; Hinderfeld, L.; Hocker, P.; Jobke, A.; Jurgens, H.; Kabisch, H.; Preusser, P.; Prindull, G.; Ramach, W.; Ritter, J.; Sekera, J.; Treuner, J.; Wust, G.; and Landbeck, G.: Neoadjuvant Chemotherapy for Osteogenic Sarcoma. Results of a Cooperative German/Austrian Study. J. Clin. Oncol., 2: 617-624,1984.

[14] Rougraff, B. T., Simon, M. A., Kneisl, J. S.,Greenberg, D. B., and Mankin, H. J. : Limb salvage compared with amputation for osteosarcoma of the distal end of the femur. A long-term oncological, functional, and quality-of-life study : J Bone Joint Surg vol. 76-a, no. 5, may 1994, pp. 649-656

[15] Van der Bijl AE, Taminiau AHM, Hermans J, Beerman H and Hogendoorn PCW. Accuracy of the Jamshidi trocar biopsy in the diagnosis of bone tumors. Clin Ortho Rel Res 1997; 334: 233-43.

[16] Bickels J, Jelinek JS, Shmookler BM, Neff RS and Malawer MM. Biopsy of musculoskeletal tumors. Clin Ortho Rel Res 1999; 368: 212-9.

[17] Mankin, Henry J., Mankin, Carole J., Simon, Michael A. : The Hazards of the Biopsy, Revisited. *J Bone Joint Surg [Am]* 1996; 78-A; 656-63

[18] Mankin, H. J.; Lange, T. A.; and Spanier, S. S.: The hazards of biopsy in patients with malignant primary bone and soft-tissue tumors. J Bone Joint Surg., 64-A: 1121-1127, Oct. 1982.

[19] Enneking, W. F.: The issue of the biopsy [editorial]. J. Bone and Joint Surg., 64-A: 1119-1120, Oct. 1982.

[20] Simon, M. A.: Current concepts review. Biopsy of musculoskeletal tumors. J. Bone and Joint Surg., 64-A: 1253-1257, Oct. 1982.

[21] Springfield DS, Rosenberg A. Biopsy: complicated and risky [editorial; comment]. J Bone Joint Surg [Am] 1996;78-A(S) :639—43.

[22] Fraser-Hill MA, Renfrew DL. Percutaneous needle biopsy of musculoskeletal lesions. 1. Effective accuracy and diagnostic utility. AJR 158: 809-812, Apr 1992.
[23] Ayala AG, Zomosa J. Primary Bone tumours: Percutaneous needle biopsy-radiologic-pathologic study of 222 biopsies. Radiology 1983; 149: 675-679.
[24] Picci P, Sangiorgi L, Rougraff BT, Neff JR, et al : Relationship of Chemotherapy induced necrosis and surgical margins to Local recurrence in Osteosarcoma. J Clin Oncol Vol 12 No 12, 1994, pp2699-2705.
[25] Wolf RE, Enneking WF. The staging and surgery of musculoskeletal neoplasms. Orthop Clin N Am 1996;27(3) :473–81.
[26] Ward WG, Yang R-S, Eckardt JJ. Endoprosthetic bone reconstruction following malignant tumor resection in skeletally immature patients. Orthop Clin N Am 1996;27(3) :493–502.31
[27] Agarwal M, Puri A, Gulia A, Reddy K. Joint-sparing or Physeal-sparing Diaphyseal Resections: The Challenge of Holding Small Fragments. Clin Orthop Relat Res. 2010 Nov;468(11):2924-32.
[28] Agarwal M, Puri A, Anchan C et al. Hemicortical Excision for Low-grade Selected Surface Sarcomas of Bone. Clin Orthop Relat Res.2007 Jun:459: 161-166
[29] Myers GJ, Abudu AT, Carter SR, et al. Endoprosthetic replacement of the distal femur for bone tumours: LONG-TERM RESULTS. J Bone Joint Surg Br. 2007 Apr;89(4):521-6.
[30] De Wilde LF, Plasschaert FS, Audenaert EA, Verdonk RC. Functional recovery after a reverse prosthesis for reconstruction of the proximal humerus in tumor surgery. Clin Orthop Relat Res. 2005 Jan;(430):156-62.
[31] Pritsch T, Bickels J, Wu CC, et al. Is A Scapular Endoprosthesis Functionally Superior to Humeral Suspension? Clin Orthop Relat Res. 2006 Sep 21
[32] Frink SJ, Rutledge J, Lewis VO, et al. Favorable long-term results of prosthetic arthroplasty of the knee for distal femur neoplasms. Clin Orthop Relat Res. 2005 Sep;438:65-70.
[33] Agarwal MG, Gulia A, Ravi B, Ghayyar R, Puri A.: Revision of Broken Knee Megaprostheses: New Solution to Old Problems. Clin Orthop Relat Res. 2010 Nov;468(11):2904-13.
[34] Abudu A, Grimer R, Tillman R, Carter S. The use of prostheses in skeletally immature patients.Orthop Clin North Am. 2006 Jan;37(1):75-84.
[35] Gupta A, Meswania J, Pollock R, et al. Non-invasive distal femoral expandable endoprosthesis for limb-salvage surgery in paediatric tumours.J Bone Joint Surg Br. 2006 May;88(5):649-54.
[36] Aisen AM, Martel W, Braunstein EM, et al: MRI and CT evaluation of primary bone and soft-tissue tumors. Am J Roentgenol 146:749-756, 1986.
[37] Cohen MD, Weetman RM, Provisor AJ, et al: Efficacy of magnetic resonance imaging in 139 children with tumors. Arch Surg 121:522-529, 1986.
[38] Gillespy T, Manfrini M, Ruggieri P, et al: Staging of intraosseous extent of osteosarcoma: Correlation of preoperative CT and MR imaging with pathologic macroslides. Radiology 167:765-767, 1988.
[39] Golfieri R, Baddeley H, Pringle JS, et al: MRI in primary bone tumors: Therapeutic implications. Eur J Radiol 12:201-207, 1991.

[40] O'Flanagan SJ, Stack JP, McGee HMJ, et al: Imaging of intramedullary tumour spread in osteosarcoma: A comparison of techniques. J Bone Joint Surg 73B:998-1001, 1991.
[41] Onikul E, Fletcher BD, Parham DM, et al: Accuracy of MR imaging for estimating intraosseous extent of osteosarcoma. Am J Roentgenol 167:1211-1215, 1996.
[42] Mankin, H. J.; Gebhardt, M. C.; Jennings, L. C.; Springfield, D.S.; and Tomford, W. W.: Long-term results of allograft replacement in the management of bone tumors. Clin. Orthop., 324: 86-97, 1996.
[43] Donald S. Garbuz, Bassam A. Masri, Andrei A. Czitrom : Biology of allografting: Orthop Clin North Am Volume 29 • Number 2 • April 1998pp199-204
[44] Enneking, WF. and Campanacci DA., Retrieved Human Allografts A Clinicopathological Study *J Bone Joint Surg(A)* 83:971-986 (2001)
[45] Hornicek FJ, Gebhardt MC, Sorger JI, Mankin HJ : Bone Graft Substitutes: Clinical Applications-Tumor Reconstruction: Orthopedic Clinics of North America Volume 30 • Number 4 • October 1999
[46] Ortiz-Cruz, E., Gebhardt, M. C., Jennings, L. C., Springfield, D. S, and Mankin, H. J: The Results Of Transplantation Of Intercalary Allografts After Resection Of Tumors. A Long-Term Follow-Up Study: J Bone Joint Surg 79-a, no. 1, january 1997, pp. 97-106
[47] Berrey, B. H., Jr.; Lord, C. F.; Gebhardt, M. C.; and Mankin, H. J.: Fractures of allografts. Frequency, treatment, and end-results. J. Bone and Joint Surg., 72-A: 825-833, July 1990.
[48] Muscolo, D. L.; Petracchi, L. J.; Ayerza, M. A.; and Calabrese, M. E.: Massive femoral allografts followed for 22 to 36 years. Report of six cases. J. Bone and Joint Surg., 74-B(6): 887-892, 1992.
[49] Thompson RC Jr; Garg A; Clohisy DR; Cheng EY: Fractures in Large Segment Allografts. Clin Orthop 2000.;370:227-235.
[50] Hazan EJ, Hornicek FJ, Tomford W, Gebhardt MC, Mankin HJ : The effect of adjuvant chemotherapy on osteoarticular allografts. Clin Orthop 2001 Apr;(385):176-81
[51] Hornicek FJ, Gebhardt MC, Tomford WW, Sorger JI, Zavatta M, Menzner JP, Mankin HJ.: Factors affecting nonunion of the allograft-host junction. Clin Orthop 2001 Jan;(382):87-98
[52] Sorger JI, Hornicek FJ, Zavatta M, Menzner JP, Gebhardt MC, Tomford WW, Mankin HJ: Allograft fractures revisited: Clin Orthop 2001 Jan;(382):66-74
[53] Donati D, Giacomini S, Gozzi E, et al. Allograft arthrodesis treatment of bone tumors: a two-center study. Clin Orthop 2002;400:217- 24.
[54] Muscolo DL, Ayerza MA, Aponte-Tinao LA. Massive allograft use in orthopedic oncology. Orthop Clin North Am. 2006 Jan;37(1):65-74.
[55] Vidyadhara S, Rao SK. Techniques in the management of juxta-articular aggressive and recurrent giant cell tumors around the knee. Eur J Surg Oncol. 2007 Mar;33(2):243-51.
[56] Harris, I. E., Leff, A. R.,Gitelis, S., Simon, M. A. Function after amputation, arthrodesis,or arthroplasty for tumors about the knee. J Bone Joint Surg VOL. 72-A, No. 10, December 1990, pp. 1477-1485.
[57] Van Nes. C.P.: Rotationplasty for congenital defects of the femur. Making use of the ankle of the shortened limb to control the knee joint of a prosthesis. JBJS., 32-B(1): 12-16, 1950.

[58] Kotz R., Salzer M.: Rotationplasty for childhood osteosarcoma of the distal part of the femur. JBJS., 64-A., 7:959, 1982.
[59] Fuchs B, Kotajarvi BR, Kaufman KR, Sim FH. Functional outcome of patients with rotationplasty about the knee. Clin Orthop Relat Res. 2003;415:52–58.
[60] Hillmann A, Hoffmann C, Gosheger G, et al. Malignant tumor of the distal part of the femur or the proximal part of the tibia: endoprosthetic replacement or rotationplasty: functional outcome and quality-of-life measurements. J Bone Joint Surg Am. 1999;81:462–468.
[61] Hillmann A, Rosenbaum D, Schroter J, et al. Electromyographic and gait analysis of forty-three patients after rotationplasty. J Bone Joint Surg Am. 2000;82:187–196.
[62] Ginsberg JP, Rai SN, Carlson CA, et al. A comparative analysis of functional outcomes in adolescents and young adults with lower-extremity bone sarcoma. Pediatr Blood Cancer. 2006 Aug 18; [Epub ahead of print]
[63] Hopyan S, Tan JW, Graham HK, Torode IP. Function and upright time following limb salvage, amputation, and rotationplasty for pediatric sarcoma of bone. J Pediatr Orthop. 2006 May-Jun;26(3):405-8.
[64] Akahane T, Shimizu T, Isobe K, et al. Evaluation of postoperative general quality of life for patients with osteosarcoma around the knee joint. J Pediatr Orthop B. 2007 Jul;16(4):269-272.
[65] Agarwal M, Puri A, Anchan C, et al. Rotationplasty for Bone Tumors: Is There Still a Role? Clin Orthop Relat Res. 2007 Jun:459: 76-81
[66] Puri A, Agarwal M. Facilitating rotationplasty.J Surg Oncol. 2007 Mar 15;95(4):351-4.
[67] Gebert C, Hardes J, Vieth V, et al. The effect of rotationplasty on the ankle joint: long-term results. Prosthet Orthot Int. 2006 Dec;30(3):316-23.
[68] Deijkers RL, Bloem RM, Kroon HM et al. Epidiaphyseal versus other intercalary allografts for tumors of the lower limb. Clin Orthop Relat Res. 2005 Oct;439:151-60.
[69] Chen CM, Disa JJ, Lee HY et al. Reconstruction of extremity long bone defects after sarcoma resection with vascularized fibula flaps: a 10-year review. Plast Reconstr Surg. 2007 Mar;119(3):915-24
[70] Pederson WC, Person DW. Long bone reconstruction with vascularized bone grafts. Orthop Clin North Am. 2007 Jan;38(1):23-35
[71] Krieg AH, Hefti F. Reconstruction with non-vascularised fibular grafts after resection of bone tumours. J Bone Joint Surg Br. 2007 Feb;89-B(2):215-221.
[72] Capanna R, Campanacci DA, Belot N, et al. A new reconstructive technique for intercalary defects of long bones: the association of massive allograft with vascularized fibular autograft. Long-term results and comparison with alternative techniques. Orthop Clin North Am. 2007 Jan;38(1):51-60.
[73] Moran SL, Shin AY, Bishop AT. The use of massive bone allograft with intramedullary free fibular flap for limb salvage in a pediatric and adolescent population. Plast Reconstr Surg. 2006 Aug;118(2):413-9.
[74] Khattak MJ, Umer M, Haroon-ur-Rasheed, Umar M. Autoclaved tumor bone for reconstruction: an alternative in developing countries. Clin Orthop Relat Res. 2006 Jun;447:138-44.
[75] Yamamoto N, Tsuchiya H, Nojima T et al. Histological and radiological analysis of autoclaved bone 2 years after extirpation. J Orthop Sci. 2003;8(1):16-9

[76] Taguchi S, Namikawa T, Ieguchi M, Takaoka K. Reconstruction of Bone Defects Using rhBMP-2-coated Devitalized Bone. Clin Orthop Relat Res. 2007 Mar 22; [Epub ahead of print]
[77] Draenert GF, Delius M. The mechanically stable steam sterilization of bone grafts. Biomaterials. 2007 Mar;28(8):1531-8.
[78] Jeon DG, Kim MS, Cho WH et al. Pasteurized Autograft for Intercalary Reconstruction: An Alternative to Allograft. Clin Orthop Relat Res. 2006 456:203–210
[79] Manabe J, Ahmed AR, Kawaguchi N, et al. Pasteurized autologous bone graft in surgery for bone and soft tissue sarcoma. Clin Orthop Relat Res. 2004 Feb;(419):258-66.
[80] Tsuchiya H, Wan S L, Sakayama K et al. Reconstruction using an autograft containing tumour treated by liquid nitrogen. J Bone Joint Surg [Br]2005;87-B:218-25
[81] Davidson AW, Hong A, McCarthy SW, Stalley PD. En-bloc resection, extracorporeal irradiation, and re-implantation in limb salvage for bony malignancies. J Bone Joint Surg Br. 2005 Jun;87(6):851-7.
[82] Chen TH, Chen WM, Huang CK. Reconstruction after intercalary resection of malignant bone tumours: comparison between segmental allograft and extracorporeally-irradiated autograft. J Bone Joint Surg Br. 2005 May;87(5):704-9.
[83] Hatano H, Ogose A, Hotta T et al. Extracorporeal irradiated autogenous osteochondral graft: a histological study. J Bone Joint Surg Br. 2005 Jul;87(7):1006-11.
[84] Muramatsu K, Ihara K, Hashimoto T, et al. Combined use of free vascularised bone graft and extracorporeally-irradiated autograft for the reconstruction of massive bone defects after resection of malignant tumour. J Plast Reconstr Aesthet Surg. 2007 May 9.
[85] Ahlmann ER, Menendez LR. Intercalary endoprosthetic reconstruction for diaphyseal bone tumours. J Bone Joint Surg Br. 2006 Nov;88(11):1487-91.
[86] Aldlyami E, Abudu A, Grimer RJ, et al. Endoprosthetic replacement of diaphyseal bone defects. Long-term results. Int Orthop. 2005 Feb;29(1):25-9.
[87] Gupta A, Pollock R, Cannon SR, et al. A knee-sparing distal femoral endoprosthesis using hydroxyapatite-coated extracortical plates. Preliminary results. J Bone Joint Surg Br. 2006 Oct;88(10):1367-72.
[88] Ozaki T, Flege S, Kevric M, Lindner N, Maas R, Delling G, Schwarz R, von Hochstetter AR, Salzer-Kuntschik M, Berdel WE, Jürgens H, Exner GU, Reichardt P,Mayer-Steinacker R, Ewerbeck V, Kotz R, Winkelmann W, Bielack SS. Osteosarcoma of the pelvis: experience of the Cooperative Osteosarcoma Study Group. J Clin Oncol.2003 Jan 15;21(2):334-41.
[89] Isakoff MS, Barkauskas DA, Ebb D, Morris C, Letson GD. Poor Survival for Osteosarcoma of the Pelvis: A Report from the Children's Oncology Group. Clin Orthop Relat Res. 2012 Feb 22. [Epub ahead of print]
[90] Grimer RJ, Carter SR, Tillman RM, Spooner D, Mangham DC, Kabukcuoglu Y.Osteosarcoma of the pelvis. J Bone Joint Surg Br. 1999 Sep;81(5):796-802.
[91] Song WS, Cho WH, Jeon DG, Kong CB, Kim MS, Lee JA, Eid AS, Kim JD, Lee SY.Pelvis and extremity osteosarcoma with similar tumor volume have an equivalent survival. J Surg Oncol. 2010 Jun 1;101(7):611-7.
[92] Hugate R Jr, Sim FH. Pelvic reconstruction techniques. Orthop Clin North Am. 2006 Jan;37(1):85-97

[93] Hoffmann C, Gosheger G, Gebert C, et al. Functional results and quality of life after treatment of pelvic sarcomas involving the acetabulum. J Bone Joint Surg Am. 2006 Mar;88(3):575-82.

[94] Beadel GP, McLaughlin CE, Wunder JS, et al. Outcome in two groups of patients with allograft-prosthetic reconstruction of pelvic tumor defects. Clin Orthop Relat Res. 2005 Sep;438:30-5.

[95] Aljassir F, Beadel GP, Turcotte RE, et al. Outcome after pelvic sarcoma resection reconstructed with saddle prosthesis. Clin Orthop Relat Res. 2005 Sep;438:36-41.

[96] Kitagawa Y, Ek ET, Choong PF. Pelvic reconstruction using saddle prosthesis following limb salvage operation for periacetabular tumour. J Orthop Surg (Hong Kong). 2006 Aug;14(2):155-62

[97] Delloye C, Banse X, Brichard B, et al. Pelvic reconstruction with a structural pelvic allograft after resection of a malignant bone tumor. J Bone Joint Surg Am. 2007 Mar;89(3):579-87

[98] Abudu A, Grimer RJ, Cannon SR, Carter SR, Sneath RS. Reconstruction of the hemipelvis after the excision of malignant tumours. Complications and functional outcome of prostheses. J Bone Joint Surg Br. 1997 Sep;79(5):773-9

[99] Müller PE, Dürr HR, Wegener B, Pellengahr C, Refior HJ, Jansson V. Internal hemipelvectomy and reconstruction with a megaprosthesis. Int Orthop. 2002;26(2):76-9.

[100] Dai KR, Yan MN, Zhu ZA, Sun YH. Computer-aided custom-made hemipelvic prosthesis used in extensive pelvic lesions. J Arthroplasty. 2007 Oct;22(7):981-6.

[101] Ozaki T, Hoffmann C, Hillmann A, Gosheger G, Lindner N, Winkelmann W. Implantation of hemipelvic prosthesis after resection of sarcoma. Clin Orthop Relat Res. 2002 Mar;(396):197-205.

[102] Guo W, Li D, Tang X, Yang Y, Ji T. Reconstruction With Modular Hemipelvic Prostheses For Periacetabular Tumor. Clin Orthop Relat Res. 2007 Apr 19;

Part 3

Osteosarcoma Research

6

Bone Formation Deregulations Are the Oncogenesis Keys in Osteosarcomas

Natacha Entz-Werlé
University of Strasbourg
France

1. Introduction

The reciprocal osteoblast-osteoclast interactions are essential in the coordinated healthy bone formation and resorption. These communications in the bone microenvironment are highly complex events and need precise regulated molecular processes to ensure constant healthy bone remodeling. (Matsuo and Irie, 2008). Malignant bone tumors seem to be mainly linked to deregulation of this osteoblast-osteoclast cooperation processes. The major malignant bone tumor in pediatrics (5% of pediatric cancers) is high-grade osteosarcoma (OS). Usually, this bone cancer is diagnosed during adolescence and represent the second most common cancer after lymphoma in this period of age. A second peak observed in life is after 50 years. During adolescence, the kids are having their puberty development and the long bones are growing then particularly fast, with a rapid cell turnover in and around the growth plate (Mathew et al., 2011; Marina et al., 2004). Then, in a not surprising way, the most common locations of OS are the long bones (frequently, distal femur, proximal tibia and humerus) and especially in these metaphyseal regions around growth plates. Furthermore, no significant improvement in prognosis for patients with OS was observed since the advent of multiagent chemotherapy, increasing the long term outcome. Even this therapeutic progress, the overall survival of the patients is now at a plateau of 70% (Le Deley et al., 2007; Mirabello et al., 2009). After increasing the patient survival, new challenges regarding chemoresistances are now appearing and are involved in the recurrence of the disease despite a successful local resection. 15 to 20% of diagnosed patients will have radiographically detectable pulmonary metastases whereas 80% will already presenting undetectable micrometastases (Bruland et al., 2009). The lack of prognostic marker at diagnosis is another key point in this cancer. The only prognostic marker is the Huvos histological grading on tumor resection after neo-adjuvant chemotherapy (Juergens et al., 1981). It is classifying patients into good responders to chemotherapy and poor responders but after 4-month-chemotherapy already done. All these epidemiologic and therapeutic characteristics initially led to develop molecular research to find new prognostic biomarkers and to define new therapeutic targets. In this context, the research focused on several genetic predisposition genes implicated in OS development even most OS tumors are sporadic cases without familial patterns. Rapidly thereafter, the OS molecular research was taking into account the worldwide well-known OS histological features, which are the presence of malignant osteoid matrix produced by the proliferating malignant osteoblastic cells. This definition underlie the fact that OS may be considered as a disease of osteoblast dedifferentiation (Haydon et al., 2007). As the normal osteoblasts derived from multipotent mesenchymal stem cells (MSCs), the several steps of this transition may be disrupted to obtain subsequently malignant osteoblasts. Based on that, multiple research teams focused, then, on osteoblast differentiation disruptions. They demonstrated that osteosarcomagenesis may result in a deregulation of normal osteogenesis signaling pathways, such as Wnt, BMP (Bone morphogenetic protein) or FGF (Fibroblast Growth Factor) (Entz-Werlé et al., 2003; Luo et al., 2007; Lau et al., 2007), and a dysexpression of several transcription factors (like Twist, Runx2, Osterix or ATF4) (Entz-werlé et al., 2005; Tang et al., 2008). These alterations result in the blockade of cells as undifferentiated precursors. The tumorigenesis seems to be also associated with disturbed bone metabolic activities, leading to the development of a penetrating tumor into the metaphyseal region of long bones and an increase in local bone destruction rates (Costa-Rodrigues et al., 2011; Avnet et al., 2008; Lamoureux et al., 2007). Osteogenesis and osteoclastogenesis signaling pathways additionally to bone microenvironment signals disruptions seem to contribute to OS development and its local or metastatic progression.

The understanding of these deregulated molecular mechanisms in osteosarcoma has and will afford new prognostic markers and new therapeutic targets. In fact, multiple phase I and II, based on all these results, are still running and including relapsed osteosarcoma patients. The recent and increase use of zoledronic acid and targeted therapies in association with standard chemotherapy has to be considered as the emerging therapies of these last decade research in osteosarcomas (Lamoureux et al., 2007; Chou et al., 2008; Broadhead et al., 2011; PosthumaDeBoer et al., 2011). However, the major problem for targeted therapies in this bone cancer is the predominant observation of frequent deletions in karyotypic and arrayCGH (microarray based comparative genomic hybridization) approaches leading to develop therapeutic approaches by-passing the absence of protein over-expression.

2. Research methodology

In such malignant tumors, 3 main models for molecular and cellular studies are available: patient tumor collections, animal models and osteosarcoma cell lines (Kim & Helman, 2009).

To optimize such high throughput molecular researches, the tumor collections have to be integrated into clinical trials to be able to collect in parallel the clinical data and to perform informative statistical correlations. These integrated translational researches have to investigate, first, homogenously treated patient cohorts in case of correlations with response to chemotherapy before any validation as independent marker(s) in several collections. In fact, the response to neo-adjuvant chemotherapy is depending on chemotherapeutic treatment itself and the percentage of response is usually modified by any chemotherapeutic changes in the protocols. Furthermore, this malignant bone tumor is having specific key problems turning around the nature of the tumor itself and its high frequency of extended spontaneous necrosis. This histological observation is impacting especially on RNA extract quality and consequently their analyses, explaining why numerous Lab focused on DNA extracts and paraffin-embedded samples for this tumor. The high complexity of chromosomal rearrangements (Sandberg et al., 2004) is also limiting the transcriptomic screening because of the difficulties in interpreting expression results. Nevertheless, genome-wide approaches to identify OS-associated genes were performed at DNA, RNA and proteomic levels during the last decade, as well as quantitative PCRs, mutation researches or sequencing, for example (Kubista et al., 2011; Luk et al., 2011; Smida et al., 2010; Lau, 2009). Wide epigenetic and polymorphism screening were also performed and allowed to detect complementary results (Sadikovic et al., 2008).

However, to by-pass the difficulties in tumor collections, *in vitro* and *in vivo* models were developed. As models, they allowed also to confirm the mechanistic conclusions obtained from patients tumors. The *in vitro* models are based on the establishment of patient cell lines and/or the use of commercial cell lines (SaOS or U2OS, for example) (Janeway & Walkley, 2011). Classical two-dimensional (2D) cultures can be done but it is lacking the mechanical and chemical features present in animal models and in the patient bone microenvironment. Therefore, three-dimensional assays were developed to create ideal conditions to study OS cell invasion and metastases (Xu et al., 2007). The 3D *in vitro* cell culture systems will allow live cell-based arrays, microfluidic cell culture systems and drug screening. The use of emerging microengineering approaches will provide repeatable 3D cell based assays and will allow large drug testing without the disadvantages and constraints of animal models (Tan et al., 2011; Xu & Burg, 2007).

The third research model will be based on animal models (mainly mouse, rodent or dog model). The mouse models can be transgenic mice or genetically engineered mice (with the controlled induction of gene over-expression or under-expression), subcutaneous implantation into immunocompromised mice or orthotopic models. OS may also be induced frequently by mouse irradiation and/or the use of chemical carcinogens. The emerging rodent model in OS seem to be progressively used in the recent lab studies and have promising advantages. The dog seem to be also in OS a promising model because of multiple similarities with human cancer and it is offering the possibilities to study autochthonous tumors (Mueller et al., 2007). The *in vivo* model has to re-create human conditions to optimize the mechanistic understanding of osteosarcomagenesis, reason why several models of localized or metastatic OS were developed (Jones, 2011; Janeway & Walkley, 2011; Entz-Werlé et al., 2010; Walkley et al., 2008; Dass et al., 2007; Ek et al., 2006; Dass et al., 2006; Luu et al., 2005). All these animal models are outstanding tools to perform *in vivo* target validation, drug optimization and pre-clinical studies. Furthermore, with the new technologies using bioluminescence, the drug testing and *in situ* tumor follow up is becoming easier (Sottnik et al., 2010 ; Rousseau et al., 2010).

3. Genetic predisposing disorders to OS development

By the past, the starting point in molecular research was frequently based on the correlation between congenital gene mutations and their associated risk of cancer development. For OS, multiple germline mutations are presenting a higher risk of OS. So, the Li and Fraumeni syndrome, an autosomal dominant disorder, is characterized by a germline mutation of *TP53* and a high risk of OS development. The *TP53* alterations (mutations, gene rearrangements or allelic loss) are frequently observed in sporadic OS (Smith-Sorensen et al., 1993) and usually associated with chemoresistance (Asada et al., 1998). The second most frequent germline mutation associated with OS initiation is the hereditary retinoblastoma (Toguchida, et al., 1989), whereas the loss of heterozygosity of *RB1* locus is also extremely frequent in sporadic OS. This *RB1* loss is lacking in case of p16 loss expression (Nielsen et al., 1998) and has been demonstrated as a poor prognosis biomarker (Feugeas et al., 1996). The third group of cancer predisposition syndromes is linked to mutations of RECQ helicases. Among them, Rothmund-Thomson syndrome (mutation of RECQL4), Bloom syndrome (mutation of BLM gene) and Werner syndrome (mutation of WRN gene) can be listed. All these syndromes are presenting similar clinical features and exhibit predispositions to develop OS (Wang, 2005). These mutations are known to increase sensitivity to DNA-damaging agents and maybe are predisposing to bone cell dedifferentiation and consequently to develop OS. Finally, the Paget disease of bone is also a heritable disorder characterized by the increased risk of OS development (approximately 1% of patients). This adult disease is defined as a rapid bone remodeling leading to abnormal bone production (McNairn et al., 2001). The pathogenesis of the Paget disease of bone was highlighting the role of FOS gene, as well as RANK or OPG, involved in bone formation. Most of these congenital disease are characterized by the alteration of genes involved in sporadic OS and most of them are part of osteoblast-osteoclast interactions, implicated in osteosarcomagenesis, as it will be developed below.

4. The role of a defective osteogenesis in osteosarcoma development

The MSCs are bone marrow stromal cells that can differentiate into osteogenic, chondrogenic, adipogenic, neurogenic or myogenic lineages (Deng et al., 2008). The osteogenic differentiation, a tightly regulated process, is needed for bone formation. At each successive stage of differentiation, the precursors are losing their proliferative ability until their terminal differentiation in mature osteoblast (Tang et al., 2008). This osteogenic differentiation is under the control of multiple markers including in particular connective tissue growth factor (CTGF), alkaline phosphatase (ALP), Osterix, Runx2, TWIST, osteopontin (OPN), osteocalcin (OCN) and collagen IaI. During the endochondral osteogenesis of long bones, the chondrogenic cascade is also needed for the bone formation and is regulated by multiple growth factors and transcription factors such as SOX9, BMP2, BMP7, and FGF2 (Deng et al., 2008). The cross-talk and feedback cycles between these two cascades are mainly based on the BMPs, PPARγ, Runx2 and the canonical Wnt signaling pathway. Several cell cycle genes are also interacting directly or indirectly at several steps of osteoblastic lineage with osteogenic differentiation genes and signaling pathways. Looking closely to these normal features, OS cells are really comparable to undifferentiated osteogenic precursors with a high proliferative capacity, a resistance to apoptosis and a differential expression of osteogenic markers, such as CTGF, Runx2, ALP, Osterix, Osteopontin and Osteocalcin. In fact, the late osteogenic markers, Osteocalcin and Osteopontin, and the early markers of osteogenesis, like ALP, are less expressed than in normal osteoblasts, whereas growth factors are up-regulated or down-regulated almost as in normal osteogenic cells (Luu et al., 2007; Rochet et al., 2003). Usually, malignant osteoblastic cells fail to undergo terminal osteoblastic differentiation. The aggressiveness and the metastatic potential of OS cells seem to depend on this dedifferentiation. Furthermore, OS cells seem to originate from mesenchymal stem cell which could involve at the initiation step cell cycle gene deregulations like p16/CDKN2 (Mohseny et al., 2009; Tang et al., 2008) or p53 (Tatria et al., 2006), followed by the defect of growth factor stimulation or their over-expression. Other pathways implicated in further osteoblastic differentiation will interfere later on. In the further paragraphs, the different biomarkers will be artificially classified depending on their potential and main roles in OS development. Therefore, cell cycle genes will be first described, followed by the major osteoblastic growth factors involved in OS dedifferentiation and in OS proliferation, as well as the Wnt signaling pathway. The main transcription factors of osteoblastic differentiation will be discussed thereafter in order to understand from the very early steps to the last one how they are acting and could interfere into OS initiation step and/or metastatic spread. Most of the growth and transcription factors listed below are precisely modulated during skeletal development and will be over-expressed or under-expressed, when needed in osteoblastic cells, in osteoclasts and/or for cell-matrix interactions. Most of the deregulations characterized in OS cells are also based on this modulated expression explaining why some of these molecular factors are at once under or over-expressed depending on the model of research and the status of OS cells.

The chapters below and the figure 1 are explaining the involvement of the multiple normal osteogenic signaling patways and their deregulations in osteosarcoma cells.

4.1 The cell cycle genes

In OS, cell cycle genes like p53, Rb, p16, MDM2, CDK4 or FOS are implicated as in most of the other cancers. In this malignant bone tumor, numerous cytogenetic studies described a variety of genetic alterations like the inactivation of Rb and/p53 pathways. These two genes are usually very frequently altered (Entz-Werlé et al., 2003) but they are functioning as co-activator of transcription factor like Runx2 (Thomas et al., 2004). MDM2 and p53 dys-expressions are also cooperating to disrupt the osteogenic differentiation into a osteoblastic precursor (Lengner et al., 2006). Because of their high frequency alterations, they were suspected to be part of the initiation step of osteosarcomagenesis, as already demonstrated in publications showing the MSC implication in the origins of OS. All these characteristics were also confirmed in genetically engineered mice where cell cycle genes are defective (Janeway & Walkley, 2011; Walkley et al., 2008).

4.2 the osteoblastic growth factors and their receptors, which are favoring the OS cell dedifferentiation

Fibroblast growth factors (FGFs) are growth factors favoring in tumor cells the increase of motility and the cell ability to microenvironment invasion. Their main receptors, FGFR1, FGFR2 and FGFR3 were described as essential osteoblastic cell surface receptors, as the inherited mutation of these genes result in skeletal dysplasia (Kan et al., 2002; Bellus et al., 2000; Bellus et al., 1996). During intramembranous ossification, FGFR4 seems to be also an important regulator of osteogenesis with involvement in preosteoblast proliferation, as well as in osteoblast functioning, explaining why it is more frequently amplified than the other FGFRs (Entz-Werlé et al., 2007a). In OS cell, alterations of the FGFs/FGFRs systems are less frequent than other genes (Entz-Werlé et al., 2007a; Mendoza et al., 2005), but they are playing a role in the activation of Runx2, which is stimulated by the activated Protein Kinase C (Kim et al., 2006), and in the modulation of OS cell interactions with thebone matrix and vessels (Georgios et al., 2011).

Connective Tissue growth Factor (CTGF), a member of the CCN family, is a modulator for osteoblast and chondrocyte differentiation and is involved in vascular endothelial cell development during endochondral ossification (Luo et al., 2004). As in uncommitted preosteoblast progenitors, CTGF is up-regulated in most of the OS cells (Luo et al., 2008; Perbal et al., 2008), contributing to maintain the undifferentiated status and may also be implicated in angiogenic pathway deregulation (mainly, VEGF and HIF1α) during OS formation (Nishida et al., 2009).

4.3 The osteoblastic growth factors and their receptors, which are also involved in OS cell proliferation

Bone Morphogenetic Proteins (BMPs) belong to the TGFβ family and are considered as pivotal growth factors of early MSC commitment to osteogenic lineage. The osteogenic BMPs include 2, 4, 6, 7 and 9 (Deng et al., 2008; Tang et al., 2008; Reddi, 1998). Even at early stages of osteogenic differentiation, these BMPs are inducing the expression of CTGF, ALP, inhibitor of DNA-binding (Id), transcription factors, like TWIST and Runx2 (Hayashi et al., 2007). The up-regulation of these specific BMPs in OS is predominantly promoting the tumor growth and OS cell proliferation (Luo et al., 2008) throughout the stimulation of most of its target genes listed above. They are also favoring the interactions between OS cells and the bone matrix.

Platelet-derived Growth factor (PDGF)/ Platelet-derived Growth factor receptor (PDGFR) signaling is preferentially playing a role in the regulation of normal osteoblastic cell proliferation and, consequently, in the deregulation of OS cell proliferation. It is also promoting malignant cell motility (Kumar et al., 2010) and it is implicated in osteoblast-osteoclast interactions (Sanchez-Fernandez et al., 2008). When the PDGF/PDGFR signaling pathway is stimulated, the patients are presenting a worst prognosis (Hassan et al., 2011; Entz-Werlé et al., 2007b).

4.4 From early to later transcriptional factors of osteoblastic differentiation

Twist, or Twist-1, and its homolog dermo1, or Twist-2, are basic helix-loop-helix (bHLH) transcription factor involved as others in osteoblastogenesis. Twist1 expression negatively regulates osteoblast differentiation and maintains osteoblastic cells in a osteoprogenitor-like state. Accordingly, Twist1 silencing enhances the osteoblast differentiation program, by acting at very early step, and mediates MSC commitment and growth (Isenman et al., 2009). This transcription factor is interacting with Id-1 and Id-2, other HLH proteins, and it is cooperating with Msx2 and BMPs. Twist1 downregulation alters usually Runx2 expression, whereas it is having at once a double effect on FGFR2 (an up-regulation or a repression activity). However, the main role of twist1 downregulation is resulting into a reduced cell apoptosis (Miraoui & Marie, 2010). These functional roles are explaining the role of Twist 1 in case of deleted and amplified gene in the OS, respectively favoring disruption of cell apoptosis and dedifferentiation of OS cells (Entz-Werlé et al., 2005 and 2007). It seem also to act at the initiation step of OS development as it was demonstrated in a double mutant mouse with Twist haploinsufficiency (Entz-Werlé et al., 2010). Dermo1 is also acting as a negative regulator of osteochondrogenesis, while promoting MSC growth and proliferation throughout the regulation of Id1 and Id-2 gene expression (Tran et al., 2010 ; Zhang et al., 2008). It is a direct transcription target of the canonical Wnt pathway and it is participating to the feedback loop of this pathway (Tran et al., 2010), but it was still yet not involved in OS development.

Runx2 is a member of the DNA-binding transcription factor family that regulates the expression of multiple genes involved in cellular differentiation and cell-cycle progression. It is genetically essential for bone development and osteoblast maturation. It is interacting with numerous transcription activators and repressors such as Rb, PTH/PTHrP, MAPLK and histone deacetylases (Deng et al., 2008; Thomas et al., 2004). It is also a critical regulator in BMP-mediated osteogenic differentiation and is having interactions during normal osteogenesis with the Wnt signaling pathway. It is physically interacting with the hypophosphorylated form of Rb to promote terminal cell cycle exit and the differentiated osteoblastic phenotype (Thomas et al., 2004). It is acting at the pre-osteoblastic step after its activation by IHH (Indian Hedge Hog). In OS tumors, Runx2 is frequently over-expressed leading to stop osteoblast maturation and to promote metastatic spread (Thomas et al., 2004; Won et al., 2009), favoring the development of a highly aggressive disease and less differentiated OS cells (Martin et al., 2011). Controversially, other publications observed Runx2 low expression in OS cells (Entz-Werlé et al., 2010; Luo et al., 2008). These opposite results are not to be oddly considered and should provoke debate around the schedule of Runx2 activation or under-expression during osteosarcomatogeneis. In fact, a higher expression is needed in case of OS initiation and at metastatic spread but in the interval period, Runx2 could have a normal expression or could be under-expressed (Thomas et al., 2004). Its counterparts Runx1 and Runx3 are also having potential but discussed roles in osteoblastic and chondrogenic differentiation, but up to date and to our knowledge no data are available on their potential implication in OS cells.

Osterix is a zinc finger-containing transcription factor, which is, as Runx2, an important regulator of osteogenic differentiation (Deng et al., 2008), it is a downstream signal after Runx2 action in osteoblastic cell lineage differentiation and seem to be regulated by Runx3. Its normal expression in osteoblastic cells is linked to less osteolysis and suppress the cell migration. It seems to have low expression in OS cells allowing to promote tumor growth and metastases (Cao et al., 2005).

All these growth and transcription factors are more or less cooperating or interacting with the canonical Wnt signaling pathway and the metabolic pathways linked to bone angiogenesis (Broadhead et al., 2011; Wan et al., 2010; Araldi & Schipani, 2010; Deng et al., 2008; Haydon et al., 2007; Luo et al., 2004), which are described below.

4.5 Wnt osteoblastic signaling pathways

The **Wnt signaling pathway** is characterized by the binding of Wnt proteins to the cell-surface receptors of the Frizzled family and its co-receptor LRP5/6, causing, then, the activation of Dishevelled (DSH) family proteins. These activated DSH proteins are inhibiting a complex of proteins, including axin, GSK3 and APC proteins. This complex normally promotes the proteolytic degradation of βcatenin. In case of Axin/GSK3/APC complex inhibition, βcatenin will be stabilized and, then, able to enter the nucleus for interactions with TCF/LEF family transcription factors and to promote specific gene expression (for example, fibronectin, c-Myc or cyclin D1). During bone formation, this pathway is predominantly linked to limb development and seems to act in the terminal differentiation of osteoblast, shunting also away cells from the chondrogenic differentiation (Monaghan et al., 2001). An increase of lytic lesions is linked with the inhibition of this canonical pathway. In OS, the Wnt/βcatenin signaling is frequently activated (Entz-Werlé et al., 2003 and 2007a; Haydon et al., 2002). This up-regulation is correlated with osteoprogenitor proliferation and OS metastases (Iwaya et al., 2003), resulting from βcatenin massive nuclear translocation and/or deletion of APC. The loss of APC at DNA and protein levels was also associated to a worst outcome and less response to pre-operative chemotherapy (Guimaraes et al., 2010; Entz-Werlé et al., 2007a). This Wnt up-regulation can also induce chemoresistance throughout the repression of a bone matrix proteoglycan, syndecan 2 (Dieudonné et al., 2010).

4.6 The angiogenic and metabolic signaling pathways:

The other central pathways are those involved in angiogenesis, which is essential in normal intramembranous and endochondral ossifications, but also for tumor growth and metastatic spread. A balance between pro-angiogenic and anti-angiogenic factors is required to regulate precisely angiogenesis. This balance is tipped towards the favor of neovasculature by tissue hypoxia. Usually, in tumor environment, hypoxic conditions are stimulating the deubiquitination of Von Hippel Landau (VHL) protein, which is releasing hypoxia-inducible factor-1 alpha (HIF-1α). The stabilized form of HIF-1α is stimulating the secretion of VEGF, which is also up-regulating via FGF and TGFα signaling. The hypoxia is also regulating processes such as apoptosis and metabolic adaptation with, in particular, the release of glycolytic enzymes. (Araldi & Schipani, 2010; Wan et al., 2010; Ishida et al., 2009). HIF-1α upstream signals is involving mTor, RAS/MAPK cascade and PTEN. The angiogenesis is also the key in OS cell-bone matrix interactions, which are described below. Among all angiogenic markers, a focus will be done on those specifically involved in OS cells from the receptor ligands to the downstream transcription factors and their target genes. The different growth factors and their receptors are rather implicated in metastatic spread (Mizobuchi et al., 2008). In the angiogenesis studies, circulating growth factors can be estimated at plasma level and could help us to appreciate the implicated circulating factors.

Cystein-X-Cystein (CXC) chemokines and their receptors (CXCR) are proteins, containing 2 highly conserved cystein residues at N-terminus, and activating usually the chemotaxis of different cells. They can be also involved in various cellular processes such as skeletal rearrangements, cell migration and cell adhesion (Fernandez et al., 2002). In OS, the circulating CXC chemokines (CXCL4, CXCL6 and CXCL12) seem to present higher concentrations (Li et al., 2011), correlated with a worst outcome in patients. They also stimulate the specific angiogenic and hypoxic signaling pathways, which are favoring the metastatic spread. Moreover, in case of circulating OS cells, the CXCR/CXC chemokine system seems to drive the homing of these cells in the metastatic locations. So, the circulating OS cells expressing CXCR4 were preferentially re-localized in lung because of CXCL12/SDF-1 (Stromal cell-Derived Factor-1) high secretions in lung (Perissinotto et al., 2005). This metastatic homing may, then, be supported by the tricky release of CXC chemokines, which is under the control of VEGF (Oda et al. 2006).

Vascular Endothelial growth factor (VEGF)-A is one of the most important members of VEGF family. There are 5 other members VEGF-B, VEGF-C, VEGF-D, VEGF-E, VEGF-F and placenta growth factor (PIGF). VEGFs are binding their receptors and consequently initiating the tyrosine kinase activation and the downstream signals. The results of this process is the vessel formation. VEGF-A was mainly involved in the angiogenic processes of OS. In this context, high levels of VEGF was regularly observed in OS and especially in metastatic forms. The VEGF combined with the proteoglycans in the bone matrix was up-regulate MMP secretion in OS and, therefore, increasing the vessel formation but also the OS cells-bone matrix interactions. It is also inducing the release via the malignant cells of anti-apoptotic factors (bcl-2 and survivin) to ensure ongoing endothelial cell proliferation and neovascularization, but it will also promote the secretion of pro-angiogenic factors like FGF or angiopoietin 1. These signaling pathway are also under control of HIF1α/mTor stimulation (Yang et al., 2011 ; Hassan et al., 2011; Broadhead et al., 2011; Haydon et al., 2007; Oda et al., 2006).

Hepatocyte Growth factor (HGF) and its receptor (MET) regulate usually mitogenesis, motility and morphogenesis. In case of deregulation, it will contribute to cell transformation and tumor progression. HGF was also described recently as part of the angiogenic pathways (Hoot et al., 2010). A over-expression of MET, inconstantly associated with HGF high secretion, was usually observed in OS confirming its role in tumor progression, in angiogenesis stimulation and its correlation with a poor outcome (Hassan et al., 2010; Patane et al., 2006; Coltella et al., 2003). Surprising results were obtained showing deletion of MET gene associated with a poor outcome and a link with metastases (Entz-Werlé et al., 2007a). The sensivity enhancement of tumor cells in case of MET/FAS concomitant activation could explain partially this difference. In fact, the deletion of MET could then be considered much more in these OS as un marker of drug resistance, which was described in other cancers (Accordi et al., 2007).

Insulin like Growth Factor (IGF) systems play a key role in cellular metabolism, differentiation, proliferation, transformation and apoptosis, during normal and malignant growth of cells. In normal bone formation, IGF-I and II are known to have effects on cell proliferation and to be inducer of collagen synthesis (Bikle &Wang, 2011; Wang et al., 2006). The recent findings demonstrated that the lack of IGF-I or its receptor in osteoblasts is enhancing the signaling between osteoblasts and osteoclasts through RANKL/RANK or PTH. Nevertheless, their roles were recently extended to the regulation of tumor angiogenesis and postnatal vasculogenesis (Orciari et al., 2009). In OS, IGF I and II are often

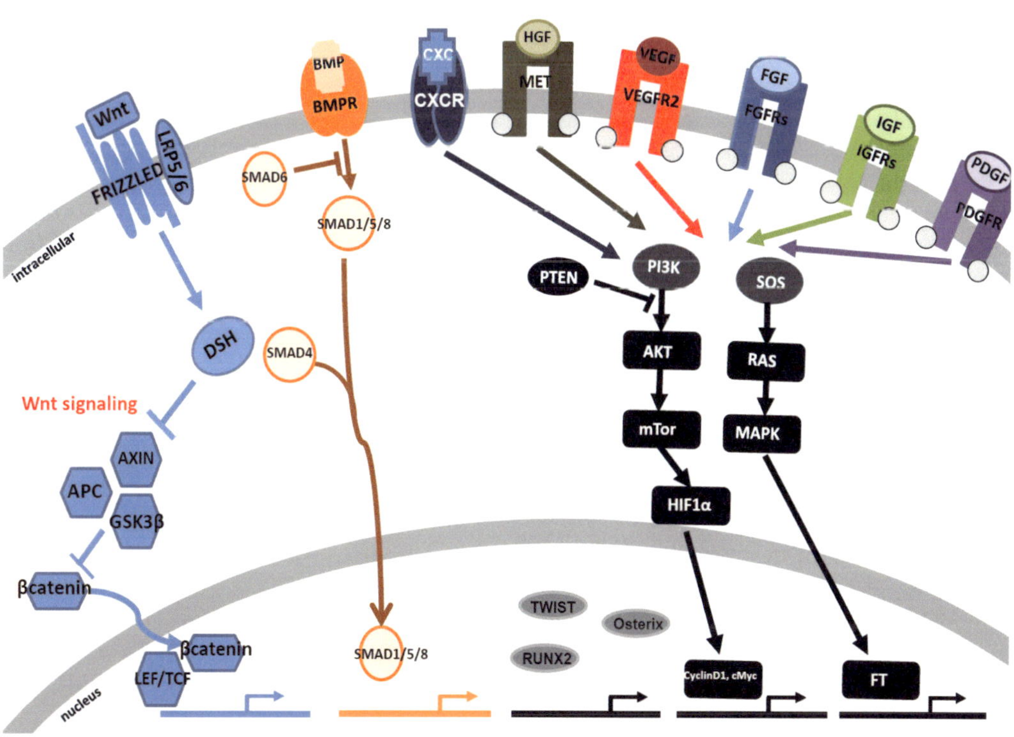

Fig. 1. A schematic summary of the major osteogenic signaling pathways involved in osteosarcomas

over-expressed. Even they are part of the osteoblastic growth regulator, they are also involved in energy homeostasis of the bone and therefore may inhibit the cell apoptosis (Hassan et al., 2011).

mTor/HIF-1α signaling and their downstream signals are playing key roles in cell proliferation and tumor hypoxia, as described above. In OS, mTor was described as an activated protein and seem to promote concomitantly with other signals the tumor progression, whereas expression of HIF-1 was mainly associated with a metastatic disease (Zhou et al., 2010; Knowles et al., 2010; Mizobuchi et al., 2010). The downstream signals like VEGF were already described as part of OS oncogenesis. Finally, few publications involved in OS the glycolytic enzymes like pyruvate kinase, for example. However, these enzymes seem to have proliferation impact (Spoden et al., 2008).

5. Deregulation of bone destruction mechanisms and cells (osteoclasts) is part of osteosarcoma progression

Osteoclasts originate from macrophage lineage and this differentiation results from a series of molecular events associating osteoclastic signals and extracellular matrix compounds. Some of these factors are required for osteoclast proliferation and differentiation, like Macrophage-Colony Stimulating factor (M-CSF), while factors like receptor activator of nuclear kβ ligand (RANKL) are more implicated in the commitment of macrophage precursors into osteoclasts and also in their survival. The RANKL/RANK activities are under the control of osteoprotegerin (OPG), which is blocking the ligand-receptor binding and subsequently the osteoclastogenesis and bone resorption (Baud'huin et al., 2011; Lamoureux et al., 2007). OPG is a potent apoptosis inhibitor of tumor necrosis factor-related apoptosis-inducing ligand (TRAIL) on tumor cells. The loss of osteoclasts in the primary tumors enhances the OS metastases (Endo-Munoz et al., 2010a). The decrease of osteoclasts is consistent with a decreased antigen-presenting activity, an enhanced chemoresistance and an impaired osteoclastogenesis (Endo-Munoz et al., 2010b). Osteoclasts are also part of the vicious cycle between bone resorption and tumor cell proliferation during tumor development. In OS, the tumor secretion of bone-modulating compounds is stimulating osteoclastic bone resorption, impacting on the release of growth factors from extracellular bone matrix. The triad RANK/RANKL/OPG seem to have play a pivotal role in this vicious cycle (Lamoureux et al., 2010). The osteoclast activity is also linked to TRACP 5A and MMP9 serum levels (Avnet et al., 2008).

The bone metabolism implicate other regulators of bone turnover like **parathyroid hormone (PTH) and parathyroid hormone related protein (PTHrP)**, which have been implicated in OS progression and especially in metastatic OS spread. PTHrP could confer also chemoresistance by blocking signaling via p53, the death receptor and the mitochondrial pathways of apoptosis (Gagiannis et al., 2009).

Upstream, the **TGFβ,** released from the degraded bone matrix, is acting on OS cells, stimulating the release of PTHrP, IL6 and IL11. These cytokines then stimulate osteoclasts, facilitating further invasion and release of pro-resorptive cytokines. After TGFβ stimulation, PTHrP and IL11 also act on osteoblasts, stimulating increased expression of RANKL (receptor activator of nuclear factor xB ligand) and M-CSF (Endo-Munoz et al., 20010b).

The normal **bone microenvironment** and **osteosarcoma matrix** during tumor development are providing optimal conditions for tumor cell proliferation and will facilitate blood vessel formation. Various protein fibrils (fibronectin, collagens, proteoglycans, integrins and laminins) and growth factors stored in matrix are contributing to tumor cell adhesion and spread. This microenvironment is usually convenient to allow detachment of OS cells from the tumor, adhesion to the extracellular matrix , local migration and invasion through stromal tissue until vascular extravasation. Extracellular matrix components such as **glycoaminoglycans** (GAGs) are also participating to the bone metabolism. In OS, GAGs over-expression is inhibiting OPG action, is acting as regulator of OPG availability and is having anti-tumor activity in bone microenvironment (Lamoureux et al., 2010). Another component of the matrix, named **Syndecan 2** (a cell surface heparin sulfate proteoglycan), can induce apoptosis and sensitize OS cells to the cytotoxic effect of chemotherapies (Orosco et al., 2007; Modrowski et al., 2005). The **integrins** are also taking part of the bone matrix role in OS progression and seem to participate to the mTor/HIF1α signaling (Kim & Helman, 2009).

Finally, the bone metabolism is regulating by the **interactions between osteoclasts and osteoblasts**, which are cell-cell contacts but are also initiating paracrine mechanisms. In fact, osteoblasts synthesize a variety of molecules important in the recruitment and survival of osteoclast precursors and these proteins will regulate the later steps of osteoclastogenesis (Costa-Rodrigues et al., 2010). As with normal osteoblasts, osteoclasts will be stimulated by the OS cells. In fact, the malignant cells are usually presenting a high osteoclastogenic-triggering capacity, which is contributing to the normal bone destruction by the tumor cells and explaining partially the "vicious cycle" described above and below in the figure 2.

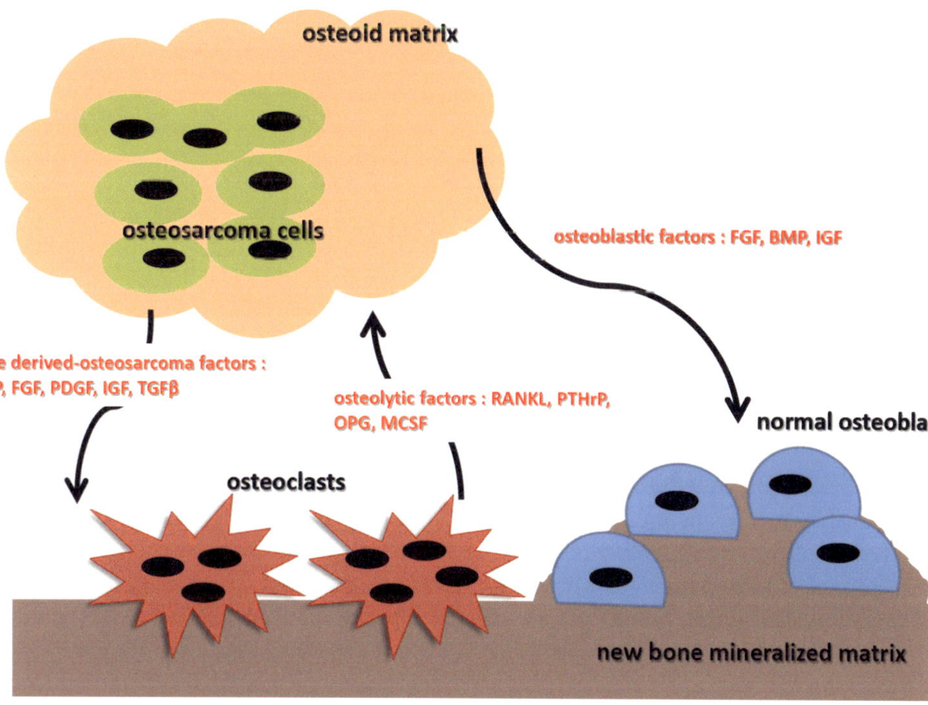

Fig. 2. A schematic summary of the bone vicious cycle involved in osteosarcoma development

6. Conclusion and future prognostic and therapeutic directions

The increase knowledge in this complex network of markers and signaling pathways involved in OS cells is now allowing to pool and extrapolate these data in a preliminary multistep osteosarcomagenesis (Figure 3).

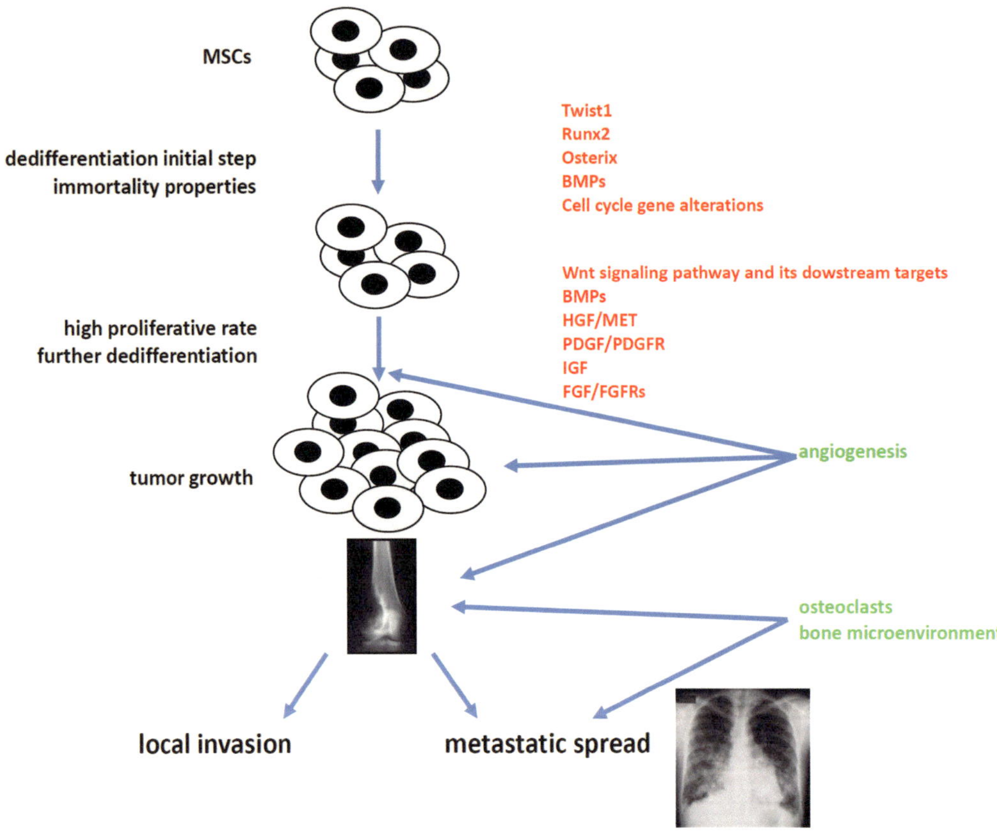

Fig. 3. An extrapolate multistep osteosarcomagenesis

Several of these biomarkers could be used as relevant prognostic factors but they have to be confirmed in larger cohorts of patients and as independent markers, like the histological Huvos grading. Among all these striking results, targeted therapies could emerge. The osteoblastic growth factors could be downregulated in case of overexpression with, for example, large spectrum inhibitors of tyrosine kinase receptors. Various PPARγ agonists may be usable to prevent proliferation and to induce terminal differentiation of malignant cells, as well as multiple anti-angiogenic approaches (antagonists of CXCR4 or VEGFR, metronomic chemotherapy, inhibition of hypoxia signaling, for example). New drugs targeting Wnt signaling pathway are also upcoming and could be usable in the next future (Chou et al., 2008; Houghton et al., 2007).

Finally, the bone destruction pathways are now considered as the larger field of innovative targeted therapies (Lamoureux et al., 2007;). The increased use of zoledronic acid in phase I and II but also in phase III is the proof of concept.

7. References

Accordi, B., Pillozzi, S., Dell'Orto, M.C., Cazzaniga, G., Arcangeli, A., Kronnie, G.T. & Basso, G. (2007). Hepatocyte growth factor receptor c-MET is associated with FAS and when activated enhances drug-induced apoptosis in pediatric B acute lymphoblastic leukemia with TEL-AML1 translocation. *J Biol Chem* 282:29384-93.

Araldi, E. & Schipani, E. (2010). Hypoxia, HIFs and bone development. *Bone* 47:190-96.

Asada, N., Tsuchiya, H. & Tomita, K. (1999). De novo deletions of p53 gene and wild-type p53 correlate with acquired cisplatin-resistance in human osteosarcoma OST cell line, *Anticancer Res* 19:5131-37.

Avnet, S., Longhi, A., Salerno, M., Halleen, J.M., Perut, F., Granchi, D., Ferrari, S., Bertoni, F., Giunti, A. & Baldini, N. (2008). Increased osteoclast activity is associated with aggressiveness of osteosarcoma. *Int J Oncol* 33:1231-38.

Bellus, G.A., Spector, E.B., Speiser, P.W., Weaver, C.A., Garber, A.T., Bryke, C.R., Israel, J., Rosengren, S.S., Webster, M.K., Donoghue, D.J. & Francomano, C.A. (2000). Distinct missense mutations of the FGFR3 lys650 codon modulate receptor kinase activation and the severity of the skeletal dysplasia phenotype. *Am J Hum Genet* 67:1411-21.

Bellus, G.A., Gaudenz, K., Zackai, E.H., Clarke, L.A., Szabo, J., Francomano, C.A. & Muenke, M. (1996). Identical mutations in three different fibroblast growth factor receptor genes in autosomal dominant craniosynostosis syndromes. *Nat Genet* 14:174-76.

Bikle, D.D. & Wang, Y. (2011). Insulin Like Growth Factor-I: A Critical Mediator of the Skeletal Response to Parathyroid Hormone. *Curr Mol Pharmacol* Jun 25. [Epub ahead of print]

Broadhead, M.L., Clark, J.C., Myers, D.E., Dass, C.R. & Choong, P.F. (2011). The molecular pathogenesis of osteosarcoma: a review. Sarcoma 2011:959248.

Bruland, O.S., Hoifodt, H., Hall, K.S., Smeland, S. & Fodstad, O. (2009). Bone marrow micrometastases studied by an immunomagnetic isolation procedure in extremity localized non-metastatic osteosarcoma patients. *Cancer Treat Res* 152:509-15.

Cao, Y., Zhou, Z., de Crombrugghe, B., Nakashima, K., Guan, H., Duan, X., Jia, S.F. & Kleinerman, E.S. (2005). Osterix, a transcription factor for osteoblast differentiation, mediates antitumor activity in murine osteosarcoma. *Cancer Res* 65:1124-28.

Chou, A.J., Geller, D.S. & Gorlick, R. (2008). Therapy for osteosarcoma: where do we go from here ? Paediatr Drugs 10:315-27.

Coltella, N., Manara, M.C., Cerisano, V., Trusolino, L., Di Renzo, M.F., Scotlandi, K. & Ferracini, R. (2003). Role of the MET/HGF receptor in proliferation and invasive behavior of osteosarcoma. *FASEB J* 17:1162-64.

Costa-Rodrigues, J., Teixeira, C.A. & Fernandes, M.H. (2011). Paracrine-mediated osteoclastogenesis by the osteosarcoma MG63 cell line: is RANKL/RANK signalling really important ? *Clin Exp Metastasis* 28:505-14.

Dass, C.R., Ek, E.T. & Choong PF. (2007). Human xenograft osteosarcoma models with spontaneous metastasis in mice: clinical relevance and applicability for drug testing. *J Cancer Res Clin Oncol* 133:193-98.

Dass, C.R., Ek, E.T., Contreras, K.G. & Choong, P.F. (2006). A novel orthotopic murine model provides insights into cellular and molecular characteristics contributing to human osteosarcoma. *Clin Exp Metastasis* 23:367-80.

Deng, Z.L., Sharff, K.A., Tang, N., Song, W.X., Luo, J., Luo, X., Chen, J., Bennett, E., Reid, R., Manning, D., Xue, A., Montag, A.G., Luu, H.H., Haydon, R.C. & He, T.C. (2008). Regulation of osteogenic differentiation during skeletal development. *Front Biosci* 13:2001-21.

Dieudonné, F.X., Marion, A., Haÿ, E., Marie, P.J. & Modrowski, D. (2010). High Wnt signaling represses the proapoptotic proteoglycan syndecan-2 in osteosarcoma cells. *Cancer Res* 70:5399-408.

Ek, E.T., Dass, C.R. & Choong, P.F. (2006). Commonly used mouse models of osteosarcoma. *Crit Rev Oncol Hematol* 60:1-8.

Endo-Munoz, L., Cumming, A., Rickwood, D., Wilson, D., Cueva, C., Ng, C., Strutton, G., Cassady, A.I., Evdokiou, A., Sommerville, S., Dickinson, I., Guminski, A. & Saunders, N.A. (2010a). Loss of osteoclasts contributes to development of osteosarcoma pulmonary metastases. *Cancer Res* 70:7063-72.

Endo-Munoz, L., Cumming, A., Sommerville, S., Dickinson, I. & Saunders, N.A. (2010b). Osteosarcoma is characterised by reduced expression of markers of osteoclastogenesis and antigen presentation compared with normal bone. *Br J Cancer* 103:73-81.

Entz-Werlé, N., Choquet, P., Neuville, A., Kuchler-Bopp, S., Clauss, F., Danse, J.M., Simo-Noumbissie, P., Guérin, E., Gaub, M.P., Freund, J.N., Boehm, N., Constantinesco, A., Lutz, P., Guenot, D. & Perrin-Schmitt, F. (2010). Targeted apc;twist double-mutant mice: a new model of spontaneous osteosarcoma that mimics the human disease. *Transl Oncol* 3:344-53.

Entz-Werle, N., Lavaux, T., Metzger, N., Stoetzel, C., Lasthaus, C., Marec, P., Kalifa, C., Brugieres, L., Pacquement, H., Schmitt, C., Tabone, M.D., Gentet, J.C., Lutz, P., Babin, A., Oudet, P., Gaub, M.P. & Perrin-Schmitt, F. (2007a). Involvement of MET/TWIST/APC combination or the potential role of ossification factors in pediatric high-grade osteosarcoma oncogenesis. *Neoplasia* 9:678-88.

Entz-Werle, N., Gaub, M.P., Lavaux, T., Marcellin, L., Metzger, N., Marec-Berard, P., Schmitt, C., Brugieres, L., Kalifa, C., Tabone, M.D., Pacquement, H., Gentet, J.C., Lutz, P., Oudet, P. & Babin, A. (2007b) KIT gene in pediatric osteosarcomas: could it be a new therapeutic target? *Int J Cancer* 120:2510-16.

Entz-Werlé, N., Stoetzel, C., Berard-Marec, P., Kalifa, C., Brugieres, L., Pacquement, H., Schmitt, C., Tabone, M.D., Gentet, J.C., Quillet, R., Oudet, P., Lutz, P., Babin-Boilletot, A., Gaub, M.P. & Perrin-Schmitt, F. (2005). Frequent genomic abnormalities at TWIST in human pediatric osteosarcomas. Int J *Cancer* 117:349-55.

Entz-Werle, N., Schneider, A., Kalifa, C., Voegeli, A.C., Tabone, M.D., Marec-Berard, P., Marcellin, L., Pacquement, H., Terrier, P., Boutard, P., Meyer, N., Gaub, M.P., Lutz, P., Babin, A., Oudet, P. (2003). Genetic alterations in primary osteosarcoma from 54 children and adolescents by targeted allelotyping. *Br J Cancer* 88:1925-31.

Fernandez, E.J. & Lolis, E. (2002). Structure, function and inhibition of chemokines. *Annu Rev Pharamcol* 42:469-99.

Feugeas, O., Guriec, N., Babin-Boilletot, A., Marcellin, L., Simon, P., Babin, S., Thyss, A., Hofman, P., Terrier, P., Kalifa, C., Brunat-Mentigny, M., Patricot, L.M. & Oberling, F. (1996). Loss of heterozygosity of the RB gene is a poor prognostic factor in patients with osteosarcoma. *J Clin Oncol* 14:467-72.

Gagiannis, S., Müller, M., Uhlemann, S., Koch, A., Melino, G., Krammer, P.H., Nawroth, P.P., Brune, M. & Schilling, T. (2009). Parathyroid hormone-related protein confers chemoresistance by blocking apoptosis signaling via death receptors and mitochondria. *Int J Cancer* 125:1551-57.

Georgios, D.A., Aikaterini, B., Dragana, N., Maria, M., Pavlos, K., Nikos, K.K. & George, T.N. (2011). Parathyroid hormone affects the fibroblast growth factor / proteoglycan signaling axis to regulate osteosarcoma cell migration. *FEBS J* Aug 11. doi: 10.1111/j.1742-4658.2011.08300.x. [Epub ahead of print]

Guimarães, A.P., Rocha, R.M., da Cunha, I.W., Guimarães, G.C., Carvalho, A.L., de Camargo, B., Lopes, A., Squire, J.A. & Soares, F.A. (2010). Prognostic impact of adenomatous polyposis coli gene expression in osteosarcoma of the extremities. *Eur J Cancer* 46:3307-15.

Hassan, S.E., Bekarev, M., Kim, M.Y., Lin, J., Piperdi, S., Gorlick, R. & Geller, D.S. (2011). Cell surface receptor expression patterns in osteosarcoma. Cancer Jul 12. doi: 10.1002/cncr.26339. [Epub ahead of print]

Hayashi, M., Nimura, K., Kashiwagi, K., Harada, T., Takaoka, K., Kato, H., Tamai, K. & Kaneda, Y. (2007). Comparative roles of Twist-1 and Id1 in transcriptional regulation by BMP signaling. *J Cell Sci* 120:1350-57.

Haydon, R.C., Lau, H.H. & He, T.C. (2007). Osteosarcoma and osteoblastic differentiation: a new perspective on oncogenesis. *Clin Orthop Relat Res* 454:237-46.

Haydon, R.C., Deyrup, A., Ishikawa, A., Heck, R., Jiang, W., Zhou, L., Feng, T., King, D., Cheng, H., Breyer, B., Peabody, T., Simon, M.A., Montag, A.G. & He, T.C. (2002). Cytoplasmic and/or nuclear accumulation of the beta-catenin protein is a frequent event in human osteosarcoma. *Int J Cancer* 102:338-42.

Hoot, K.E., Oka, M., Han, G., Bottinger, E., Zhang, Q. & Wang, X.J. (2010). HGF upregulation contributes to angiogenesis in mice with keratinocyte-specific Smad2 deletion. *J Clin Invest* 120:3606-16.

Houghton, P.J., Morton, C.L., Tucker, C., Payne, D., Favours, E., Cole, C., Gorlick, R., Kolb, E.A., Zhang, W., Lock, R., Carol, H., Tajbakhsh, M., Reynolds, C.P., Maris, J.M., Courtright, J., Keir, S.T., Friedman, H.S., Stopford, C., Zeidner, J., Wu, J., Liu, T., Billups, C.A., Khan, J., Ansher, S., Zhang, J. & Smith, M.A. (2007). The pediatric preclinical testing program: description of models and early testing results. *Pediatr Blood Cancer* 49:928-40.

Isenmann, S., Arthur, A., Zannettino, A.C., Turner, J.L., Shi, S., Glackin, C.A. & Gronthos, S. (2009). TWIST family of basic helix-loop-helix transcription factors mediate human mesenchymal stem cell growth and commitment. *Stem Cells* 27:2457-68.

Iwaya, K., Ogawa, H., Kuroda, M., Izumi, M., Ishida, T. & Makai K. (2003). Cytoplasmic and/or nuclear staining of beta-catenin is associated with lung metastases. *Clin Exp Metast* 6:525-29.

Janeway, K.A. & Walkley, C.R. (2011). Modeling human osteosarcoma in mouse: from bedside to bench. *Bone* 47:859-65.

Jones KB. Osteosarcomagenesis: modeling cancer initiation in the mouse. Sarcoma 2011:694136.

Juergens, H., Kosloff, C., Nirenberg, A., Mehta, B.M., Huvos, A.G. & Rosen, G. (1981). Prognostic factors in the response of primary osteogenic sarcoma to preoperative chemotherapy (high-dose methotrexate with citrovorum factor). *Natl Cancer Inst Monogr* 56:221-26.

Kan, S.H., Elanko, N., Johnson, D., Cornejo-Roldan, L., Cook, J., Reich, E.W., Tomkins, S., Verloes, A., Twigg, S.R., Rannan-Eliya, S., McDonald-McGinn, D.M., Zackai, E.H., Wall, S.A., Muenke, M. &, Wilkie, A.O. (2002). Genomic screening of fibroblast growth-factor receptor 2 reveals a wide spectrum of mutations in patients with syndromic craniosynostosis. *Am J Hum Genet* 70:472-86.

Kim, S.Y. & Helman, L.I. (2009). Strategies to explore new approaches in the investigation and treatment of osteosarcoma. *Cancer Treat Res* 152:517-28..

Kim, B.G., Kim, H.J., Park, H.J., Kim, Y.J., Yoon, W.J., Lee, S.J., Ryoo, H.M. & Cho, J.Y. (2006). Runx2 phosphorylation induced by fibroblast growth factor-2/protein kinase C pathways. *Proteomics* 6:1166-74.

Knowles, H.J., Schaefer, K.L., Dirksen, U. & Athanasou, N.A. (2010). Hypoxia and hypoglycaemia in Ewing's sarcoma and osteosarcoma: regulation and phenotypic effects of Hypoxia-Inducible Factor. *BMC Cancer* 10:372.

Kubista, B., Klinglmueller, F., Bilban, M., Pfeiffer, M., Lass, R., Giurea, A., Funovics, P.T., Toma, C., Dominkus, M., Kotz, R., Thalhammer, T., Trieb, K., Zettl, T. & Singer, C.F. (2011). Microarray analysis identifies distinct gene expression profiles associated with histological subtype in human osteosarcoma. *Int Orthop* 35:401-11.

Kumar, A., Salimath, B.P., Stark, G.B. & Finkenzeller, G. (2010). Platelet-derived growth factor receptor signaling is not involved in osteogenic differentiation of human mesenchymal stem cells. *Tissue Eng Part A* 16:983-93.

Lamoureux, F, Moriceau, G., Picarda, G., Rousseau, J., Trichet, V. & Redini, F. (2010). Regulation of osteoprotegerin pro- or anti-tumoral activity by bone tumor microenvironment. *Biochim Biophys Acta* 1805(1):17-24.

Lamoureux, F., Richard, P., Wittrant, Y., Battaglia, S., Pilet, P., Trichet, V., Blanchard, F., Gouin, F., Pitard, B., Heymann, D. & Redini, F. (2007). Therapeutic relevance of osteoprotegerin gene therapy in osteosarcoma: blockade of the vicious cycle between tumor cell proliferation and bone resorption. *Cancer Res* 67:7308-18.

Lau, C.C. (2009). Molecular classification of osteosarcoma. *Cancer Treat Res* 152:459-65.

Lau, H.H., Song, W.X., Lao, X., Manning, D, Luo, J., Deng, Z.L., Sharff, K.A., Montag, A.G., Haydon, R.C. & He, T.C. (2007). Distinct roles of bone morphogenetic proteins in osteogenic differentiation of mesenchymal stem cells. *J Orthop Res* 25:665-77.

Le Deley, M.C., Guinebretière, J.M., Gentet, J.C., Pacquement, H., Pichon, F., Marec-Bérard, P., Entz-Werlé, N., Schmitt, C., Brugières, L., Vanel, D., Dupoüy, N., Tabone, M.D., Kalifa, C. & Société Française d'Oncologie Pédiatrique (SFOP). (2007). SFOP OS94: a randomised trial comparing preoperative high-dose methotrexate plus doxorubicin to high-dose methotrexate plus etoposide and ifosfamide in osteosarcoma patients. *Eur J Cancer* 43:752-61.

Lengner, C.J., Steinman, H.A., Gagnon, J., Smith, T.W., Henderson, J.E., Kream, B.E., Stein, G.S., Lian, J.B. & Jones, S.N. (2006). Osteoblast differentiation and skeletal development are regulated by Mdm2-p53 signaling. *J Cell Biol* 172:909-21.

Li, Y., Flores, R., Yu, A., Okcu, M.F., Murray, J., Chintagumpala, M., Hicks, J., Lau, C.C. & Man, T.K. (2011). Elevated expression of CXC chemokines in pediatric osteosarcoma patients. *Cancer* 117:207-17.

Luk, F., Yu, Y., Dong, H.T., Walsh, W.R. & Yang, J.L. (2011). New gene groups associated with dissimilar osteoblastic differentiation are linked to osteosarcomagenesis. *Cancer Genomics Proteomics* 8:65-75.

Luo, J., Chen, J., Deng, Z.L., Lao, X., Song, W.X., Sharff, K.A, Tang, N., Haydon, R.C., Lau, H.H. & He, T.C. (2007). Wnt signaling and human diseases, what are the therapeutic implications ? *Curr Gene Ther* 5:167-79.

Luo, Q., Kang, Q., Si, W., Jiang, W., Park, J.K., Peng, Y., Li, X., Luu, H.H., Luo, J., Montag, A.G., Haydon, R.C. & He, T.C. (2004). Connective tissue growth factor (CTGF) is regulated by Wnt and bone morphogenetic proteins signaling in osteoblast differentiation of mesenchymal stem cells. *J Biol Chem* 279:55958-68.

Luo X, Chen J, Song WX, Tang N, Luo J, Deng ZL, Sharff KA, He G, Bi Y, He BC, Bennett E, Huang J, Kang Q, Jiang W, Su Y, Zhu GH, Yin H, He Y, Wang Y, Souris JS, Chen L, Zuo GW, Montag AG, Reid RR, Haydon RC, Luu HH, He TC. (2008). Osteogenic BMPs promote tumor growth of human osteosarcomas that harbor differentiation defects. *Lab Invest* 88:1264-77.

Luu, H.H., Song, W.X., Luo, X., Manning, D., Luo, J., Deng, Z.L., Sharff, K.A., Montag, A.G., Haydon, R.C. & He, T.C. (2007). Distinct roles of bone morphogenetic proteins in osteogenic differentiation of mesenchymal stem cells. *J Orthop Res* 25:665-77.

Luu, H.H., Kang, Q., Park, J.K., Si, W., Luo, Q., Jiang, W., Yin, H., Montag, A.G., Simon, M.A., Peabody, T.D., Haydon, R.C., Rinker-Schaeffer, C.W. & He, T.C. (2005). An orthotopic model of human osteosarcoma growth and spontaneous pulmonary metastasis. *Clin Exp Metastasis* 22:319-29.

Marina, N., Gebhardt, M., Teot, L. & Gorlick, R. (2004). Biology and therapeutic advances for pediatric osteosarcoma, *Oncologist* 9:422-41.

Martin, J.W., Zielenska, M., Stein, G.S., van Wijnen, A.J. & Squire, J.A. (2011). The Role of RUNX2 in Osteosarcoma Oncogenesis. *Sarcoma* 2011:282745. Epub 2010 Dec 9.

Matsuo, K. & Irie, N. (2008). Osteoclast-osteoblast communication. Arch Biochem Biophys 473:201-9.

Mizobuchi, H., García-Castellano, J.M., Philip, S., Healey, J.H. & Gorlick, R. (2008) Hypoxia markers in human osteosarcoma: an exploratory study. *Clin Orthop Relat Res* 466:2052-9.

McNairn, J.D., Damron, T.A., Landas, S.K., Ambrose, J.L. & Shrimpton, A.E. (2001). Inheritance of osteosarcoma and Paget's disease of bone: a familial loss of heterozygosity study. *J Mol Diagn* 3:171-77.

Mendoza, S., David, H., Gaylord, G.M. & Miller, C.W. (2005). Allelic loss at 10q26 in osteosarcoma intthe region of BUB3and FGFR2 genes. *Cancer Genet Cytogenet* 158:142-17.

Mirabello, L., Troisi, R.J. & Savage, S.A. (2009). Osteosarcoma incidence and survival rates from 1973 to 2004: data from the Surveillance, Epidemiology, and End Results Program. *Cancer* 115:1531-43.

Miraoui, H. & Marie, P.J. (2010). Pivotal role of Twist in skeletal biology and pathology. *Gene* 458:1-7.

Modrowski, D., Orosco, A., Thévenard, J., Fromigué, O. & Marie, P.J. (2005). Syndecan-2 overexpression induces osteosarcoma cell apoptosis: Implication of syndecan-2 cytoplasmic domain and JNK signaling. *Bone* 37:180-9.

Mohseny, A.B., Szuhai, K., Romeo, S., Buddingh, E.P., Briaire-de Bruijn, I., de Jong, D., van Pel, M., Cleton-Jansen, A.M. & Hogendoorn, P.C. (2009). Osteosarcoma originates from mesenchymal stem cells in consequence of aneuploidization and genomic loss of Cdkn2. *J Pathol* 219:294-305.

Monaghan, H., Bubb, V.J., Sirimujalin, R., Millward-Sadler, S.J. & Salter, D.M. (2001). Adenomatous polyposis coli (APC), beta-catenin, and cadherin are expressed in human bone and cartilage. *Histopathology* 39:611-9.

Mueller, F., Fuchs, B. & Kaser-Hotz, B. (2007). Comparative biology of human and canine osteosarcoma. *Anticancer Res* 27:155-64.

Nielsen, G.P., Burns, K.L., Rosenberg, A.E. & Louis, D.N. (1998). CDKN2A gene deletions and loss of p16 expression occur in osteosarcomas that lack RB alterations. *Am J Pathol* 153:159-163.

Nishida, T., Kondo, S., Maeda, A., Kubota, S., Lyons, K.M. & Takigawa, M. (2009). CCN family 2/connective tissue growth factor (CCN2/CTGF) regulates the expression of Vegf through Hif-1alpha expression in a chondrocytic cell line, HCS-2/8, under hypoxic condition. Bone 44:24-31.

Oda, Y., Yamamoto, H., Tamiya, S., Matsuda, S., Tanaka, K., Yokoyama, R., Iwamoto, Y. & Tsuneyoshi, M. (2006). CXCR4 and VEGF expression in the primary site and the metastatic site of human osteosarcoma: analysis within a group of patients, all of whom developed lung metastasis. *Mod Pathol* 19:738-45.

Orciari, S., Di Nuzzo, S., Lazzarini, R., Caprari, P., Procopio, A. & Catalano, A. (2009). The effects of insulin and insulin-like growth factors on tumor vascularization: new insights of insulin-like growth factor family in cancer. *Curr Med Chem* 16:3931-42.

Orosco, A., Fromigué, O., Bazille, C., Entz-Werle, N., Levillain, P., Marie, P.J. & Modrowski, D. (2007). Syndecan-2 affects the basal and chemotherapy-induced apoptosis in osteosarcoma. *Cancer Res* 8:3708-15.

Patanè, S., Avnet, S., Coltella, N., Costa, B., Sponza, S., Olivero, M., Vigna, E., Naldini, L., Baldini, N., Ferracini, R., Corso, S., Giordano, S., Comoglio, P.M. & Di Renzo, M.F. (2006). MET overexpression turns human primary osteoblasts into osteosarcomas. *Cancer Res* 66:4750-57.

Perbal, B., Zuntini, M., Zambelli, D., Serra, M., Sciandra, M., Cantiani, L., Lucarelli, E., Picci, P. & Scotlandi, K. (2008). Prognostic value of CCN3 in osteosarcoma. *Clin Cancer Res* 14:701-9.

Perissinotto, E., Cavalloni, G., Leone, F., Fonsato, V., Mitola, S., Grignani, G., Surrenti, N., Sangiolo, D., Bussolino, F., Piacibello, W. & Aglietta, M. (2005). Involvement of chemokine receptor 4/stromal cell-derived factor 1 system during osteosarcoma tumor progression. *Clin Cancer Res* 11:490-7.

PosthumaDeBoer, J., Witlox, M.A., Kaspers, G.J. & van Royen, B.J. (2011). Molecular alterations as target for therapy in metastatic osteosarcoma: a review of literature. *Clin Exp Metastasis* 28:493-503.

Reddi, A.H. (1998). Role of morphogenetic proteins in skeletal tissue engineering and regeneration. *Nature Biotech* 3:247-252.

Rochet, N., Loubat, A., Laugier, J.P., Hofman, P., Bouler, J.M., Daculsi, G., Carle, G.F. & Rossi, B. (2003). Modification of gene expression induced in human osteogenic and osteosarcoma cells by culture on a biphasic calcium phosphate bone substitute. *Bone* 32:602-10.

Rousseau, J., Escriou, V., Perrot, P., Picarda, G., Charrier, C., Scherman, D., Heymann, D., Rédini, F. & Trichet, V. (2010). Advantages of bioluminescence imaging to follow siRNA or chemotherapeutic treatments in osteosarcoma preclinical models. *Cancer Gene Ther* 17:387-97.

Sadikovic, B., Yoshimoto, M., Al-Romaih, K., Maire, G., Zielenska, M. & Squire, J.A. (2008). In vitro analysis of integrated global high-resolution DNA methylation profiling with genomic imbalance and gene expression in osteosarcoma. *PLoS One* 3:e2834.

Sanchez-Fernandez, M.A., Gallois, A., Riedl, T., Jurdic, P. & Hoflack, B. (2008). Osteoclasts control osteoblast chemotaxis via PDGF-BB/PDGF receptor beta signalling. *PLoS One* 3:e3537.

Smida, J., Baumhoer, D., Rosemann, M., Walch, A., Bielack, S., Poremba, C., Remberger, K., Korsching, E., Scheurlen, W., Dierkes, C., Burdach, S., Jundt, G., Atkinson, M.J. & Nathrath, M. (2010). Genomic alterations and allelic imbalances are strong prognostic predictors in osteosarcoma. *Clin Cancer Res* 16:4256-67.

Smith-Sorensen, B., Gebhardt, M;C;, Kloen, P., McINtyre, J., Aguilar, F., Cerruti, P. & Borresen, A.L. (1993). Screening for TP53 mutations in osteosarcomas using constant denaturant gel electrophoresis (CDGE). *Hum Mutant* 2:274-285.

Sottnik, J.L., Duval, D.L., Ehrhart, E.J. & Thamm, D.H. (2010). An orthotopic, postsurgical model of luciferase transfected murine osteosarcoma with spontaneous metastasis. *Clin Exp Metastasis* 27:151-60.

Spoden, G.A., Mazurek, S., Morandell, D., Bacher, N., Ausserlechner, M.J., Jansen-Dürr, P., Eigenbrodt, E. & Zwerschke, W. (2008). Isotype-specific inhibitors of the glycolytic key regulator pyruvate kinase subtype M2 moderately decelerate tumor cell proliferation. *Int J Cancer* 123:312-21.

Tan, P.H., Aung, K.Z., Toh, S.L., Goh, J.C. & Nathan, S.S. (2011). Three-dimensional porous silk tumor constructs in the approximation of in vivo osteosarcoma physiology. *Biomaterials* 32:6131-7.

Tang, N., Song, W.X., Luo J., Haydon, R.C. & He, T.C. (2008). Osteosarcoma development and stem cell differentiation. *Clin Orthop Relat Res* 466:2114-2130.

Tataria, M., Quarto, N., Longaker, M.T. & Sylvester, K.G. Absence of the p53 tumor suppressor gene promotes osteogenesis in mesenchymal stem cells. *J Pediatr Surg* 41:624-32; discussion 624-32.

Thomas, D.M., Johnson, S.A., Sims, N.A., Trivett, M.K., Slavin, J.L., Rubin, B.P., Waring, P., McArthur, G.A., Walkley, C.R., Holloway, A.J., Diyagama, D., Grim, J.E., Clurman, B.E., Bowtell, D.D., Lee, J.S., Gutierrez, G.M., Piscopo, D.M., Carty, S.A. & Hinds, P.W. (2004). Terminal osteoblast differentiation, mediated by runx2 and p27KIP1, is disrupted in osteosarcoma. *J Cell Biol* 167:925-34.

Toguchida, J., Ishizaki, K., Sasaki, M.S., Nakamura, Y., Ikenaga, M., Kato, M., Sugimot, M., Kotoura, Y. & Yamamuro T. (1989). Preferential mutation of paternally derived RB gene as the initial event in sporadic osteosarcoma. *Nature* 338:156-8.

Tran, T.H., Jarrell, A., Zentner, G.E., Welsh, A., Brownell, I., Scacheri, P.C. & Atit, R. (2010). Role of canonical Wnt signaling/ß-catenin via Dermo1 in cranial dermal cell development. *Development* 137:3973-84.

Walkley, C.R., Qudsi, R., Sankaran, V.G., Perry, J.A., Gostissa, M., Roth, S.I., Rodda, S.J., Snay, E., Dunning, P., Fahey, F.H., Alt, F.W., McMahon, A.P. & Orkin, S.H. (2008).

Conditional mouse osteosarcoma, dependent on p53 loss and potentiated by loss of Rb, mimics the human disease. *Genes Dev* 22:1662-76.
Wan, C., Shao, J., Gilbert, S.R., Riddle, R.C., Long, F., Johnson, R.S., Schipani, E. & Clemens, T.L.(2010). Role of HIF-1alpha in skeletal development. *Ann N Y Acad Sci* 1192:322-6.
Wang, Y., Nishida, S., Elalieh, H.Z., Long, R.K., Halloran, B.P. & Bikle, D.D. (2006). Role of IGF-I signaling in regulating osteoclastogenesis. *J Bone Miner Res* 21:1350-58.
Wang, L.L. (2005). Biology of osteosarcoma. *Cancer J* 11:294-305.
Won, K.Y., Park, H.R. & Park Y.K. (2009). Prognostic implication of immunohistochemical Runx2 expression in osteosarcoma. *Tumori* 95:311-316.
Xu, F., Wu, J., Wang, S., Durmus, N.G., Gurkan, U.A. & Demirci, U. (2011). Microengineering methods for cell-based microarrays and high-throughput drug-screening applications. *Biofabrication* 3:034101.
Xu, F. & Burg, K.J. (2007). Three-dimensional polymeric systems for cancer cell studies. *Cytotechnology* 54:135-43.
Yang, J., Yang, D., Sun, Y, Sun, B., Wang, G., Trent, J., Araujo, D., Chen, K. & Zhang, W. (2011). Genetic amplification of the vascular endothelial growth factor (VEGF) pathway genes, including VEGFA, in human osteosarcoma. *Cancer* Apr 14. doi: 10.1002/cncr.26116. [Epub ahead of print]
Zhang, Y., Hassan, M.Q., Li, Z.Y., Stein, J.L., Lian, J.B., van Wijnen, A.J. & Stein, G.S. (2008). Intricate gene regulatory networks of helix-loop-helix (HLH) proteins support regulation of bone-tissue related genes during osteoblast differentiation. *J Cell Biochem* 105:487-96.

7

The Retinoblastoma Protein in Osteosarcomagenesis

Elizabeth Kong and Philip W. Hinds
Molecular Oncology Research Institute, Tufts Medical Center, Boston, MA USA

1. Introduction

Osteosarcoma is one of the most common primary non-hematologic bone tumors present in both children and adults. The etiology of most cases of osteosarcoma is unknown although a genetic predisposition is suspected. Most osteosarcomas are diagnosed before the age of 20, where the pathology is likely distinct from osteosarcoma diagnosed over the age of 60, which is associated with bone diseases such as Paget disease or Rothmund-Thomson syndrome. Although rare, osteosarcoma is a complication in survivors of childhood cancers treated with radiation therapy. Tumors from patients diagnosed early in life are reported to have a broad range of genetic and molecular factors that are potential targets in disease formation. However, *RB1* and/or *TP53* mutations are consistently detected in the majority of osteosarcomas. This chapter will focus on understanding the potential links between disruption of genetic components in osteogenic differentiation and osteosarcoma.

Osteosarcoma is the most frequent primary bone tumor, but is relatively rare with less than 900 new cases diagnosed each year in the United States (Sandberg and Bridge, 2003). There is considerable diversity in histologic features and grade, but osteosarcoma is defined as a malignant tumor of mesodermal origin, where tumor cells produce bone or osteoid (Schajowicz et al., 1995). There are two peaks of occurrence for osteosarcoma. The first peak is during adolescence, when approximately 70% of osteosarcomas are diagnosed (Hauben et al., 2003), but the disease is rarely diagnosed before the age of five. The second peak, accounting for approximately 10% of osteosarcomas, is observed in patients over the age of 60, and is associated with individuals with underlying non-cancerous bone diseases such as Paget, Werner or Rothmund-Thomson Syndrome or in patients previously exposed to radiation therapy (McNairn et al., 2001; Wang et al., 2001; Nellissery et al., 1998; Lindor et al., 2000; Picci, 2007; Paulino and Fowler, 2005).

Although osteosarcoma can develop in any part of the skeleton, in younger patients, areas of rapid bone growth such as the lower long bones have a higher frequency of occurrence (Mirabello et al., 2009). Osteosarcoma in the mandible or skull is more frequently seen in patients diagnosed after the 6th decade of life (Caron et al., 1971) and is often a secondary lesion (Longhi et al., 2008). Irrespective of age, approximately 80% of patients have either detectable metastasis, primarily to the lung, or sub-clinical micro-metastasis (Kaste et al., 1999). The disease is seen globally and more frequently in males compared to females (Stiller et al., 2006), but is observed earlier in females correlating to growth spurts. Osteosarcoma diagnosed during the first two decades of life is often poorly differentiated, and cells from these tumors have characteristics of early osteoprogenitor or mesenchymal progenitor cells (Dahlin, 1988; Huvos, 1993; Hopyan et al., 1999; Klein and Siegal, 2006). Correlations between early markers of osteogenesis in conventional osteosarcoma with periods of rapid cell division infer that the disease may be associated with defects in osteoblast differentiation.

Most osteosarcomas are de novo, but inherited predispositions for osteosarcoma have provided insight into possible genetic factors associated with the disease. Mouse models and *in vitro* studies have proven to be powerful tools in elucidating molecular mechanisms and the genetic pathology of osteosarcoma. Interestingly only *RB1* and/or *TP53* mutations are consistently detected in the majority of human osteosarcomas despite a broad range of reported factors associated with the disease. Presented here are some of the genetic aspects of osteosarcoma with a focus on the tumor suppressor protein, pRB, in tumor formation and metastasis.

2. The retinoblastoma tumor suppressor and osteosarcoma

Loss of *RB1* was the first genetic predisposition associated with osteosarcoma development. The predominant tumor types seen in patients with a germline mutation in the *RB1* gene are retinoblastoma, osteosarcoma and rarely small cell lung, bladder and breast carcinomas (Gurney et al., 1995). This suggests that tumors exhibiting the highest frequency of pRb loss, such as osteosarcoma, may require pRb function in multiple cell cycle exit programs and differentiation. Children with hereditary retinoblastoma have a 69-fold increased risk of osteosarcoma. Previous radiation treatment to the primary tumor site increases the risk of osteosarcoma by 406-fold (Mohney et al., 1998; Savage and Mirabello, 2011; Kitchin and Ellsworth, 1974; Gonzalez-Vasconcellos et al., 2011). Although heterozygous loss of *RB1* predisposes to tumor formation, *RB1* loss is also consistently observed in 60% of sporadic osteosarcomas (Friend et al., 1986; Hansen, 1991; Wadayama et al., 1994) and loss of *RB1* heterozygosity is associated with poor patient prognosis (Marina et al., 2004; Tang et al., 2008).

The retinoblastoma protein, pRb, is part of a regulatory pathway that is targeted in most human cancers Weinberg, 1994 Mulligan and Jacks, 1998. pRb functions in every cell type to control the exit from G1 by regulating the E2F family of transcription factors. This process is facilitated by the recruitment of histone deacetylase enzymes (HDACs), SWI/SNF and histone methyltransferases at the promoter of cell cycle genes (Alland et al., 1997; Hassig et al., 1997; Grunstein, 1997; Luo et al., 1998) to repress E2F family member activity and prevent S-phase progression. This repression promotes cell cycle exit during differentiation and senescence programs (Alexander and Hinds, 2001; Chen et al., 1996; Schneider et al., 1994; Sellers et al., 1998; Tiemann and Hinds, 1998). Regulation of pRb and thus cell cycle progression from G1 to S begins with mitogenic signals that induce activation of cell-cycle dependent kinase complexes Cdk4/Cdk6-cyclin D and Cdk2-cyclin E (Hinds et al., 1992; Kato et al., 1993; Hatakeyama et al., 1994; Sherr and Roberts, 1999; Takaki et al., 2005). These complexes phosphorylate pRb on multiple serine and threonine residues. When pRb is sufficiently hyperphosphorylated, repression of E2F is released and transcription of genes important in S-phase progression occurs (Buchkovich et al., 1989; Sherr, 1996; Dyson, 1998; Trimarchi and Lees, 2002; Bracken et al., 2004). Mechanisms that police premature entry into S phase focus on inhibition of the cyclin-Cdk complexes. These inhibitors include members of the INK4 family ($p15^{INK4b}$, $p16^{INK4a}$, $p18^{INK4c}$ and $p19^{INK4d}$), which specifically interact with Cdk4/6 and impair interaction with D-type cyclins, and CIP/KIP ($p21^{CIP1}$, $p27^{KIP1}$ and $p57^{KIP2}$) family members, that act on cyclin/CDK by forming a ternary complex (Shapiro et al., 1995; Sherr, 1996; Stiegler et al., 1998). Mutation of genes encoding members of the retinoblastoma pathway is associated with osteosarcoma, although with far less frequency than mutation of *RB1* itself.

Studies have shown that inactivation of *CDKN2A*, the gene encoding $p16^{INK4a}$, is observed in osteosarcomas (Miller et al., 1996; Benassi et al., 1999) and loss of $p27^{KIP1}$ expression has been correlated with high-grade osteosarcomas (Thomas et al., 2004). $p15^{INK4b}$ loss has been reported in osteosarcomas at a low frequency, and animals mutant for this gene develop osteosarcoma at low penetrance (Miller et al., 1996; Sharpless et al., 2001; Krimpenfort et al., 2007). Of note, increased expression of CDK4 is associated mainly with low-grade osteosarcomas (Dujardin et al., 2011).

Early *in vivo* evidence of pRb's involvement in osteosarcoma was observed in transgenic mice that expressed SV40 large T-antigen (Knowles et al., 1990). pRb can be inactivated by viral oncoproteins such as human adenovirus E1A, SV40 large T antigen, and the E7 protein of human papillomavirus type-16 (Whyte et al., 1988; DeCaprio et al., 1988; Dyson et al., 1989). By binding to pRb, the viral proteins interfere with its normal function, thus mimicking the loss of pRb (Stabel et al., 1985; Harlow et al., 1986; Lee et al., 1987; Whyte et al., 1988; DeCaprio et al., 1988; Munger et al., 1989; Vousden and Jat, 1989; Dyson et al., 1989). These animals developed metastatic osteosarcoma at about 15 months of age.

A paradox is that targeted disruption of one allele of *RB1* in mice does not lead to cancer. In addition, studies of conditional *RB1* knockout mice have shown that loss of *RB1* in mouse photoreceptor cells does not result in retinoblastoma or any other phenotypic changes in these cells (Vooijs et al., 2002). Instead, mice that are heterozygous for *RB1* show an increased predisposition to pituitary and thyroid tumors within one year of age, which are associated with a loss of heterozygosity at the *RB1* locus (Jacks et al., 1992; Williams et al., 1994). Often tumor formation in mouse models requires the loss of p107 or p130, pRb related pocket protein family members, which may account for the phenotypes seen in $RB1^{-/-}$ animals (Dannenberg et al., 2004). Contrary to osteosarcoma seen in humans, where only the loss of *RB1* appears to be required for tumor formation. $RB1^{-/+}$; $p107^{-/-}$ or $RB1^{-/+}$;$p130^{-/-}$ animals do develop retinoblastoma and osteosarcoma mimicking the loss of *RB1* in humans (Dannenberg et al., 2004). Neither $p107^{-/-}$ nor $p130^{-/-}$ mutant mouse strains have apparent phenotypes (Cobrinik et al., 1992; Lee et al., 1996). Additional mouse models of osteosarcoma include animals with the loss of both *RB1* and *Trp53*.

A significant proportion of osteosarcomas have mutations in p53, thus identifying p53 loss as a predisposition to the disease. p53 mutations were initially observed in sporadic osteosarcoma, and then discovered in approximately 3% of patients diagnosed with Li-Fraumeni syndrome, an autosomal dominant disorder characterized by a germline mutation of *TP53* (Li and Fraumeni, 1969; Hisada et al., 1998; Porter et al., 1992; Upton et al., 2009). Mice bearing germline disruption of Trp53 (which encodes p53 in mice) develop a wide variety of tumors, including osteosarcoma, which is observed in up to 32% of heterozygous Trp53 mutant animals (Harvey et al., 1993; Olive et al., 2004). Significantly, when *Trp53* is deleted from *RB1* heterozygous mice, the animals develop retinal dysplasia (Morgenbesser et al., 1994). Work from two separate groups generated an animal model with conditional targeted mutations in the bone of both *RB1* and *Trp53*. The combined loss of both tumor suppressors greatly enhances the formation of osteosarcomas and additional neoplasms not observed to be associated with the loss of *RB1* in humans such as rhabdomyosarcoma, neuroendocrine tumors and hibernomas (Berman et al., 2008; Walkley et al., 2008). This indicates that loss of p53 could be a rate-limiting event in the initiation of this tumor in mice in the context of germline *RB1* mutations, but not in humans. Although the loss of p53 or variants of p53 are observed in 22% of osteosarcomas, these occurrences have yet to consistently correlate with disease stage or prognosis (Wunder et al., 2005; Ta et al., 2009). Tumor cells from both human and mouse osteosarcomas have characteristics of early osteoprogenitor and arguably mesenchymal progenitor cells. These cells are multipotent, have some self-renewal capacity, and often lack late markers of osteogenesis. This absence of differentiation and progenitor-like phenotype in conventional osteosarcoma suggests that disruption of osteoblast differentiation may be a critical event in tumor formation.

3. Osteogenesis

The transition from mesenchymal stem cell to osteoprogenitor and preosteoblast requires activation of the transcription factor Runx2 (AML3; Osf2; Cbfa1; PEBP2aA; Pebp2a1). Runx2 (runt-related transcription factor 2) is a transcription factor that belongs to the Runx family (Komori, 2002) and acquires DNA binding activity by heterodimerizing with Cbfβ (Kundu et al., 2002; Miller et al., 2002; Yoshida et al., 2002). *Runx2*$^{-/-}$ mice lack bone formation due to the absence of osteoblast differentiation, and die just after birth (Komori et al., 1997; Otto et al., 1997). Runx2 is found to be restricted to the mesenchymal condensations that form bone (Ducy et al., 1997). Thus, Runx2 is termed the master regulator/platform protein of osteoblast differentiation and is essential to bone formation. In rare cases, *RUNX2* amplification is observed in osteosarcoma, but Runx2 function in tumorigenesis has yet to be identified. Preliminary reports suggest that an increased level of Runx2 is associated with chemoresistance (Kurek et al., 2010; Longhi et al., 2006) and that high expression of Runx2 may be related to metastasis in osteosarcoma (Won et al., 2009). However, other studies suggest that Runx2 function may be impaired during the process of osteosarcomagenesis, despite its elevated expression in these tumors (Thomas et al., 2004).

Early evidence for a role for pRb in osteogenesis came from the discovery that osteoblast differentiation can be inhibited in cells by the viral oncoproteins SV40 large T antigen and E1A, which specifically target the pocket proteins (Feuerbach et al., 1997). These studies showed that osteoblasts immortalized by temperature sensitive SV40 large T antigen targeting pRb demonstrate reduced expression of late markers of differentiation. This process can be reversed by deactivation of the viral oncoproteins (Feuerbach et al., 1997). The reintroduction of a pRb variant (R661W), discovered in a patient tumor sample that lacks canonical E2F binding capacity, is capable of arresting and differentiating osteosarcoma cells (SAOS2) (Sellers et al., 1998). Thus, the ability of pRb to promote osteoblast differentiation may be separable from its role as a regulator of the E2F family of transcription factors. These observations established a clear connection between pRb and osteogenesis.

pRb has been shown to directly bind to Runx2 in osteoblasts. The pRb-Runx2 complex can localize to the promoter of a late bone specific marker, osteocalcin, and promote transcriptional activity. In the absence of pRb, expression of osteocalcin is significantly reduced. The pRb-Runx2 complex also involves the transcription factor HES1. This process appears to be specific to pRb and not the other pocket protein family members, p107 and p130 (Thomas et al., 2001; Lee et al., 2006). In osteosarcoma cell lines, pRb was shown to be necessary for displacement of RBP2 (KDM5A/JARID1A), a histone demethylase, from the osteocalcin promoter to relieve repression (Benevolenskaya et al., 2005). Thus, pRb is required for the transcriptional activation of the osteocalcin promoter and in removing repressive components late in differentiation. Increasing evidence suggests that pRb may also be important in early osteogenesis and osteoblast lineage commitment (Figure 1).

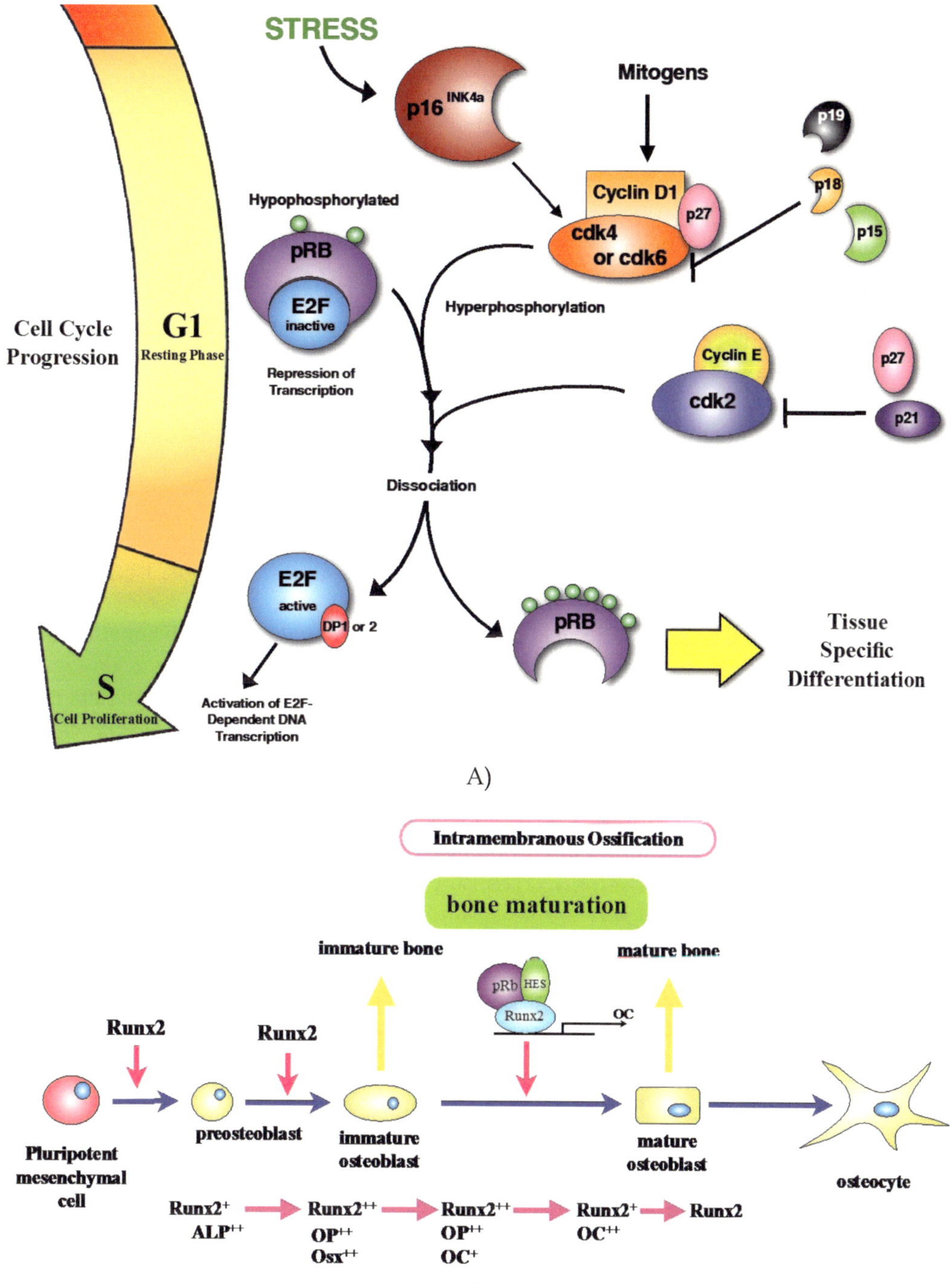

Fig. 1. Schematic of the retinoblastoma pathway and osteoblast differentiation

A) Progression through the cell cycle from G1 to S begins with mitogenic signals that induce activation of cell-cycle dependent kinase complexes Cdk4/Cdk6-cyclin D and Cdk2-cyclin E.

These complexes phosphorylate pRb and other substrates important for cell cycle progression. Cyclin D-cdk4/6 phosphorylates pRb early in G1, while cyclin E-cdk2 phosphorylates the protein near the end of G1, and cyclin A–cdk2 maintains phosphorylation of pRb during S phase. When pRb is sufficiently hyperphosphorylated, E2F is released and transcription of genes important in S-phase progression occurs. Mechanisms that police premature entry into S phase focus on inhibition of the cyclin-Cdk complexes. These inhibitors include members of the INK4 family (p15, p16, p18 and p19), which specifically interact with Cdk4/6 and impair interaction with D-type cyclins, and CIP/KIP (p21, p27 and p57) family members, that act on cyclin-Cdk complexes. p27 also stimulates the formation of cyclin D-Cdk4/6 complexes, which titrates it away from inhibiting cyclin E-Cdk2 complexes. This seemingly contradictory process permits further phosphorylation of pRb. B) During the development of intramembranous bones, Runx2 is strongly detected in preosteoblasts, immature osteoblasts, and early mature osteoblasts. Increased expression of osterix (Osx) and alkaline phosphatase (ALP) is detected in the transition between preosteoblasts to immature osteoblasts. Osteoblasts express high levels of osteocalcin (OC), which is transcriptionally regulated by the pRb-HES1-Runx2 complex.

Gene expression profiles of different stages in osteogenesis suggest that increased expression of ALP is seen early in osteoprogenitors (Narisawa et al., 1997; Komori, 2005). Recent work showed that pRb is required to recruit BRG1, an activating SWI/SNF chromatin-remodeling complex, to the alkaline phosphatase promoter (Flowers et al., 2010). Unlike the osteocalcin system, pRb does not appear to be required for removal of suppressive proteins. Thus in the absence of pRb, progression both at early and late stages of differentiation may be disrupted. Moreover, mouse embryos conditionally deleted for pRb display defects in bone ossification in part due to an increased progenitor population (Gutierrez et al., 2008). Recent work has suggested that pRb may be important in progenitor cell fate between bone and adipose tissue (Calo et al., 2010). Together, these data imply an important role for pRb in promoting tissue-specific differentiation and early lineage commitment. Recently the hedgehog and the Wnt/beta-catenin pathways have been shown to be important in osteoblast differentiation and are associated with osteosarcoma. The hedgehog signaling pathway is crucial for proliferation, cell fate and differentiation during embryonic development (McMahon et al., 2003). This pathway functions through several components including the transmembrane proteins PATCHED (PTCH1) and SMOOTHENED (SMO) to activate the GLI zinc-finger transcription factors (Ingham and McMahon, 2001; Ruiz i Altaba et al., 2002). Evidence of hedgehog pathway activation early in tumor development has been reported in basal cell carcinomas and medulloblastoma (Gupta et al., 2010), but the role of this pathway in osteosarcoma is not clear. The first association between Ihh and Runx2 came with the finding that Runx2 can directly bind to the promoter of *Ihh* and induce promoter activity (Yoshida et al., 2004). Further, Ihh expression is significantly reduced in *Runx2*$^{-/-}$ animals, which are devoid of any osteoblast formation. Work done in C3H10T1/2 mouse embryonic fibroblasts showed that Ihh regulates osteoblast differentiation of mesenchymal cells through up-regulation of the expression and function of Runx2 by Gli2 (Shimoyama et al., 2007). This suggests a possible feed-forward loop between hedgehog signaling and Runx2 expression early in lineage commitment.

Studies of conditional *Ihh*$^{-/-}$ mice showed that Ihh is required for epithelial stem cell proliferation and differentiation in the gut (Ramalho-Santos et al., 2000; Mao et al., 2010).

Additional work in the intestinal epithelium showed conditional *RB1*$^{-/-}$ animals have an increased proliferation of enteroendocrine, differentiated cells (Yang and Hinds, 2007) and elevated levels of Ihh expression. Recent *in vitro* data suggests that in some osteosarcoma cell lines the hedgehog pathway is overexpressed and that inactivation of SMO may prevent tumor cell growth (Hirotsu et al., 2010). Thus it is possible that pRb and Runx2 may complex to regulate hedgehog signaling early in osteoblast differentiation, but this has yet to be established.

Aberrations in the Wnt/Beta-catenin signaling pathway, important in osteoblast differentiation, have been associated with osteosarcoma (Haydon et al., 2002; Iwaya et al., 2003). The canonical Wnt pathway involves binding of the Wnt glycoprotein to the transmembrane Frizzled receptor and LRP5/6 co-receptors. Ligand-receptor binding prevents downstream phosphorylation of beta-catenin, allowing it to translocate to the nucleus and activate downstream genes that mediate cell proliferation and differentiation [Reviewed in Luo et al., 2007]. Members of the Wnt pathway are expressed in early osteoprogenitors (Luo et al., 2007; Glass and Karsenty, 2007). Increased nuclear localization of beta-catenin and atypical localization of adherens junction proteins, such as cadherins, are detected in osteosarcoma and correlate with metastasis (Iwaya et al., 2003; Kashima et al., 1999; Park et al., 2006; Hunter, 2004). Cadherins mediate cell-to-cell attachments, and osteoprogenitor cells express cadherins that stimulate differentiation into mature osteoblasts (Cheng et al., 2000; Hynes and Lander, 1992; Hay et al., 2000; Stains and Civitelli, 2005). An important component of adherens junction complexes includes the RhoA GTPases, Rac1 and RhoA. High Rac1 expression suppresses RhoA, which prevents merlin activation and cadherin, beta-catenin junction assembly. Recent work has shown that pRb is important in repressing Rac1, and thus regulates the assembly of adherens junctions for cell adhesion (Sosa-Garcia et al., 2010). Therefore the loss of *RB1* may not only disrupt cell cycle regulation and lineage commitment, but also cell-cell interactions that may lead to metastasis in osteosarcoma.

4. Other genetic factors in osteosarcoma

Although LOH of *RB1* is strongly associated with osteosarcoma and may be responsible for several important phenotypes as discussed above, pRB loss manifests these properties in the context of many other genetic and epigenetic alterations. Allelic amplification and/or loss at many chromosomal sites have been reported in as many as 70% of all osteosarcomas (Yamaguchi et al., 1992; Kruzelock et al., 1997; Sandberg and Bridge, 2003). This implies other potential genes involved in osteosarcoma development and progression. Overexpression of oncogenes such as c-MYC and HER2/neu (c-erbB-2) have been reported in osteosarcoma and have been associated with early pulmonary metastases (Barrios et al., 1993; Ladanyi et al., 1993; Onda et al., 1996; Gorlick et al., 1999; Zhou et al., 2003). In rare cases telomerase activity has been reported in osteosarcoma and may also be associated with pulmonary metastases (Scheel et al., 2001). In addition, amplification of MDM2, a suppressor of p53, is related to progression and metastasis of osteosarcoma (Ladanyi et al., 1993). These and other genetic mutations aside from pRb and p53 may be key to the properties of discrete forms of osteosarcoma.

Patients with bone diseases such as Rothmund-Thomson or Werner syndrome, which are associated with RECQ helicases, important for double strand break repair, are predisposed to developing osteosarcoma (Wang et al., 2003; Hickson, 2003; Chu and Hickson, 2009). About a third of the patients diagnosed with these bone diseases will develop osteosarcoma. Recently, a possibly *RB1*-independent mouse model for spontaneous osteosarcoma was reported that involves the transcription factor Twist and the APC complex in Wnt signaling (Entz-Werle et al., 2010). Twist and APC loss have been reported in several cases of human osteosarcoma where the loss of Twist and APC are associated with a poor patient prognosis (Entz-Werle et al., 2007). Neither Twist nor APC loss alone in murine models results in development of osteosarcoma, but *in vitro* assays suggest that Twist and APC/Beta-catenin/GSK complex coordinate to activate Runx2 expression (Entz-Werle et al., 2010; Stein et al., 2004). The molecular mechanism associated with these factors remains unclear as the heterogeneity of the tumors compounded with the rare occurrence of the disease hinders a clear definition for the pathology of osteosarcoma.

5. Conclusion

Functional heterogeneity is a widely recognized trait of osteosarcoma tumor cells. Osteosarcoma is a broad terminology for a tumor that arises from bone and consists of dozens of sub-classes. While the full etiological spectrum of the disease remains unclear due to its rare occurrence, various reports suggest environmental factors, bone syndromes that predispose a patient to osteosarcoma, signaling pathways and multiple genetic factors may be involved in tumor formation. Although environmental factors such as radiation therapy and bone disorders such as Paget and Rothmund-Thomas syndrome may help explain some occurrences of osteosarcoma later in life, it does not account for patients diagnosed with the disease before the age of 25. Studies of germline mutations, such as those in *RB1,* that predispose individuals to osteosarcoma may provide clues to the molecular pathology of the disease. Emerging evidence suggests osteosarcoma is a disease of differentiation caused by genetic changes that disrupt lineage progression (Haydon et al., 2007).

Growing *in vivo* and *in vitro* data reveal an increasingly complex role for pRb both in early and late osteoblast differentiation, and possibly in cell fate and metastasis (Calo et al., 2010; Gutierrez et al., 2008; Sosa-Garcia et al., 2010). Loss of *RB1* at different stages of lineage commitment could account for the various phenotypes observed in sporadic osteosarcomas. The progenitor phenotype observed in conventional osteosarcomas raises the question of whether committed osteoblasts "back up" following the loss of *RB1* to display properties of progenitor cells and/or whether the loss of *RB1* predominantly acts to delay the progression of multipotent progenitors. An increased population of progenitor-like cells that are delayed in differentiation would then be susceptible to additional transforming events (Figure 2). Although the loss or mutation of p53 is reported in some osteosarcomas (Papachristou and Papavassiliou, 2007) the question remains if p53 is essential in initiation or strictly in tumor progression. Increased understanding of the retinoblastoma gene and protein in osteogenesis presents a more complex role of this tumor suppressor as a target in tumorigenesis. Through an understanding of the molecular mechanism underlying osteogenic differentiation, we may begin to unravel the molecular pathogenesis of human osteosarcoma and identify possible co-activators or repressors that may become key targets for treating the disease.

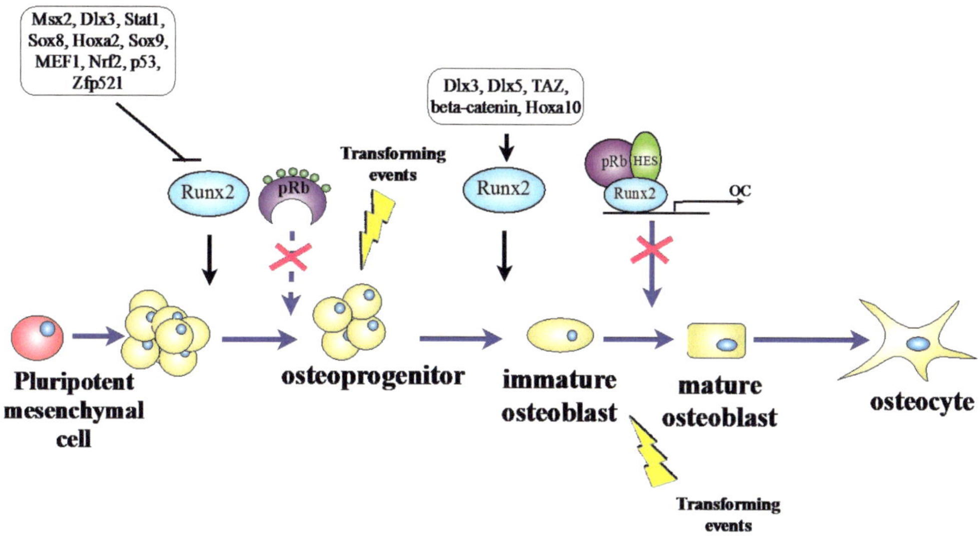

Fig. 2. Disruption of genetic components in osteoblast differentiation and osteosarcoma.

The presence of only early markers of osteoblast differentiation in osteosarcoma with periods of rapid cell division infer that the disease may be associated with genetic defects in osteoblast differentiation. Loss of *RB1* early in differentiation may result in an increased progenitor-like population that is conceivably susceptible to transforming events that may result in poorly differentiated and aggressive osteosarcoma. Genetic alterations at different stages of differentiation may be one explanation for the heterogeneity of the disease. It is unclear if genetic defects and transforming events late in differentiation generate a situation where committed osteoblasts can "back up" to display the progenitor-like phenotype observed in aggressive osteosarcomas.

6. Acknowledgements

The authors thank all members of the Hinds lab for discussion and comment. Work described in this article was supported by NIH grant AG020208 to PWH.

7. References

Alexander, K and PW Hinds (2001), 'Requirement for p27(KIP1) in retinoblastoma protein-mediated senescence.', *Mol Cell Biol*, 21 (11), 3616-31.

Alland, L, et al. (1997), 'Role for N-CoR and histone deacetylase in Sin3-mediated transcriptional repression.', *Nature*, 387 (6628), 49-55.

Barrios, C, et al. (1993), 'Amplification of c-myc oncogene and absence of c-Ha-ras point mutation in human bone sarcoma.', *J Orthop Res*, 11 (4), 556-63.

Benassi, MS, et al. (1999), 'Alteration of pRb/p16/cdk4 regulation in human osteosarcoma.', *Int J Cancer*, 84 (5), 489-93.

Benevolenskaya, EV, et al. (2005), 'Binding of pRB to the PHD protein RBP2 promotes cellular differentiation.', *Mol Cell*, 18 (6), 623-35.

Berman, SD, et al. (2008), 'Metastatic osteosarcoma induced by inactivation of Rb and p53 in the osteoblast lineage.', *Proc Natl Acad Sci U S A*, 105 (33), 11851-56.

Bracken, AP, et al. (2004), 'E2F target genes: unraveling the biology.', *Trends Biochem Sci*, 29 (8), 409-17.

Buchkovich, K, LA Duffy, and E Harlow (1989), 'The retinoblastoma protein is phosphorylated during specific phases of the cell cycle.', *Cell*, 58 (6), 1097-105.

Calo, E, et al. (2010), 'Rb regulates fate choice and lineage commitment in vivo.', *Nature*, 466 (7310), 1110-14.

Caron, AS, SI Hajdu, and EW Strong (1971), 'Osteogenic sarcoma of the facial and cranial bones. A review of forty-three cases.', *Am J Surg*, 122 (6), 719-25.

Chen, PL, et al. (1996), 'Retinoblastoma protein positively regulates terminal adipocyte differentiation through direct interaction with C/EBPs.', *Genes Dev*, 10 (21), 2794-804.

Cheng, SL, et al. (2000), 'A dominant negative cadherin inhibits osteoblast differentiation.', *J Bone Miner Res*, 15 (12), 2362-70.

Chu, WK and ID Hickson (2009), 'RecQ helicases: multifunctional genome caretakers.', *Nat Rev Cancer*, 9 (9), 644-54.

Cobrinik, D, et al. (1992), 'The retinoblastoma protein and the regulation of cell cycling.', *Trends Biochem Sci*, 17 (8), 312-15.

Dahlin, DC (1988), 'Malignant bone tumors: improvement in prognosis.', *Mayo Clin Proc*, 63 (4), 414-15.

Dannenberg, JH, et al. (2004), 'Tissue-specific tumor suppressor activity of retinoblastoma gene homologs p107 and p130.', *Genes Dev*, 18 (23), 2952-62.

DeCaprio, JA, et al. (1988), 'SV40 large tumor antigen forms a specific complex with the product of the retinoblastoma susceptibility gene.', *Cell*, 54 (2), 275-83.

Ducy, P, et al. (1997), 'Osf2/Cbfa1: a transcriptional activator of osteoblast differentiation.', *Cell*, 89 (5), 747-54.

Dujardin, F, et al. (2011), 'MDM2 and CDK4 immunohistochemistry is a valuable tool in the differential diagnosis of low-grade osteosarcomas and other primary fibro-osseous lesions of the bone.', *Mod Pathol*, 24 (5), 624-37.

Dyson, N, et al. (1989), 'The cellular 107K protein that binds to adenovirus E1A also associates with the large T antigens of SV40 and JC virus.', *Cell*, 58 (2), 249-55.

Dyson, N (1998), 'The regulation of E2F by pRB-family proteins.', *Genes Dev*, 12 (15), 2245-62.

Entz-Werle, N, et al. (2007), 'Involvement of MET/TWIST/APC combination or the potential role of ossification factors in pediatric high-grade osteosarcoma oncogenesis.', *Neoplasia*, 9 (8), 678-88.

Entz-Werle, N, et al. (2010), 'Targeted apc;twist double-mutant mice: a new model of spontaneous osteosarcoma that mimics the human disease.', *Transl Oncol*, 3 (6), 344-53.

Feuerbach, D, et al. (1997), 'Establishment and characterization of conditionally immortalized stromal cell lines from a temperature-sensitive T-Ag transgenic mouse.', *J Bone Miner Res*, 12 (2), 179-90.

Flowers, S, GR Jr Beck, and E Moran (2010), 'Transcriptional activation by pRB and its coordination with SWI/SNF recruitment.', *Cancer Res*, 70 (21), 8282-87.

Friend, SH, et al. (1986), 'A human DNA segment with properties of the gene that predisposes to retinoblastoma and osteosarcoma.', *Nature*, 323 (6089), 643-46.

Glass, DA 2nd and G Karsenty (2007), 'In vivo analysis of Wnt signaling in bone.', *Endocrinology*, 148 (6), 2630-34.

Gonzalez-Vasconcellos, I, et al. (2011), 'Differential effects of genes of the Rb1 signalling pathway on osteosarcoma incidence and latency in alpha-particle irradiated mice.', *Radiat Environ Biophys*, 50 (1), 135-41.
Gorlick, R, et al. (1999), 'Expression of HER2/erbB-2 correlates with survival in osteosarcoma.', *J Clin Oncol*, 17 (9), 2781-88.
Grunstein, M (1997), 'Histone acetylation in chromatin structure and transcription.', *Nature*, 389 (6649), 349-52.
Gupta, S, N Takebe, and P Lorusso (2010), 'Targeting the Hedgehog pathway in cancer.', *Ther Adv Med Oncol*, 2 (4), 237-50.
Gurney, JG, et al. (1995), 'Incidence of cancer in children in the United States. Sex-, race-, and 1-year age-specific rates by histologic type.', *Cancer*, 75 (8), 2186-95.
Gutierrez, GM, et al. (2008), 'Impaired bone development and increased mesenchymal progenitor cells in calvaria of RB1-/- mice.', *Proc Natl Acad Sci U S A*, 105 (47), 18402-07.
Hansen, MF (1991), 'Molecular genetic considerations in osteosarcoma.', *Clin Orthop Relat Res*, (270), 237-46.
Harlow, E, et al. (1986), 'Association of adenovirus early-region 1A proteins with cellular polypeptides.', *Mol Cell Biol*, 6 (5), 1579-89.
Harvey, M, et al. (1993), 'Spontaneous and carcinogen-induced tumorigenesis in p53-deficient mice.', *Nat Genet*, 5 (3), 225-29.
Hassig, CA, et al. (1997), 'Histone deacetylase activity is required for full transcriptional repression by mSin3A.', *Cell*, 89 (3), 341-47.
Hatakeyama, M, et al. (1994), 'Collaboration of G1 cyclins in the functional inactivation of the retinoblastoma protein.', *Genes Dev*, 8 (15), 1759-71.
Hauben, EI, et al. (2003), 'Multiple primary malignancies in osteosarcoma patients. Incidence and predictive value of osteosarcoma subtype for cancer syndromes related with osteosarcoma.', *Eur J Hum Genet*, 11 (8), 611-18.
Hay, E, et al. (2000), 'N- and E-cadherin mediate early human calvaria osteoblast differentiation promoted by bone morphogenetic protein-2.', *J Cell Physiol*, 183 (1), 117-28.
Haydon, RC, et al. (2002), 'Cytoplasmic and/or nuclear accumulation of the beta-catenin protein is a frequent event in human osteosarcoma.', *Int J Cancer*, 102 (4), 338-42.
Haydon, RC, HH Luu, and TC He (2007), 'Osteosarcoma and osteoblastic differentiation: a new perspective on oncogenesis.', *Clin Orthop Relat Res*, 454 237-46.
Hickson, ID (2003), 'RecQ helicases: caretakers of the genome.', *Nat Rev Cancer*, 3 (3), 169-78.
Hinds, PW, et al. (1992), 'Regulation of retinoblastoma protein functions by ectopic expression of human cyclins.', *Cell*, 70 (6), 993-1006.
Hirotsu, M, et al. (2010), 'Smoothened as a new therapeutic target for human osteosarcoma.', *Mol Cancer*, 9 5.
Hisada, M, et al. (1998), 'Multiple primary cancers in families with Li-Fraumeni syndrome.', *J Natl Cancer Inst*, 90 (8), 606-11.
Hopyan, S, et al. (1999), 'Expression of osteocalcin and its transcriptional regulators core-binding factor alpha 1 and MSX2 in osteoid-forming tumours.', *J Orthop Res*, 17 (5), 633-38.
Hunter, KW (2004), 'Ezrin, a key component in tumor metastasis.', *Trends Mol Med*, 10 (5), 201-04.
Huvos, AG (1993), 'Osteosarcoma in adolescents and young adults: new developments and controversies. Commentary on pathology.', *Cancer Treat Res*, 62 375-77.

Hynes, RO and AD Lander (1992), 'Contact and adhesive specificities in the associations, migrations, and targeting of cells and axons.', *Cell*, 68 (2), 303-22.

Ingham, PW and AP McMahon (2001), 'Hedgehog signaling in animal development: paradigms and principles.', *Genes Dev*, 15 (23), 3059-87.

Iwaya, K, et al. (2003), 'Cytoplasmic and/or nuclear staining of beta-catenin is associated with lung metastasis.', *Clin Exp Metastasis*, 20 (6), 525-29.

Jacks, T, et al. (1992), 'Effects of an Rb mutation in the mouse.', *Nature*, 359 (6393), 295-300.

Kashima, T, et al. (1999), 'Anomalous cadherin expression in osteosarcoma. Possible relationships to metastasis and morphogenesis.', *Am J Pathol*, 155 (5), 1549-55.

Kaste, SC, et al. (1999), 'Metastases detected at the time of diagnosis of primary pediatric extremity osteosarcoma at diagnosis: imaging features.', *Cancer*, 86 (8), 1602-08.

Kato, J, et al. (1993), 'Direct binding of cyclin D to the retinoblastoma gene product (pRb) and pRb phosphorylation by the cyclin D-dependent kinase CDK4.', *Genes Dev*, 7 (3), 331-42.

Kitchin, FD and RM Ellsworth (1974), 'Pleiotropic effects of the gene for retinoblastoma.', *J Med Genet*, 11 (3), 244-46.

Klein, MJ and GP Siegal (2006), 'Osteosarcoma: anatomic and histologic variants.', *Am J Clin Pathol*, 125 (4), 555-81.

Knowles, BB, et al. (1990), 'Osteosarcomas in transgenic mice expressing an alpha-amylase-SV40 T-antigen hybrid gene.', *Am J Pathol*, 137 (2), 259-62.

Komori, T, et al. (1997), 'Targeted disruption of Cbfa1 results in a complete lack of bone formation owing to maturational arrest of osteoblasts.', *Cell*, 89 (5), 755-64.

Komori, T (2002), 'Runx2, a multifunctional transcription factor in skeletal development.', *J Cell Biochem*, 87 (1), 1-8.

Komori, T (2005), 'Regulation of skeletal development by the Runx family of transcription factors.', *J Cell Biochem*, 95 (3), 445-53.

Krimpenfort, P, et al. (2007), 'p15Ink4b is a critical tumour suppressor in the absence of p16Ink4a.', *Nature*, 448 (7156), 943-46.

Kruzelock, RP, et al. (1997), 'Localization of a novel tumor suppressor locus on human chromosome 3q important in osteosarcoma tumorigenesis.', *Cancer Res*, 57 (1), 106-09.

Kundu, M, et al. (2002), 'Cbfbeta interacts with Runx2 and has a critical role in bone development.', *Nat Genet*, 32 (4), 639-44.

Kurek, KC, et al. (2010), 'Frequent attenuation of the WWOX tumor suppressor in osteosarcoma is associated with increased tumorigenicity and aberrant RUNX2 expression.', *Cancer Res*, 70 (13), 5577-86.

Ladanyi, M, et al. (1993), 'MDM2 gene amplification in metastatic osteosarcoma.', *Cancer Res*, 53 (1), 16-18.

Lee, JS, et al. (2006), 'HES1 cooperates with pRb to activate RUNX2-dependent transcription.', *J Bone Miner Res*, 21 (6), 921-33.

Lee, MH, et al. (1996), 'Targeted disruption of p107: functional overlap between p107 and Rb.', *Genes Dev*, 10 (13), 1621-32.

Lee, WH, et al. (1987), 'The retinoblastoma susceptibility gene encodes a nuclear phosphoprotein associated with DNA binding activity.', *Nature*, 329 (6140), 642-45.

Li, FP and JF Jr Fraumeni (1969), 'Soft-tissue sarcomas, breast cancer, and other neoplasms. A familial syndrome?', *Ann Intern Med*, 71 (4), 747-52.

Lindor, NM, et al. (2000), 'Rothmund-Thomson syndrome due to RECQ4 helicase mutations: report and clinical and molecular comparisons with Bloom syndrome and Werner syndrome.', *Am J Med Genet*, 90 (3), 223-28.

Longhi, A, et al. (2006), 'Primary bone osteosarcoma in the pediatric age: state of the art.', *Cancer Treat Rev*, 32 (6), 423-36.

Longhi, A, et al. (2008), 'Osteosarcoma in patients older than 65 years.', *J Clin Oncol*, 26 (33), 5368-73.

Luo, J, et al. (2007), 'Wnt signaling and human diseases: what are the therapeutic implications?', *Lab Invest*, 87 (2), 97-103.

Luo, RX, AA Postigo, and DC Dean (1998), 'Rb interacts with histone deacetylase to repress transcription.', *Cell*, 92 (4), 463-73.

Mao, J, et al. (2010), 'Hedgehog signaling controls mesenchymal growth in the developing mammalian digestive tract.', *Development*, 137 (10), 1721-29.

Marina, N, et al. (2004), 'Biology and therapeutic advances for pediatric osteosarcoma.', *Oncologist*, 9 (4), 422-41.

McMahon, AP, PW Ingham, and CJ Tabin (2003), 'Developmental roles and clinical significance of hedgehog signaling.', *Curr Top Dev Biol*, 53 1-114.

McNairn, JD, et al. (2001), 'Inheritance of osteosarcoma and Paget's disease of bone: a familial loss of heterozygosity study.', *J Mol Diagn*, 3 (4), 171-77.

Miller, CW, et al. (1996), 'Alterations of the p15, p16,and p18 genes in osteosarcoma.', *Cancer Genet Cytogenet*, 86 (2), 136-42.

Miller, J, et al. (2002), 'The core-binding factor beta subunit is required for bone formation and hematopoietic maturation.', *Nat Genet*, 32 (4), 645-49.

Mirabello, L, RJ Troisi, and SA Savage (2009), 'Osteosarcoma incidence and survival rates from 1973 to 2004: data from the Surveillance, Epidemiology, and End Results Program.', *Cancer*, 115 (7), 1531-43.

Mohney, BG, et al. (1998), 'Second nonocular tumors in survivors of heritable retinoblastoma and prior radiation therapy.', *Am J Ophthalmol*, 126 (2), 269-77.

Morgenbesser, SD, et al. (1994), 'p53-dependent apoptosis produced by Rb-deficiency in the developing mouse lens.', *Nature*, 371 (6492), 72-74.

Mulligan, G and T Jacks (1998), 'The retinoblastoma gene family: cousins with overlapping interests.', *Trends Genet*, 14 (6), 223-29.

Munger, K, et al. (1989), 'Complex formation of human papillomavirus E7 proteins with the retinoblastoma tumor suppressor gene product.', *EMBO J*, 8 (13), 4099-105.

Narisawa, S, N Frohlander, and JL Millan (1997), 'Inactivation of two mouse alkaline phosphatase genes and establishment of a model of infantile hypophosphatasia.', *Dev Dyn*, 208 (3), 432-46.

Nellissery, MJ, et al. (1998), 'Evidence for a novel osteosarcoma tumor-suppressor gene in the chromosome 18 region genetically linked with Paget disease of bone.', *Am J Hum Genet*, 63 (3), 817-24.

Olive, KP, et al. (2004), 'Mutant p53 gain of function in two mouse models of Li-Fraumeni syndrome.', *Cell*, 119 (6), 847-60.

Onda, M, et al. (1996), 'ErbB-2 expression is correlated with poor prognosis for patients with osteosarcoma.', *Cancer*, 77 (1), 71-78.

Otto, F, et al. (1997), 'Cbfa1, a candidate gene for cleidocranial dysplasia syndrome, is essential for osteoblast differentiation and bone development.', *Cell*, 89 (5), 765-71.

Papachristou, DJ and AG Papavassiliou (2007), 'Osteosarcoma and chondrosarcoma: new signaling pathways as targets for novel therapeutic interventions.', *Int J Biochem Cell Biol*, 39 (5), 857-62.

Park, HR, et al. (2006), 'Ezrin in osteosarcoma: comparison between conventional high-grade and central low-grade osteosarcoma.', *Pathol Res Pract*, 202 (7), 509-15.

Paulino, AC and BZ Fowler (2005), 'Secondary neoplasms after radiotherapy for a childhood solid tumor.', *Pediatr Hematol Oncol*, 22 (2), 89-101.

Picci, P (2007), 'Osteosarcoma (osteogenic sarcoma).', *Orphanet J Rare Dis*, 2 6.

Porter, DE, et al. (1992), 'A significant proportion of patients with osteosarcoma may belong to Li-Fraumeni cancer families.', *J Bone Joint Surg Br*, 74 (6), 883-86.

Ramalho-Santos, M, DA Melton, and AP McMahon (2000), 'Hedgehog signals regulate multiple aspects of gastrointestinal development.', *Development*, 127 (12), 2763-72.

Ruiz i Altaba, A, P Sanchez, and N Dahmane (2002), 'Gli and hedgehog in cancer: tumours, embryos and stem cells.', *Nat Rev Cancer*, 2 (5), 361-72.

Sandberg, AA and JA Bridge (2003), 'Updates on the cytogenetics and molecular genetics of bone and soft tissue tumors: osteosarcoma and related tumors.', *Cancer Genet Cytogenet*, 145 (1), 1-30.

Savage, SA and L Mirabello (2011), 'Using epidemiology and genomics to understand osteosarcoma etiology.', *Sarcoma*, 2011 548151.

Schajowicz, F, HA Sissons, and LH Sobin (1995), 'The World Health Organization's histologic classification of bone tumors. A commentary on the second edition.', *Cancer*, 75 (5), 1208-14.

Scheel, C, et al. (2001), 'Alternative lengthening of telomeres is associated with chromosomal instability in osteosarcomas.', *Oncogene*, 20 (29), 3835-44.

Schneider, JW, et al. (1994), 'Reversal of terminal differentiation mediated by p107 in Rb-/- muscle cells.', *Science*, 264 (5164), 1467-71.

Sellers, WR, et al. (1998), 'Stable binding to E2F is not required for the retinoblastoma protein to activate transcription, promote differentiation, and suppress tumor cell growth.', *Genes Dev*, 12 (1), 95-106.

Shapiro, GI, et al. (1995), 'Multiple mechanisms of p16INK4A inactivation in non-small cell lung cancer cell lines.', *Cancer Res*, 55 (24), 6200-09.

Sharpless, NE, et al. (2001), 'Loss of p16Ink4a with retention of p19Arf predisposes mice to tumorigenesis.', *Nature*, 413 (6851), 86-91.

Sherr, CJ (1996), 'Cancer cell cycles.', *Science*, 274 (5293), 1672-77.

Sherr, CJ and JM Roberts (1999), 'CDK inhibitors: positive and negative regulators of G1-phase progression.', *Genes Dev*, 13 (12), 1501-12.

Shimoyama, A, et al. (2007), 'Ihh/Gli2 signaling promotes osteoblast differentiation by regulating Runx2 expression and function.', *Mol Biol Cell*, 18 (7), 2411-18.

Sosa-Garcia, B, et al. (2010), 'A role for the retinoblastoma protein as a regulator of mouse osteoblast cell adhesion: implications for osteogenesis and osteosarcoma formation.', *PLoS One*, 5 (11), e13954.

Stabel, S, P Argos, and L Philipson (1985), 'The release of growth arrest by microinjection of adenovirus E1A DNA.', *EMBO J*, 4 (9), 2329-36.

Stains, JP and R Civitelli (2005), 'Cell-cell interactions in regulating osteogenesis and osteoblast function.', *Birth Defects Res C Embryo Today*, 75 (1), 72-80.

Stein, GS, et al. (2004), 'Runx2 control of organization, assembly and activity of the regulatory machinery for skeletal gene expression.', *Oncogene*, 23 (24), 4315-29.

Stiegler, P, M Kasten, and A Giordano (1998), 'The RB family of cell cycle regulatory factors.', *J Cell Biochem Suppl*, 30-31 30-36.

Stiller, CA, et al. (2006), 'Bone tumours in European children and adolescents, 1978-1997. Report from the Automated Childhood Cancer Information System project.', *Eur J Cancer*, 42 (13), 2124-35.

Ta, HT, et al. (2009), 'Osteosarcoma treatment: state of the art.', *Cancer Metastasis Rev*, 28 (1-2), 247-63.

Takaki, T, et al. (2005), 'Preferences for phosphorylation sites in the retinoblastoma protein of D-type cyclin-dependent kinases, Cdk4 and Cdk6, in vitro.', *J Biochem*, 137 (3), 381-86.

Tang, N, et al. (2008), 'Osteosarcoma development and stem cell differentiation.', *Clin Orthop Relat Res*, 466 (9), 2114-30.

Thomas, DM, et al. (2001), 'The retinoblastoma protein acts as a transcriptional coactivator required for osteogenic differentiation.', *Mol Cell*, 8 (2), 303-16.

Thomas, DM, et al. (2004), 'Terminal osteoblast differentiation, mediated by runx2 and p27KIP1, is disrupted in osteosarcoma.', *J Cell Biol*, 167 (5), 925-34.

Tiemann, F and PW Hinds (1998), 'Induction of DNA synthesis and apoptosis by regulated inactivation of a temperature-sensitive retinoblastoma protein.', *EMBO J*, 17 (4), 1040-52.

Trimarchi, JM and JA Lees (2002), 'Sibling rivalry in the E2F family.', *Nat Rev Mol Cell Biol*, 3 (1), 11-20.

Upton, B, Q Chu, and BD Li (2009), 'Li-Fraumeni syndrome: the genetics and treatment considerations for the sarcoma and associated neoplasms.', *Surg Oncol Clin N Am*, 18 (1), 145-56, ix.

Vooijs, M, et al. (2002), 'Tumor formation in mice with somatic inactivation of the retinoblastoma gene in interphotoreceptor retinol binding protein-expressing cells.', *Oncogene*, 21 (30), 4635-45.

Vousden, KH and PS Jat (1989), 'Functional similarity between HPV16E7, SV40 large T and adenovirus E1a proteins.', *Oncogene*, 4 (2), 153-58.

Wadayama, B, et al. (1994), 'Mutation spectrum of the retinoblastoma gene in osteosarcomas.', *Cancer Res*, 54 (11), 3042-48.

Walkley, CR, et al. (2008), 'Conditional mouse osteosarcoma, dependent on p53 loss and potentiated by loss of Rb, mimics the human disease.', *Genes Dev*, 22 (12), 1662-76.

Wang, LL, et al. (2001), 'Clinical manifestations in a cohort of 41 Rothmund-Thomson syndrome patients.', *Am J Med Genet*, 102 (1), 11-17.

Wang, LL, et al. (2003), 'Association between osteosarcoma and deleterious mutations in the RECQL4 gene in Rothmund-Thomson syndrome.', *J Natl Cancer Inst*, 95 (9), 669-74.

Weinberg, RA (1994), 'Oncogenes and tumor suppressor genes.', *CA Cancer J Clin*, 44 (3), 160-70.

Whyte, P, et al. (1988), 'Association between an oncogene and an anti-oncogene: the adenovirus E1A proteins bind to the retinoblastoma gene product.', *Nature*, 334 (6178), 124-29.

Williams, BO, et al. (1994), 'Extensive contribution of Rb-deficient cells to adult chimeric mice with limited histopathological consequences.', *EMBO J*, 13 (18), 4251-59.

Won, KY, HR Park, and YK Park (2009), 'Prognostic implication of immunohistochemical Runx2 expression in osteosarcoma.', *Tumori*, 95 (3), 311-16.

Wunder, JS, et al. (2005), 'TP53 mutations and outcome in osteosarcoma: a prospective, multicenter study.', *J Clin Oncol*, 23 (7), 1483-90.

Yamaguchi, T, et al. (1992), 'Allelotype analysis in osteosarcomas: frequent allele loss on 3q, 13q, 17p, and 18q.', *Cancer Res*, 52 (9), 2419-23.

Yang, HS and PW Hinds (2007), 'pRb-mediated control of epithelial cell proliferation and Indian hedgehog expression in mouse intestinal development.', *BMC Dev Biol*, 7 6.

Yoshida, CA, et al. (2002), 'Core-binding factor beta interacts with Runx2 and is required for skeletal development.', *Nat Genet*, 32 (4), 633-38.

Yoshida, CA, et al. (2004), 'Runx2 and Runx3 are essential for chondrocyte maturation, and Runx2 regulates limb growth through induction of Indian hedgehog.', *Genes Dev*, 18 (8), 952-63.

Zhou, H, et al. (2003), 'Her-2/neu expression in osteosarcoma increases risk of lung metastasis and can be associated with gene amplification.', *J Pediatr Hematol Oncol*, 25 (1), 27-32.